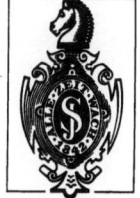

Treatment of
Male Infertility

Edited by
Jerald Bain, Wolf-Bernhard Schill
and Luis Schwarzstein

With 98 Figures

Springer-Verlag
Berlin Heidelberg New York 1982

Jerald Bain, M.D.
Division of Endocrinology and Metabolism
University of Toronto and Mount Sinai Hospital
600 University Avenue; Suites 639–640
Toronto, Ontario M5G 1X5; Canada

Prof. Dr. Wolf-B. Schill
Dermatologische Klinik und Poliklinik
der Universität München
Frauenlobstr. 9–11
8000 München 2, West Germany

Dr. Luis Schwarzstein
Grupo de Estudio en Fertilidad y Endocrinologia de Rosario
Cordoba 1764
2000 Rosario (SF), Argentina

ISBN-13:978-3-642-68225-4   e-ISBN-13:978-3-642-68223-0
DOI: 10.1007/978-3-642-68223-0

Library of Congress Cataloging in Publication Data.

Main entry under title: Treatment of male infertility. Includes bibliographies
and index. 1. Infertility, Male—Treatment. I. Bain, Jerald. II. Schill, W.-B.
(Wolf-Bernhard), 1939–. III Schwarzstein, Luis, 1938–. [DNLM: 1. Sterility,
Male—Therapy. WJ 709 T784]
RC889.T73   616.6′92   82-3349
ISBN-13:978-3-642-68225-4 (U.S.) AACR2

2121/3321   543210

Contents

III. Surgical Treatment

IV. Cryopreservation and Insemination

List of Contributors

Aparicio, N.
Grupo de Estudio en Fertilidad y Endocrinologia de Rosario
(G.E.F.E.R), Cordoba 1764, 2000 Rosario, Argentina

Bain, J.
Department of Medicine and Obstetrics and Gynecology, Division
of Endocrinology, University of Toronto, Mount Sinai Hospital, 600
University Avenue, Suites 639–640, Toronto, Ontario M5G 1X5,
Canada

Barkay, J.
Male Fertility Institute, Department of Obstetrics and Gynecology,
Central Emek Hospital, Afula, Israel

Barwin, B. N.
Department of Obstetrics and Gynecology, University of Ottawa,
Ottawa General Hospital, 501 Smyth Road, Ottawa, Ontario
K1N 8L6, Canada

de Castro, M. P. P.
Rua Pernambuco, 190-1° and, 01240 São Paulo, Brasil

Collins, J. P.
Department of Urology, University of Ottawa, Ottawa Civic Hospital, 1053 Carling Avenue, Ottawa, Ontario K1Y 4E9, Canada

Comhaire, F.
Department of Internal Medicine, Section of Endocrinology, State
University Hospital, Academisch Ziekenhuis, 185, De Pintelaan,
B-9000 Gent, Belgium

Fenster, H.
Department of Surgery, Division of Urology, University of British
Columbia, Shaughnessy Hospital, 4500 Oak Street, Vancouver,
B. C. V6H 3N1, Canada

Freischem, C. W.
Max Planck Clinical Research Unit for Reproductive Medicine,
University Women's Hospital, Domagkstr. 11, D-4400 Münster,
Federal Republic of Germany

Friberg, J.
Division of Reproductive Endocrinology and Infertility, Department of Obstetrics and Gynecology, Mount Sinai Hospital, Medical Center of Chicago, Rush Medical College, California Avenue at 15th Street, Chicago, Illinois 60608, USA

Glezerman, M.
Division of Obstetrics and Gynecology, The Soroka Medical Center and Ben-Gurion-University of the Negev, Beer Sheva, Israel

Kelâmi, A.
Department of Urology, Klinikum Steglitz, Free University of Berlin, Hindenburgdamm 30, D-1000 Berlin 45, Federal Republic of Germany

Kockott, G.
Department of Psychiatry, Technical University of Munich, Möhlstr. 26, D-8000 München 80, Federal Republic of Germany

Mariani, M.
University of Pisa, Postgraduate School of Andrology, 1 Clinica Medica, Policlinico S. Chiara, I-56100 Pisa, Italy

McLoughlin, M. G.
University of British Columbia, Urology Clinic, Vancouver General Hospital, 855 West 10th Avenue, Vancouver, B.C. V6H 3N1, Canada

Menchini-Fabris, G. F.
University of Pisa, Postgraduate School of Andrology, 1 Clinica Medica, Policlinico S. Chiara, I-56100 Pisa, Italy

Nahoum, C. R. D.
Grupo de Estudos de Fertilidade e Esterilidade do Rio de Janeiro, Rua Tavares de Macedo 157, CEP 24220, Niteroi RJ, Brasil

Nieschlag, E.
Max Planck Clinical Research Unit for Reproductive Medicine, University Women's Hospital, Domagkstr. 11, D-4400 Münster, Federal Republic of Germany

del Pozo, E.
Experimetal Therapeutics Department, Clinical Research Division, Sandoz AG, CH-4002 Basle, Switzerland

Schellen, A. M. C. M.
Ch. Beltjenslaan 23, 6132 Ae Sittard, The Netherlands

Schill, W. B.
University of Munich, Department of Dermatology, Andrology Unit, Frauenlobstr. 9–11, D-8000 München 2, Federal Republic of Germany

Schwarzstein, L.
Grupo de Estudio en Fertilidad y Endocrinologia de Rosario (G.E.F.E.R.), Cordoba 1764, 2000 Rosario, Argentina

Shuber, J.
Department of Obstetrics and Gynecology, University of Toronto, Mount Sinai Hospital, 600 University Avenue, Suite 457, Toronto, Ontario M5G 1X5, Canada

Troen, P.
University of Pittsburgh School of Medicine, Department of Medicine, Montefiori Hospital, 3459 Fifth Avenue, Pittsburgh, Pa 15213, USA

Vermeulen, L.
Department of Internal Medicine, Section of Endocrinology, State University Hospital, Academisch Ziekenhuis, 185, de Pintelaan, B-9000 Gent, Belgium

Wagenknecht, L. V.
Department of Urology, University of Hamburg, Martinistr. 52, D-2000 Hamburg 20, Federal Republic of Germany

Winters, S. J.
University of Pittsburgh School of Medicine, Department of Medicine, Montefiori Hospital, 3459 Fifth Avenue, Pittsburgh, Pa 15213, USA

Zegers-Hochschild, F.
Department of Obstetrics and Gynecology, Hospital Jose Joaquim Aquirre, Universidad de Chile, P.P.Box 6637, Casilla, Santiago, Chile

Zuckerman, H.
Male Fertility Institute, Department of Obstetrics and Gynecology, Central Emek Hospital, Afula, Israel

Preface

Our insight into the mechanisms of the physiology of reproduction has experienced a swift and constant development these last few years. The advent of more sophisticated diagnostic methods and their relatively easy clinical application allow for the incorporation of that knowledge into the evaluation of the infertile couple. These facts, together with an obvious change in social psychology, have facilitated the development of different specialities dealing with the problems of infertility. It is now possible in medical centers all around the world to undertake a better disposition of the infertile husband to look for advice, to be studied, and treated.

Confronted with this situation we are still unable to offer specific therapy in most cases; however, empirically based therapy abounds. Advances in therapy have not kept pace with our increased physiological knowledge and improved diagnostic techniques. Pathophysiological mechanisms and etiological factors in male infertility are largely unknown. This has significantly hampered both clinical evaluation and advances in treatment allowing for frequent non-scientific therapeutic incursions into the armamentarium of the andrologist.

Several factors have given birth to therapeutic "fashions", which are bound to survive as long as this state of lack of knowledge continues. For example, we may ask whether the treatment of varicocele constitutes a fashion? Though we accept the treatment of varicocele as the best available treatment of male infertility, we do not know its mechanism of action and so we cannot predict a therapeutic result. This is also true of the majority of the treatments currently in use.

This book, which aims to present the widest, most up-to-date information available about the state of the art, is an outcome of the editorial efforts of a Canadian, a German, and an Argentinian, with the invaluable collaboration or authors from Europe, North and South America, and Israel. The multicentric international authorship of this book has brought together current ideas and opinions about male infertility and its management as viewed by different andrologists from around the world. This has contributed greatly to promoting a better understanding of the whole spectrum of male infertility and has manifested an international cooperation so vital to the development of science and knowledge.

Because of the many gaps in our knowledge, because of the relatively poor results with any form of therapy for the subfertile male, and because there is so much research yet to be done, this book can only represent a continuum and not an end. Much more needs to be studied and written and we, the editors, hope that we can continue to be part of exciting new developments in an exciting and blossoming area of human reproduction.

The Editors, 1982

I. General Considerations

Male Infertility: Problems in Assessing Response to Treatment

Jerald Bain

In attempting to evaluate the infertile male the first problem is the definition of infertility. We must recognize that with the current state of our knowledge no clear definition exists. We know that oligozoospermia, a term used to denote a low sperm count, means different things to different people. If oligozoospermia means a sperm count of less than 40×10^6/ml in one center and less than 20×10^6/ml in another, how then can we agree that treatment is appropriate let alone effective?

It is known that extreme variations in sperm count occur over a protracted period in any young healthy individual. How many counts do we need to determine what his mean sperm production is? Because of the great ebb und flow of spermatogenesis is it even appropriate to calculate a "mean" sperm count? What is the true meaning of such a figure? We may logically reason that today a man is fertile because of a wave of spermatogenesis and he is subfertile next week because sperm production has waned to a degree that reduces the chances of fertility.

Sperm count, in itself, is not the all-encompassing parameter that dictates fertilizing capacity. There are many other factors to consider. One of these is sperm morphology. Morphologists have taken great pains to describe a multitude of spermatozoal shapes and sizes. Some spermatozoa have large heads, small heads, two heads, no heads, two tails, or no tails. What do these descriptions mean when it comes to understanding the fertilizability of an individual spermatozoon? We believe that the common oval-headed spermatozoon with one tail which moves, is the spermatozoon that has the potential of penetrating and fertilizing an ovum. How many such spermatozoa must be present before fertility can be presumed? Once again there are no firm data. Is it 50% of the total number of mature spermatozoa? 60%? 65%? If we don't know what "normal" is, how can we relate "improvement" of a sperm parameter after treatment to possible subsequent pregnancy?

Sperm motility is another parameter upon which we focus with great care and compulsion. We not only count the number of motile spermatozoa, but we grade the motility on some sort of scale (e.g., 0, 1+, 2+, 3+) that gives us an idea of the degree of motility with purposeful forward progression. We have made a number of technical and electronic advances in our attempt to quantify motility, but to what avail? There is no one motility "index" that we can unequivocally relate to improved fertility.

In one of the chapters of this book, a technique that separates the more motile from the less motile sperm is discussed. This is an interesting technological advance which may allow us to actually demonstrate the increased fertilizing capacity of spermatozoa with purposeful movement by using such sperm preparations for artificial insemination. This kind of an experiment might then give us a better understanding of the relationship between enhanced sperm motility and subsequent pregnancy.

The life of andrologists is made all the more complicated when they attempt to get an overview of spermatozoal fertilizing capacity by somehow inter-relating sperm count, morphology, motility, and semen volume, plus or minus a variety of other parameters that this or that laboratory may assess. To add to our troubles, nature occasionally plays a dirty trick on us by producing a pregnancy from a semen specimen that we would have given up as hopeless.

Against this confusing background, scientists are expected to produce data on the results of treatment in male infertility that have meaning and validity. In the majority of cases the cause of the subfertility is unknown, and consequently we have no specific therapy and are forced to use drugs which we believe will affect certain metabolic processes. How frustrating our task is! But the frustration of our task must not make us any less vigilant over what we do to patients and how we interpret the results of what we do.

The rationale of some of the therapies is based on a logical appreciation of normal physiology. We know that the pituitary gland stimulates testicular function. It is reasonable then to use drugs like tamoxifen or clomiphene citrate in an attempt to stimulate pituitary secretion and thus enhance sperm production. It is reasonable to look for infection of the reproductive tract in the hopes that treatment will provide the optimal milieu for sperm function. It makes good sense to attempt to increase the intratesticular androgen level for enhanced spermatogenesis because we know that androgen is needed for normal sperm production. These treatments are based on known physiological phenomena. That they aren't universally effective or even highly effective illustrates the difficulty of applying physiology to poorly understood pathophysiological states.

Other therapies may have less valid rationales, but have crept into use because of presumed positive metabolic effects or because of the supposed beneficial results in some subfertile men. Hence, testosterone suppression and subsequent occasional rebound is still with us after many years of use. Newer methods invoke an attempt at enhancing spermatozoal metabolism; kallikrein, caffeine, and nucleotides fall into this category. Unfortunately, the great array of therapeutic modes attests to our inability to find the one, two, or three treatments that really work in a significant number of cases. Nonetheless, we must continue to try various methods, not only for the intrinsic value of helping subfertile men achieve fertility, but also because our attempts at therapy may help uncover some of the mysteries of pathophysiology. And when we have a better understanding of pathophysiology, we'll be better able to direct our attentions toward the development of specific therapies that hopefully will have a high degree of efficacy.

In attempting to assess the therapeutic value of a particular form of treatment, the clinician is often unaware that he or she may be instilling a bias that will influence interpretation of the results; for example, it is widely observed that 15%–20% of oligozoospermic men or men with derangements of sperm morphology or motility will eventually induce a pregnancy spontaneously without the intervention of any specific therapy. If this is so, then reported pregnancy rates of 30%, 40%, or more after treatment of infertile men must be readjusted downward to take into account pregnancies that would be expected to occur by chance. One of the factors to which andrologists have paid very little attention is the time to pregnancy with or without treatment of male subfertility. It might be argued that a success rate of 30% is reasonable, because without therapy it may have taken a much longer time for the spontaneous success rate of 20%. The statisticians will have to help us with these complicated manipulations.

Most of us share in the guilt of perpetrating yet another bias; i.e., the unconscious bias of not reporting lack of success. How often in the literature do we read the success of compound "X" in effecting a pregnancy rate of 35%, yet in our hands we see no positive effect above that of chance alone? Are the first author's data in question? Did we give the right dose? Was our patient population similar? Are there geographical or ethnic differences that might account for his success and our failure? If we had published our negative results and put them alongside his positive results, the accumulated success rate might presumably be scaled down from 35% to half that figure or to what chance alone might have produced.

In most reports describing treatment of male infertility, we are given either no data regarding the status of the female partner or we are simply told that she was found to be "normal". What does this mean? To know how successful a man might be in inducing a pregnancy we need to know how successful his female partner might be. Rarely are we told about menstrual pattern, proof of ovulation (e.g., by temperature charting or luteal phase progesterone levels), tubal patency by hysterosalpingography, or pelvic health by laparoscopy. In no other branch of medicine does successful treatment of one individual depend on the good health and normal physiological functioning of another individual as it does in the field of infertility. How much meaning can reported pregnancy rates of 20%, 30%, or 40% have under such adverse circumstances?

When we treat the infertile male we make certain assumptions. We assume (hopefully, based on objective data) that his female partner is normally fertile and continues to maintain that normal fertility throughout the course of his therapy. We assume that there are no cyclic variations in the degree of spermatogenesis based either on the time of day or month of the year. We assume the subject takes his medication if it is of the self-administering kind. We assume that intercourse with ejaculation is taking place frequently enough for the chance of conception to be reasonably high. We assume that the reported pregnancy was really induced by the male subject we are treating. We have no choice but to make some of these assumptions, but others may be amenable to some degree of control. How often do we exercise this control?

In animal experiments we insist upon controls and we are rigid about it. We relax our obsession about controls when we come to treating human beings. We do this because we want to offer our patients every benefit. We don't want to deprive them of the possibility of a therapeutic success. It may seem ludicrous, but we don't really know whether an incision into the groin by itself or incision into the groin plus ligation of the internal spermatic vein is the real reason for the perceived, but relatively small increase in pregnancy rate after varicocelectomy. Who would do such an experiment? But that's the control we need if we are to know with certainty that eliminating varicocele enhances fertility.

Male infertility is undoubtedly a heterogenous phenomenon, yet we rarely even consider this when embarking upon a research program to assess therapy. Generally, we paint all subfertile with the same broad brush and the same color paint. We tend to lump all oligozoospermic men into one category and look at a mean increase in sperm count for this whole group, rather than for subgroups based on differences in sperm count. Occasionally we separate those with a varicocele from those without a varicocele, but not often. Usually we pay little or no attention to possible influencing factors such as smoking, alcohol intake, ingestion of drugs, and exposure to chemicals or environmental pollutants. We almost completely ignore one of the factors that may play the greatest role in reproductive function; namely, the psyche and emotional parameters.

One of the difficulties in creating subsets of patients is the fact that each subset would need a large enough number of patients to assure statistical validity of the results. Many published reports would not have been published if these criteria had to be met.

Finally, let us return to the sperm count question. Extreme variations occur within one individual. This is readily observed if enough semen analyses are performed over a long period of time. We know that sperm production may be transiently suppressed by assorted acute illnesses, such as a viral infection which may manifest itself as the common cold. The common cold is common. If it can induce transient suppression of sperm production then there must be a period of time when sperm production recovers and sperm count gradually drifts upward. How often do we look for trends in sperm counts? Do we do enough semen analyses to determine whether what we are interpreting as oligozoospermia is really the low ebb of spermatogenesis reduced by an illness or environmental factor? Is that the moment when we institute therapy and do we ascribe a successful outcome to the therapy or to what would have happened spontaneously? Could this kind of phenomenon explain why 20% of oligozoospermic men eventually produce a pregnancy?

The problems we face in treating and evaluating treatment of the infertile male are enormous. Usually we have no specific disease entity to treat, we have no treatment that has a very high success rate, and we need a second human being (the female partner) whose fertility is hopefully normal to be our guidepost for proof of pregnancy induced by a successfully treated infertile male subject. All of these factors are enough to deter us from any further attempt at studying possible therapeutic regimens for the subfertile male. Thankfully, we are not deterred. Thankfully there are those from many areas of the world who are willing to venture into new and old areas to study the therapy and pathophysiology of the infertile male.

The questions raised in this essay may be applicable to some or all of the contributions to this text, but the work must still be done, patients must be evaluated, and we must be critical. The editors of this book consider this effort to be a continuum in the long, arduous process of finding meaningful treatment for the subfertile male. From that perspective, this book does not represent an end in itself, but rather an extension from the past and present and a projection into the future. More, much more, is yet to come in our understanding of and in our ability to treat the infertile male.

II. Medical Treatment

1 Inflammation and Infection

C. R. D. Nahoum

The inflammatory response is a beneficial process, but inflammatory injury of male accessory sex organs can reduce fertility by the following pathophysiological mechanisms: increased sperm agglutination (Derrick and Dahlberg 1976); reduced sperm motility and viability (Eliasson 1975); and obstruction of the ejaculatory ducts (Pomerol 1978). Disturbances in epididymal sperm maturation (Bedford 1975) affecting motility (Gaddum 1968) and the fertilizing ability of spermatozoa (Bedford et al. 1973) may also be sequelae of inflammation. Inflammation and infection are often mistakenly considered to be interchangeable terms. Infections by microorganisms are just one among several causes of inflammation (Woolf 1977). Diagnostic and therapeutic criteria for the management of the inflammatory state of male accessory genital organs are the subjects of this chapter.

1.1 Inflammation of Male Accessory Sex Organs

1.1.1 Genital and Rectal Examination

An inflammatory process may cause disease in the epididymis. Abnormalities in size, shape, and consistency of the epididymides may be appreciated by scrotal palpation or, less often, pathology may be assessed by direct visualization during testicular biopsy.

The prostate gland and seminal vesicles are palpated by rectal examination. Normal seminal vesicles are seldom felt. If abnormal they may become palpable and occasionally painful. One method to visualize and detect changes in prostate and seminal vesicle sizes is through computorized tomography (Fig. 1). Visualization and estimation of the size of the seminal vesicles by means of ultrasonic beta-scanning has also been described (Rönnberg et al. 1978). The prostate is a fibromuscular organ containing 30–50 small tubuloalveolar glands with about 25 excretory ducts opening into the urethra. The gland is composed of five lobes; two lateral, one anterior, one posterior, and one median. Only the lateral lobes of the prostate are easily palpable. The anterior lobe cannot be felt and only rarely the median lobe. When normal, the prostate has a uniform, firm, elastic consistency with the median furrow clearly palpable. Before massaging the prostate the examiner must analyze the size, surface abnormalities, shape, mobility, and consistency of the gland. Fixation of the gland to surrounding tissues and stony indurations are indications for a malignancy evaluation. Enlargement of the prostate gland by in-

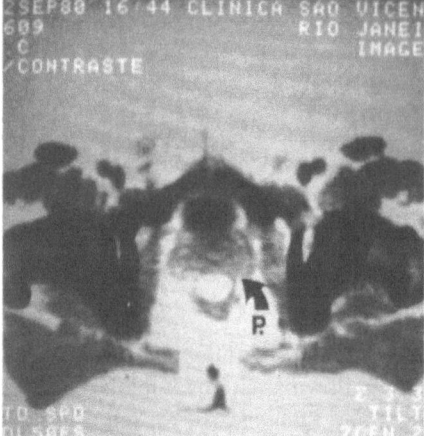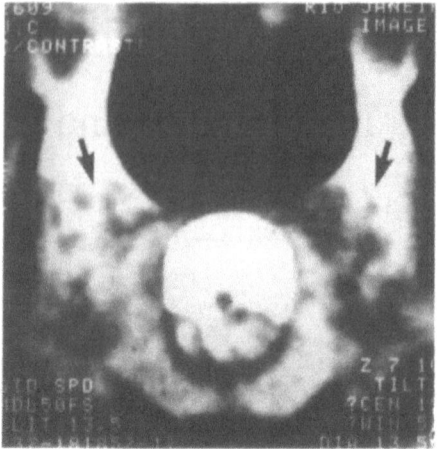

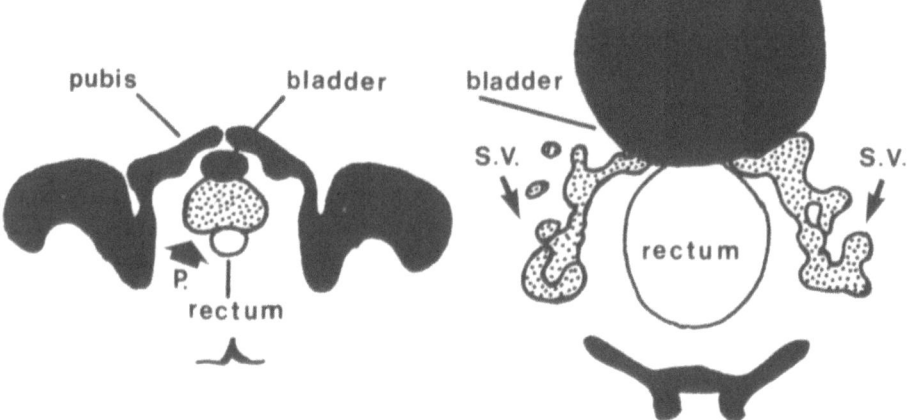

Fig. 1. Prostate and seminal vesicles (*top*) identified through computerized tomography (*arrows*) (courtesy of Dr. P. A. Andreiuolo, Rio de Janeiro)

flammation usually accentuates the median furrow. Sometimes, changes in shape and volume can only be detected through endoscopic examination of the posterior urethra. During chronic inflammation the prostate appears congested with an irregular and mildly indurated surface.

Palpatory findings in andrological practice are often normal or inconclusive, in spite of abnormal exfoliative cytology (Mears 1973, Eliasson 1976 b).

1.1.2 Collection and Processing of the Prostatic Vesicular Fluid (PVF)

For massage, patients must observe the following instructions: sexual abstinence for 3–5 days (the latter is especially indicated in those patients with low testosterone levels); emptying of the rectal ampulla several hours before the examination; urinary continence 2–3 h prior to the massage. Immediately before examination, patients must empty the bladder to remove excess desquamated urethral epithelial cells. The knee-chest position on an appropriate table is one of the postures recommended for examination. To collect PVF, patients must keep a clean plastic vial against the glans penis until the massage is stopped. After collection of one or two drops in a container and with the patient still kneeling, any further drops are smeared directly onto microscopic slides. The drops collected in the receptacle are fixed with an equal volume of 75% alcohol in normal saline. An assessment of the number of polymorphonuclear (PMN) leukocytes in this fluid is made (Nahoum and Cardozo 1980). Additional drops may be produced by repeated anal contractions. In most cases it is not necessary to milk the urethra downwards.

The slides are immediately fixed by gentle immersion in a jar containing an alcohol-ether mixture (1:1). Care must be taken to avoid air drying. The smear should be left in the fixative for at least 1 h. Coating sprays composed of polyethylene glycol and alcohol as fixatives can also be used, but are not as satisfactory. It is recommended to routinely prepare two pairs of slides. The Papanicolaou-stained pair is used for analysis of qualitative changes of epithelial cells and for slide counting of neutrophils. The other pair can be used for the acridine orange technique (Turner 1960) used for the detection of malignant changes of the cells, or the presence of bacteria, fungi, and Trichomonas (the latter requiring examination in a fluorescence microscope).

Even if an adequate volume of excretory fluid has been obtained, it is beneficial to collect the first 15–30 ml of the postmassage urine directly into a vial, half filled with the alcohol-ether mixture. As urine is a medium containing essentially no protein, the cells will not ordinarily adhere to the slide.

For the preparation of urinary smears, following centrifugation (2000 rpm, 10–15 min), either albumin is added to the pellet (0.1 ml 22% bovine serum albumin) or the smears of sediment are prepared on previously albuminized slides. When desired, filtering membrane techniques can be applied (Lillie and Fullmer 1976). The smears from urinary sediments, however, are usually satisfactory, cheaper, and easier to prepare.

1.1.3 Cytological Examination of PVF

Exfoliative cytology of PVF has been the most accepted method for screening inflammation of male accessory genital organs. Some fundamental limitations of the method, however, must be kept in mind: (1) it is limited to evaluation of fluid only from the prostate and seminal vesicles; (2) PVF samples are not always readily obtained; (3) the number of exfoliated cells often has little relation to the size of the lesion; (4) the exfoliated cells may not represent the true nature of the entire lesion (Naib 1970); (5) sometimes excessive mucus in prostatic vesicular fluid may hinder a uniform spreading of the inflammatory cells on the slides; (6) some of the diagnostic criteria of male accessory sex organ secretions are still controversial.

1.1.3.1 Cellular Elements of the PVF

Prostatic cells are rare in fluids obtained by massage of healthy prostates. Their size and shape are usually regular: most are cuboidal or columnar showing a basophilic and clear cytoplasm with the Papanicolaou's stain. In most cases prostatic cells appear in clusters. Normal seminal vesicle cells are also cuboidal or columnar and can be found in less than 10% of the specimens obtained by massage. These cells appear singly or in small clusters. They are more irregular in shape and size than those from prostate origin. A yellowish or golden-orange lipochrome pigment found in their cytoplasm is considered characteristic of these cells. Cells of the transitional epithelium of the urinary tract are commonly seen. They are larger in size than the cells of the prostate and seminal vesicles. Cells of the squamous epithelium resemble vaginal squamous cells and are commonly seen in PVF. The number of these cells greatly increases with mechanical trauma of the urethra. The round cells of late spermatogenesis are not always easily recognized and may be mistaken for leukocytes in Papanicolaou's stain. Special techniques may be required for their identification (Endtz 1972; Couture et al. 1976; Nahoum and Cardozo 1980). Spermatozoa, when present, are easily recognized. A few PMN are normally seen in normal PVF. In abnormal smears, however, increased number of neutrophils, macrophages, lymphocytes, and plasma cells combine to form different kinds of inflammatory patterns. Eosinophils are rarely found.

1.1.3.2 Quantitative Changes of the PVF Cells During Inflammation

Neutrophils are usually the only inflammatory cells quantified during cytological examination. Their number is determined by counting at least ten different fields of the smear. When these cells are extensively clumped they cannot be accurately counted and the smear is described as showing *massive infiltration* of PMN (Johannisson 1976). Smears with less than 5 PMN/HPF (high power field) are considered to be normal (class I). To the other extreme, those with more than 20 PMN/HPF (class III) are abnormal. Smears with counts of 5–20 PMN/HPF, do not exclude or confirm the presence of an inflammatory process (class II). In such cases, a repeated prostatic massage is recommended.

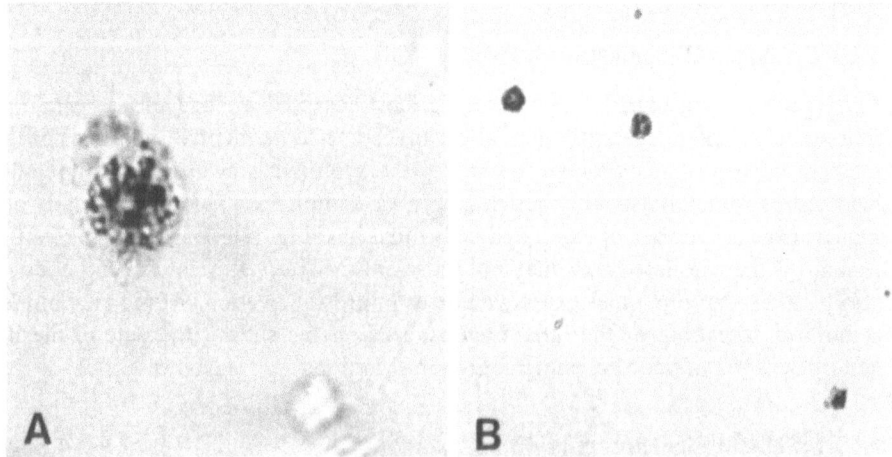

Fig. 2. **A** Granules of neutrophil peroxidase by the o-toluidine technique (×400). **B** Stained neutrophils in semen as visualized during chamber counting (×100)

There is no agreement in the literature about the upper limit for the number of PMN in samples of normal PVF (Johannisson and Eliasson 1978). The irregular escape of the neutrophils from the prostate during massages, and imprecisions of the slide counting method are at least in part responsible.

A simple and inexpensive method for counting neutrophils in small quantities of PVF has been described (Nahoum and Cardozo 1980). O-Toluidine is used for the identification of PMN, because it changes from a colorless to a brownish compound by the action of the neutrophils' peroxidase upon hydrogen peroxide. The stained granules of peroxidase easily identify the neutrophils (Fig. 2).

Semen or PVF samples are fixed in 75% alcohol-normal saline (1 : 1), allowing it to act for at least 10 min. A white blood cell pipette is filled with fixed material (level 1.0) or with unfixed material (level 0.5). In both situations the pipette must be filled to 11.0 with the working solution.

Table 1. Volumetric count of PMN leukocytes in semen and PVF according to the o-toluidine technique ($\times 10^3$/ML)

	Normal men (n = 14)	Infertile patients (n = 50)
Semen		
Mean ± 2 SD	160 ± 195	770 ± 1 345
Range	0 – 350	0 – 2 300
PVF		
Mean ± 2 SD	380 ± 510	5 230 ± 6 460
Range	50 – 900	0 – 12 800

To prepare the working solution, the following are mixed immediately before use: 10 ml 0.15% o-toluidine in normal saline and 0.02 ml of 1.5% hydrogen peroxide.

The test solution in the pipette is shaken for 2–5 min, after which the pipette is put aside at 37 °C for 20–30 min. Counts, as for blood neutrophils, are made in the leukocyte chamber and expressed per milliliter of material analyzed.

In 14 selected men with a mean age of 31.2 years (range 21–48), without a previous history of genital disease, with normal palpatory findings, normal semen analysis, and exfoliative cytology showing less than 5 PMN/HPF and absence of qualitative inflammatory changes of the epithelial cells, the volumetric counting of neutrophils gave the results presented in Table 1.

In 50 infertile patients with suspected male adnexitis, the volumetric technique revealed binomially distributed values, excluding six patients with clearly normal results. The group with less than 3×10^6 cells/ml and a central tendency of 1×10^6 cells/ml included 68.5% (27/38) of the cases. On the other hand, 31.5% (12/38) of the samples showed obviously augmented values, with PMN leukocytes varying from 5 to 12.8×10^6 cells/ml PVF. Only a few cases (n = 5) were found to be between the limits of the two groups.

Table 2. Volumetric count of PMN leukocytes in split ejaculates $(\times 10^3/\text{ml})$ $(n = 17)$

	First fraction	Second fraction
Normal men	200	100
(n = 10)	50	150
	0	150
	0	50
	0	50
	450	200
	350	50
	150	0
	100	50
	50	0
Prostatitis	2 700	400
(n = 5)	3 600	600
	650	100
	1 000	150
	1 200	300
Vesiculitis	1 900	5 950
(n = 2)	500	1 100

All the cases classified as class III by the traditional method showed more than 5×10^6 neutrophils/ml PVF samples. Those Papanicolaou-stained smears considered to be of class II (doubtfully inflamed) revealed PMN above the limit of 5×10^6 cells/ml in 25% of the cases. Such findings seem to indicate that the o-tolui-dine technique may reduce the number of doubtful or even false-negative smears, as classified by traditional exfoliative cytology.

There was no significant correlation (n = 30, p > 0.5) between the number of neutrophils in semen and PVF samples of infertile patients. However, when considering 1×10^6 PMN/ml for semen and 5×10^6 PMN/ml for PVF as the upper nor-

Table 3. Qualitative changes of the epithelial cells during inflammation. Squamous metaplasia is commonly found in samples from prostate with chronic processes

Discrete changes	Increased cytoplasmic eosinophilia
	Increased nuclear basophilia
	Inclusions, pigments and vacuoles
Moderate changes	Cellular swelling
	Irregularities of the cell margins
	Disturbed nuclear-cytoplasmic relationship
	Pyknosis
	Karyorrhexis
Severe changes	Cytoplasmic autolysis
	Karyolysis

mal limits for neutrophils in such fluids, matched values were in concordance. Parallelism between seminal and PVF neutrophil values, was found in 73% of the cases.

The o-toluidine technique can also be used for the volumetric counting of PMN in split ejaculates. Preliminary findings (n = 20) seem to anticipate the profitable utility of this procedure in the diagnosis of single or prostate-combined vesiculitis (Table 2).

1.1.3.3 Qualitative Changes of Epithelial Cells During Inflammation

Inflammation increases the number of normal or disease-altered epithelial cells exfoliated. Epithelial cells of PVF show typical changes during inflammation of accessory sex organs (Johannisson 1976). The qualitative changes are best analyzed using Papanicolaou's or acridine orange-stained smears. The most common cellular injuries are graded arbitrarily (Table 3).

In the group of patients with more than 5×10^6 PMN/ml PVF, qualitative changes of the epithelial cells were observed in 83.3% (10/12) of the cases. Otherwise, only 16.7% (1/6) of the patients under the limit of 1×10^6 neutrophils/ml PVF exhibited qualitative changes of the epithelial cells. The epithelial alterations varied from discrete (47.8%) to moderate (39.1%) or intense (20.3%) degrees.

PVF is considered inflamed if there are fewer than 1×10^6 neutrophils/ml, but PVF shows intense epithelial cellular changes; samples with $1-5 \times 10^6$ neutrophils/ml exhibit epithelial cell changes of moderate or intense degrees; the number of PMN leukocytes is above 5×10^6 cells/ml, independent of the presence of qualitative changes of the epithelial cells.

1.1.3.4 Cellular Patterns of the Smears

The relationship between the cellular patterns of the infiltrates and male infertility is still unclear. In our series of 50 patients, cytological patterns were found to be nonspecific in 12%. Of the smears, 59% presented a specific pattern in which the predominant cell type was PMN in 51%, macrophagic in 3%, and lymphoplasmocytic in 5% of the cases. Combined types occurred in 29% of the samples.

1.1.4 Molecular Tracers of the Inflammatory Process

If a severe degree of damage occurs, all the levels of the microcirculation may be involved in the inflammatory process with resultant injury of the endothelial cells producing an exudate. Only after hemodynamic and vascular permeability changes does leukocytic emigration occur. Therefore, emigration of PMN cells is essentially a phasic phenomenon during the inflammatory reaction. Molecular indicators of exudation and chemical mediators of the inflammatory process would be more reliable tracers of tissue reaction to injury. Semen, instead of PVF, and chemical substances, rather than inflammatory cells, may be preferable in screening for inflammation of the male reproductive tract.

In an attempt to diagnose male genital inflammation on a molecular basis (Fig. 3), several substances involved in the biology of the inflammatory process were assayed. The study included infertile men with and without inflammation of the ac-

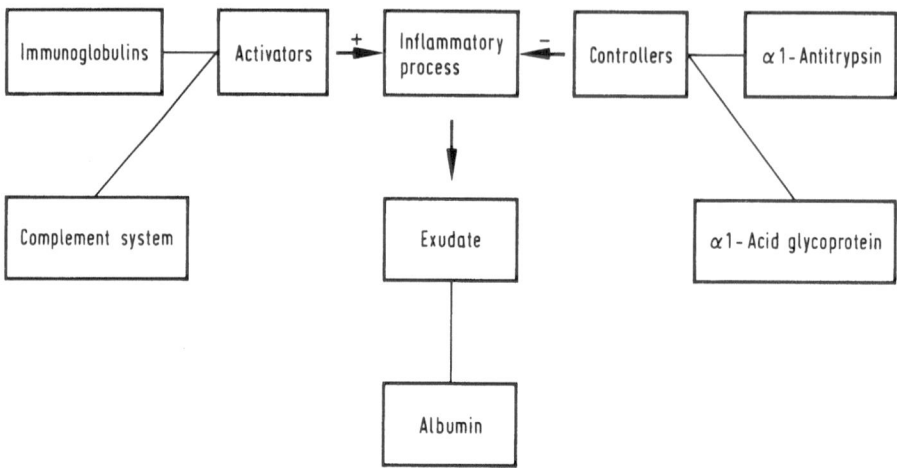

Fig. 3. Some molecular events in the inflammatory reaction

cessory sex organs according to the clinical and cytological criteria previously referred to here. Quantitative determinations were performed employing the radial immunodiffusion method (M-partigen plates for α_1-antitrypsin and α_1-acid glycoprotein and LC-partigen plates for IgA, IgG, and albumin; Behringwerke AG, Marburg, West Germany). Results are presented in Table 4.

1.1.4.1 Immunoglobulins

IgA and IgG can both be considered activators of the inflammatory process and their seminal levels in normal men have been previously reported; 0–6 and 7–22 mg/dl, respectively (Friberg 1974; Rümke 1974). Infertile patients without inflammation demonstrate similar values.

Rümke (1974) found that the distribution of these immunoglobulins in the split ejaculate corresponds to that of acid phosphatase. In our experience the highest IgA and IgG levels are observed during acute or subacute epididymitis; therefore, it may be that at least during inflammation these immunoglobulins reach the seminal fluid from organs other than prostate. Infertile men with inflammation of the genital tract have increased levels of IgA and IgG in about 70% and 60% of the cases, respectively, with few false-positive results.

1.1.4.2 C_3 Factor of the Complement System

The upper normal limit of the C_3 factor of complement first demonstrated in pooled human seminal plasma by Herrmann and Hermann (1969), is 1.4 mg/dl (Blenk et al. 1974). The seminal plasma levels in prostatitis and epididymitis are 3.2–12.0 mg/dl. High levels of C_3 component of complement in PVF are also found in patients with prostatitis, benign prostatic hyperplasia, and carcinoma of the prostate (Grayhack 1980). It is usually undetectable in the semen of normal men (Quinlivan and Sullivan 1976). The overall incidence of detectable amounts of C_3 in our infertile

Table 4. Molecular tracers of inflammation: Seminal levels in normal men and infertile patients. All values measured are expressed in mg/dl. False-positive and false-negative results are expressed in percentages

	IgA	IgG	C_3	Albumin	α^1-Anti-trypsin	α^1-Acid Glyco-protein
Upper limits in normal men (n=10)	5.8	20.0	1.8	120.0	18.5	18.5
Infertile patients without inflammation						
(n)	(33)	(133)	(63)	(127)	(134)	(79)
Mean	3.1	10.2	–	70.5	–	–
Mode	–	–	<0.7	–	13.5	<10.0
Range	1.4 – 5.8	0.3 – 19.4	<0.7 – 1.8	12.2 – 160.3	<6.1 – 18.3	<10.0 – 18.5
False-positivity (%)	3.3	0.0	3.2	6.3	0.0	5.2
Infertile patients with inflammation						
(n)	(23)	(111)	(78)	(104)	(103)	(101)
Mean	10.2	27.1	–	166.5	23.8	69.3
Mode	–	–	2.0	–	–	–
Range	2.5 – 54.2	3.0 – 116.5	<0.7 – 12.3	56.0 – 918.0	9.1 – 72.6	10.5 – 229.6
False-negativity (%)	30.4	37.8	25.6	35.1	47.6	47.5

patients was almost 70%, while it was above the upper normal limit of 1.8 mg/dl in about 75% of the cases with genital inflammation.

1.1.4.3 Albumin

Albumin, a normal constituent of human seminal plasma (Li and Shulman 1971; Quinlivan and Sullivan 1972), is present in increased amounts during inflammation. In normal men the mean seminal plasma concentration of this protein is 63 mg/dl (range 30–97 mg/dl) (Zaneveld et al. 1971). In infertile men the mean concentration is 143 mg/dl (range 27–720 mg/dl, n = 23) (Lindholmer et al. 1974). However, Lindholmer's group probably included patients with inflammatory disease of the male genital tract. Our patients with inflammation showed abnormal amounts of albumin in 65% of the cases.

   Important functions have been attributed to albumin in seminal plasma. It can initiate the progressive motility of epididymal spermatozoa, interfere with the sperm nuclear chromatin stability, and alter membrane permeability to eosin Y (Lindholmer 1974). Because albumin can trap zinc ions it may be that the mid-piece respiratory and/or glycolytic metalloenzymes might be affected by inflammatory changes of the seminal plasma.

1.1.4.4 α_1-Antitrypsin

Acrosomal hydrolytic enzymes allow the spermatozoa to penetrate the outer layers of the ovum. Acrosin, a proteinase belonging to this group of enzymes, allows spermatozoa to penetrate the zona pellucida. For capacitation to occur proteinase inhibitors normally found in seminal plasma, must be removed from spermatozoa before fertilization (Polakoski and Zaneveld 1976). Proteinase inhibitors with high and low molecular weight are present in human seminal plasma. Those with high molecular weight include α_1-antitrypsin and α_1-antichymotrypsin, and those with low molecular weight include human seminal plasma inhibitor I or trypsin-chymotrypsin inhibitor (HUSI-I, mol. wt. 11,000) and the human seminal plasma inhibitor II or trypsin-acrosin inhibitor (HUSI-II, mol. wt. 6200) (Fink et al. 1971; Zaneveld et al. 1971). α_1-Antitrypsin is most likely part of a defensive mechanism to protect spermatozoa and basal membranes of the genital tract against the lytic action of leukocytic and bacterial proteinases. The trypsin-acrosin inhibitor or HUSI-II may be considered as a natural antagonist of human acrosin. It forms complexes with acrosin very rapidly even in relatively low concentrations (Fritz et al. 1975). Inflammatory processes of the genital tract may increase the level of acrosin-blocking substances, thus affecting the fertilizing ability of spermatozoa. However, it is not known if inflammation increases the concentration of HUSI-II in male accessory organs secretions.

   Like Blenk et al. (1974), we have found markedly augmented levels of α_1-antitrypsin in semen of some infertile patients with proved accessory sex organ inflammation (mean concentration 23.8 mg/dl, range 9.1–72.6 mg/dl, n = 103). Blenk's values, however, were lower than ours since, when affected by prostatitis or epididymitis, their patients showed values of 12.0–22.0 mg/dl.

   In normal men, Blenk et al. (1974) found a mean concentration of 8.0 mg/dl with an upper normal limit of 11.0 mg/dl. Schill (1976) analyzed the seminal levels of α_1-antitrypsin in 129 andrological patients (23–53 years old) without clinical or seminal signs of chronic or acute genital tract inflammation. He found the average concentration of the enzyme as being 9.8 mg/dl (range 0.5–27.5 mg/dl).

In a group of 134 infertile patients without clinical or cytological signs of inflammation of the genital tract, we found the mean value of α_1-antitrypsin in this group to be 13.5 mg/dl (range 6.1–18.3 mg/dl). In patients with inflammation, α_1-antitrypsin was found to be increased above the limit of 18.5 mg/dl in 52.4% of the cases. At concentrations found in seminal plasma of healthy men this enzyme has weak antifertility properties. However, the velocity of inhibition of acrosin runs parallel to the increase of α_1-antitrypsin concentration (Fritz et al. 1972). The potential correlation between high levels of α_1-antitrypsin in seminal plasma of patients with genital inflammation and male infertility remains to be investigated.

1.1.4.5 α_1-Acid Glycoprotein

α_1-acid glycoprotein (α_1-AG) belongs to the group of the acute phase enzymes occurring in human serum during inflammation and neoplasm. Several hypotheses have been elicited to explain the role of α_1-AG. This enzyme is supposed to be involved in the healing of wounds and tissue repair (Jayle et al. 1971; Zeineh and Kukral 1970), as well as in the inhibition of lysosomal proteolytic enzymes (Koj 1974) and in the immunosuppression of tumor cells (Apffel and Peters 1969). α_1-AG might, in some way, influence the inflammatory or cell proliferative processes in situ: based on this, the seminal level of α_1-AG was estimated in 180 infertile patients attending our clinical unit. In those patients without inflammation of the male genital accessory organs (n = 79) undetectable amounts of the substance were found in most of the cases (maximal value 18.5 mg/dl). On the other hand, 52.5% of the patients with genital inflammation presented values above this limit. The mean seminal concentration in this group was 69.3 mg/dl (range 10.5–229.6 mg/dl). Also in relation to α_1-AG, the highest values were seen in epididymitis, with a low occurrence of false-positive results.

The leukocytic origin of α_1-AG would categorize it as a promising indicator of the presence of inflammatory disease in the male genital tract.

1.2 Infectious Male Adnexitis

1.2.1 General Considerations

The prostatitis syndromes include three forms: acute prostatitis; chronic bacterial prostatitis; and nonacute or abacterial prostatitis (also called prostatosis). Infertile patients in an andrological practice rarely present the acute form. Patients with acute prostatitis are febrile with acute urinary symptoms. Chronic bacterial prostatitis occurs in about 10%–15% of patients (Fritjoffsson et al. 1973; Ulstein et al. 1976). The acute and chronic bacterial forms of the disease are almost always caused by Escherichia coli. The commonest type of prostatitis, nonacute (NAP), has an unknown etiology.

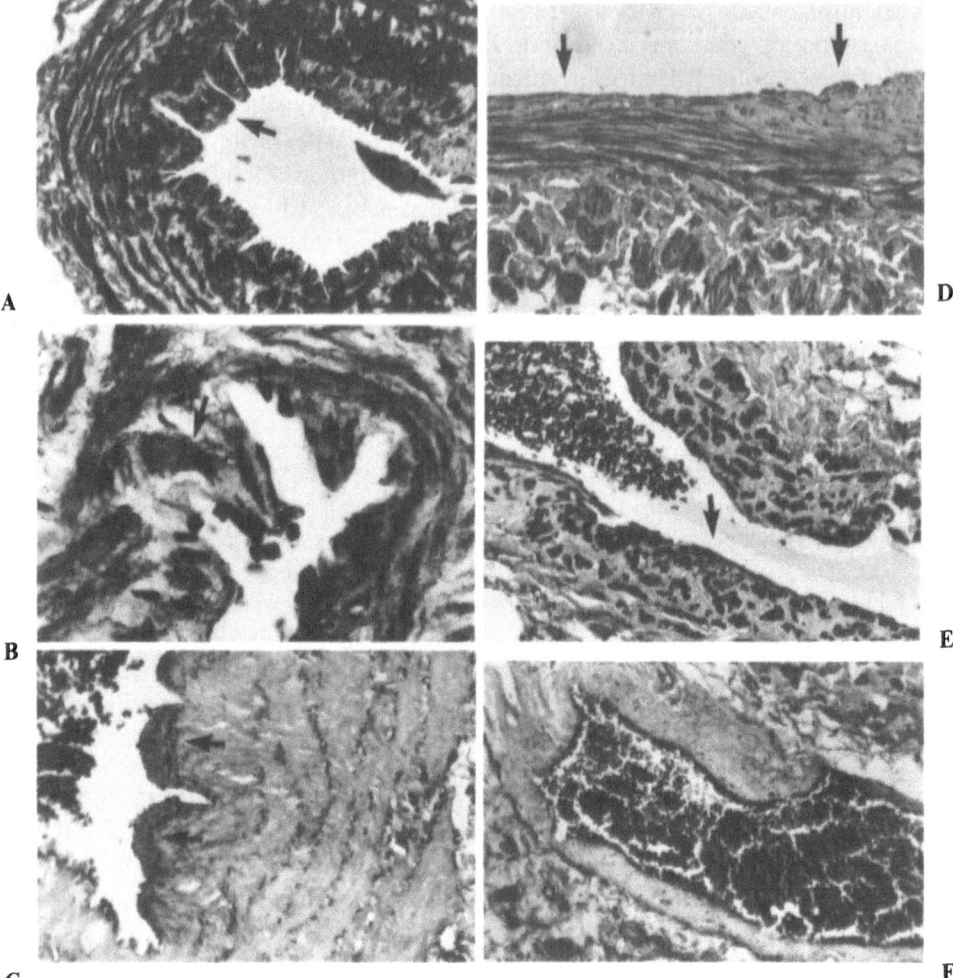

Fig. 4. A. Section of a pampiniforme plexus vein from a normal man (Gomori trichrome stain, ×400). Projections of the intimal layer into the lumen (polsters) are seen (*arrows*). Similar structures are also found in prostatic and hemorrhoidal veins. **B** Muscular fibers from the tunica media are axially projected along normal polsters (Masson trichrome stain, ×400). **C** A band of normal elastic fibers placed in the basis of the polsters (acetic orcein stain, ×100). **D** Section of a pampiniform plexus vein in a varicocele patient. An area with loss of polsters is seen beside preserved ones (*arrows*) (Gomori trichrome stain, ×100). **E** Section of a rectal vein of a patient with hemorrhoids and varicocele showing total loss of intimal polsters and elastic fibers (acetic orcein stain, ×100). **F** Section of a varicose vein of prostatic plexus (Santorini's plexus) from a patient with varicocele and chronic abacterial prostatitis, also showing total loss of intimal polsters (Masson trichrome stain, ×100)

The finding of increased numbers of leukocytes in semen or PVF does not always correlate with identification of pathogenic microorganisms in cultures (Mears 1973). Trichomonas vaginalis (Colleen and Mårdh 1975 a), L-phase saprophitic and opportunistic bacteria (Eliasson 1976 b), mycoplasmas (Colleen and Mårdh 1975 a), chlamydia (Mårdh et al. 1972), viruses and fungi (Mårdh and Colleen 1975 a) have been described as potentially related to NAP. The data, however, are inconclusive.

In this context the possibility of noninfectious etiologies for NAP must be considered. Congestive prostatitis in which no bacteria have been isolated may occur in 50% of young symptomatic patients (Frick 1976).

The author and co-workers have found varices and congestion of the prostatic venous plexus in patients with varicoceles which may occur as frequently as hemorrhoids in such patients. These findings (Fig. 4) suggest the existence of a true pelvic venopathy in some infertile patients. The same histopathologic changes (mostly rupture of elastic fibers and loss of intimal polsters) were found in the venous wall of hemorrhoidal, prostatic, and testicular vein plexus of varicocele patients. The frequent finding of prostatic congestion during rectal examination of varicocele patients and the mild increase of neutrophils in their, otherwise abacterial, PVF could be explained by chronic congestion of the prostate with sustained hypoxia of the gland. Hypoxia is one of the well-established causes of inflammation (Woolf 1977).

1.2.2 Qualitative and Quantitative Data on Genital Infection in Infertile Patients

Several microorganisms have been identified in genital secretions of infertile patients but their pathogenicity has not been established (Chernov 1978; Gnarpe and Friberg 1973; Moberg et al. 1979, 1980; Swenson et al. 1980). Adding an E. coli suspension to fresh ejaculates results in sperm clumping and inhibition of sperm motility (Wu 1957; Teague et al. 1971). A low molecular weight spermatozoal immobilization factor has been isolated from E. coli cultures (Paulson and Polakoski 1977). Mycoplasma colonies adhere to the junction between the sperm head and the midpiece of the spermatozoa causing sperm agglutination (Taylor-Robinson and Manchee 1967) and reduced motility (Fowlkes et al. 1975; O'Leary and Frick 1975; Hofstetter et al. 1978). Chlamydia trachomatis, a microorganism implicated as the major cause of "idiopathic" epididymitis in humans (Berger et al. 1978) also induces epididymal infection in monkeys (Moller and Mårdh 1980). There are no consistent data about Trichomonas infection as related to male fertility.

Efforts have been made to establish the critical limits of significance for bacteriospermia (Fari et al. 1977; Comhaire et al. 1980). Prescribed limits were 3×10^3 gram-negative pathogens/ml semen or more than 10^4 gram-positive nonpathogenic bacteria/ml in 1:2 diluted seminal plasma, respectively. Seminal dilution recommended by Comhaire et al. (1980) would neutralize the recognized bacteriostatic capacity of the seminal plasma (Mårdh and Colleen 1975 b).

In 230 seminal plasma cultures of infertile patients with abnormal exfoliative cytology, we observed bacterial growth above 10^3 colonies/ml in 54% of the cases, but established urinary tract pathogens were only detected in 27% of the cases. Saprophitic and opportunistic bacteria, mostly Staphylococcus epidermidis, predominated in those cultures with less than 10^3 microorganisms/ml semen. Gram-negative pathogens growing above 10^3 colonies/ml were found in only 9% of the cases. In view of these findings, routine cultures of semen are not likely to be rewarding.

Criteria for selection of semen specimens for microbiological analysis are: counting PMN cells in genital secretions (Comhaire et al. 1977; Ulstein et al. 1976) and the acridine-orange staining techniques applied to prostatic fluid smears (Lillie and Fullmer 1976). Stained by acridine-orange, coliforms, cocci, fungi, and gonococcus make reddish fluorescence that become readily detected. Smears showing such microorganisms can be better selected for specific culture techniques. Trichomonas vaginalis stains red with a yellow nucleus. Atypical dyskaryotic and hyperplastic epithelial cells are easily identified by color changes of nuclear and cytoplasmic material. Neutrophils fluoresce as bright green or greenish yellow. Acridine-orange staining of prostatic fluid smears is a very useful procedure in the study of inflammatory or infectious states of the prostatic gland (Turner 1960). A short procedure, also called the 10-sec acridine-orange staining technique, may be used (Derrick 1977). One or two drops of the prostatic fluid are smeared and thinned on a slide and air-dried. For staining, the slide is immersed successively about five times in a 0.025% solution of acridine orange. It is washed in 2% alcohol in normal saline by agitation for 3 s, followed by agitation for at least 4 s in normal saline. The saline solutions must be renewed daily. Mounting of the slides is made with a droplet of saline under the cover glass. Cytological examination is done at $100\times$ magnification and bacteriological identification at $400\times$ magnification. The slide may be restained in 50% alcohol for 5 min and restained by the Papanicolaou's stain technique. To prepare the acridine-orange solution 0.25 g of the stain is dissolved in 1000 ml 2% acetic acid solution to which 0.2 ml Tween-80 is added. The solution is protected from light and changed weekly.

1.3 Secretory Function of Accessory Glands and Male Adnexitis

A high incidence of reduced seminal levels of zinc and acid phosphatase was reported in patients with male adnexitis (Eliasson et al. 1966, 1970). These findings encouraged routine seminal plasma assays of biochemical tracers of prostatic and seminal vesicular function in the screening of male adnexal inflammation. However, accessory gland inflammation is not necessarily associated with seminal biochemical changes. It is known that zinc and acid phosphatase reflect only the degree of epithelial activity of those glands. They are not specific indicators of an inflammatory process. Moreover, Kerr et al. (1960) have found remarkable variations of zinc content within the normal human prostate. The seminal plasma concentration of zinc is at least partially dependent on the affected area. In addition, prostatic epithelium is highly dependent on circulating androgen levels and castration has been shown to result in prostatic epithelial atrophy (Hoare et al. 1956; Mackenzie et al. 1962). Thus, reduced testosterone levels could be responsible for noninflammatory changes in seminal concentrations of zinc. Zinc seems to inhibit phagocytic activity of PVF granulocytes (Stankova et al. 1976); it inhibits histamine release from mast cells (Kazimierczak and Maslinski 1974), serotonin release from platelets (Chvapil et al. 1975), and it also inactivates peritoneal macrophages (Chvapil 1976). It seems reasonable that zinc in PVF might limit the release of various mediators of inflammation by leukocytes (Stankova et al. 1976). However, daily testosterone excretion by patients with chronic prostatitis is reduced (Yunda and Imshinetskaya 1977). Because of these facts, an increase of leukocytes in abacterial PVF may reflect a reduction in the inhibitory action of zinc upon granulocytes, secondary to low androgen concentrations in prostatic tissue. This would explain the proposed benefit of testosterone therapy in the management of some types of chronic prostatitis (Kobelev 1971; Yunda 1972).

A significant difference between seminal zinc and magnesium concentrations in patients with nonacute prostatitis and normal individuals could not be found (Colleen et al. 1975). However, in patients with gonococci in PVF, zinc concentrations were significantly low. This suggests that a significant fall of this ion in semen is achieved only after extensive or severe damage of the prostatic epithelium. In the author's experience almost 75% of the patients with mild inflammation (class II) show zinc values in the ejaculate similar to those found in normal men. On the other hand, the degree of zinc reduction in semen parallels the severity of the PVF cytological changes. Biochemical prostatic tracers of epithelial secretory function as well as seminal vesicular markers, such as fructose, have shown little diagnostic value in the screening of male adnexitis. They are, however, useful indicators of gland dysfunction. Comhaire et al. (1980) clearly distinguish among infection, inflammation, and disturbed secretory function. Inflammation speaks for the process itself; infection is associated with a causative agent and secretory activity with the degree of loss of function by the gland. Important functions have now been attributed to zinc ions in seminal plasma (Eliasson 1976 b; Eliasson et al. 1971; Eliasson and Kvist 1976).

1.4 Treatment of Male Adnexitis

1.4.1 Introduction

Only in those situations in which pathogenic microorganisms are observed in semen or prostatic-vesicular fluid, can the presence of infectious male adnexitis be considered. Abnormal rectal examination, altered exfoliative cytology, pyospermia, and decreased secretory function of accessory glands (Eliasson et al. 1966) are only indicative of an inflammatory response whatever the causative agent. Frequently, however, patients with inflammation or infections are incorrectly considered together (Comhaire et al. 1980).

Whenever possible, medical treatment should be directed towards the causative agents of the diseases. Adequate criteria to select patients for treatment as well as appropriate therapy in the management of adnexitis in fertile men remain to be established.

1.4.2 Therapeutic Procedures

Although prostatic massage may have some clinical benefit and rectal examination reverts to normal in patients with congestive prostatitis, seminal quality and pregnancy rate seem to show no improvement (Homonnai et al. 1979).

Table 5. Current antimicrobial therapeutics in the management of male adnexitis

Generic name	Trademark name	Action spectrum[a]	Preparations	Dose interval	Daily dose	Presence in genital secretions
Ampicillin	Polycillin (Bristol)	G+ G−	Capsules (250 or 500 mg)	Every 6 h	2.0 – 4.0 g	First fraction of split ejaculates (Malmborg et al. 1975)
Erythromycin	Ilosone (Lilly)	G+ G−	Tablets (125, 250, or 500 mg)	Every 6 h	1.0 – 4.0 g	First and second fractions of split ejaculates (Malmborg et al. 1975)
Doxycycline	Vibramycin (Pfizer)	G+ G− M C	Capsules (5 or 100 mg)	100 mg every 12 h during the first 24 h followed by 100 mg once a day	100–200 mg	First fraction of split ejaculates (Malmborg et al. 1975) Prostatic tissue (Oosterlinck et al. 1976)
Minocycline	Minocin (Lederle)	G+ G− M C	Capsules (50 or 100 mg)	200 mg for the first dose and 200 mg, then 100 mg every 12 h	200 mg	Prostatic tissue (Homonnai et al. 1975) (Hensle et al. 1977)
Methacycline	Rondomycin (Cyanamid)	G+ G− M C	Capsules (50 or 150 mg)	150 mg every 6 h or 300 mg every 12 h	600 mg	PVF (Colleen and Maroh 1975b)
Cephalexin	Keflex (Lilly)	G+ G−	Capsules (50 or 500 mg)	Every 6 h	1.0–4.0 g	Total ejaculate (Dalet et al. 1978) (Symes et al. 1974)
Thiamphenicol	Glitisol (Zambon)	G+ G− M C	Capsules (250 mg)	500 mg Every 8 h	1.5 g	Total ejaculate (Plomp et al. 1978)

Trimethoprim + Sulfamethoxazole	Bactrim (Roche)	G+ G−	Tablets (400 mg Sulfamethoxazole + 800 mg Trimethoprim)	Every 12 h[b]	800–1600 mg Sulfamethoxazole, 60–320 mg Trimethoprim	First and second fractions of split ejaculates (Eliasson and Dornbusch 1977) (Schirren and Schaller 1971)
Metronidazole	Flagyl (Rhodia)	TV AB	Tablets (250 mg)	250 mg every 8 h or 1.25 g twice after meals with 12 h interval	750–2500 mg	First and second fractions of split ejaculates (Eliasson and Dornbusch 1980)

[a] G+ (gram positive); G− (gram negative); M (Mycoplasmas other than T-strain); C (Chlamydia); TV (*Trichomonas vaginalis*); AB (anerobic bacteria); [b] Both short-term therapy (two tablets twice a day for 2 weeks) and long-term therapy (two tablets twice a day for 2 months, followed by one tablet twice a day for 2–9 months) for chronic prostatitis have been recommended regarding the sulfamethoxazole-trimethoprim combination (Weinstein 1975)

Table 6. Currently available anti-inflammatory drugs in andrological practice (Woodbury and Fingl 1975)

Generic name	Trade name	Preparations	Dose interval	Daily dose
Aspirin	Ronal (Rhodia)	Tablets (65–650 mg) Capsules (300 mg) Suppositories (65–1300 mg)	4 h	3 000–6 000 mg
Phenylbutazone	Butazolidin (Geigy)	Coated tablets (100 mg)	4 h	400–600 mg
Oxyphenbutazone	Tanderil (Geigy)	Tablets (100 mg)	6 h	400–600 mg
Indomethacin	Indocin (Merck, Sharp & Dohme)	Capsules (25 or 50 mg)	12 h	100–150 mg
Ibuprofen	Motrin (Upjohn)	Coated tablets (400 mg)	6–12 h	800–1 600 mg
Naproxen	Naprosyn (Syntex)	Tablets (250 mg)	12 h	500–750 mg

Mucolytic agents like N-cyclohexy^1-N-methylchloridrate (Bysolvon, Boehringer Ingelheim) and N-acetylcysteine (Fluimucyl, Zambon) may be tried in order to reduce seminal hyperviscosity presented by some patients with adnexial glandular inflammation (Schoysman et al. 1978).

Bracci et al. (1978) combined an antiandrogen with anti-inflammatory drugs in the management of prostatitis: orally administered cyproterone acetate (12.5 mg Androcur) were given on alternate days for 40–60 days. Treatment was considered successful in 78.5% of the cases (11/16) with respect to the reduction of the prostatic volume and the relief of subjective symptoms. Oligozoospermia, reduced sperm motility and decreased libido, however, were undesirable side effects in an unacceptable number of cases.

A remarkable reduction of clinical symptoms occurred in five of six patients with prostatitis or epididymitis who underwent treatment with levamisole (150 mg twice weekly for 12 weeks) (Jecht and Haneke 1978). Levamisole seems to stimulate the function of immunodeficient cells, mostly macrophages, PMN leukocytes and T lymphocytes (Symoens and Rosenthal 1977). A proposed schedule for its use is 2.5 mg/kg/day orally for 3 consecutive days, repeated every other week. Higher doses may be immunosuppressive (Wybran 1976).

Antibiotics and anti-inflammatory drugs are currently the commonest combination utilized in the treatment of chronic bacterial and chronic abacterial nonacute types of prostatitis. Culture and sensitivity studies indicate the drug of choice for treatment of bacterial prostatitis. However, some authors have reported improvement of seminal quality after antibiotic treatment, even when pathogenic microorganisms were not found (Baker et al. 1979; Nikkanen et al. 1979). Recommended dosages of several antibiotics excreted in effective concentrations in male genital secretions are indicated in Table 5 (Woodbury and Fingl 1975). Monitoring of patients under treatment is imperative. The commonest causes of failure of therapy are inadequate dosage and inappropriate duration of therapy. Antibiotics must be used whenever indicated, but their indiscriminate use is to be avoided. The deleterious effect of nitrofurans upon spermatozoa is well known (Albert et al. 1975; Gomes 1970). There is no evidence that trimethoprim-sulfamethoxazole, when given in the recommended doses, induces folate deficiency in normal persons. Mammalian cells are considered to utilize preformed folates from the diet and do not synthesize the compound (Weinstein 1975). However, Mathur et al. (1977) was able to induce inhibition of spermatogenesis in adult male albino rats through the injection of a folic acid antagonist. Sulfonamide inhibits the incorporation of PABA into folic acid and trimethoprim prevents the reduction of dihydrofolate to tetrahydrofolate. The potentially harmful effect of this commonly used and highly effective combination on human spermatogenesis needs to be investigated.

The anti-inflammatory drugs most commonly used in the treatment of infertile men with accessory gland inflammation are showed in Table 6 (Eliasson and Johannisson 1978; Homonnai et al. 1975). The antiphlogistic action of salicylates, indomethacin, and other anti-inflammatory drugs are due primarily to an inhibition of prostaglandin synthesis. Other mechanisms, like inhibition of leukocyte phagocytosis and stabilization of lysosomal membranes may also be involved (Ferreira and Vane 1974).

Indomethacin is more potent than aspirin, but toxicity often limits its use. Oxyphenbutazone (Tanderil, Geigy) has the same spectrum of activity, therapeutic uses, interaction and toxicity as salicylates. Ibuprofen (Motrin, Upjohn) compared with aspirin, seems to have an inferior anti-inflammatory effect but causes less gastrointestinal distress. Naproxen (Naprosyn, Syntex) is well-tolerated during long-term therapy. It appears to be more effective than Ibuprofen and is better tolerated than aspirin. A new terpenyl-pyrazolidinedione derivate (Metrazone, Boehringer Ingelheim), has been shown to have effective anti-inflammatory action (Bianchi 1972): because of good gastric tolerance and the rarity of untoward effects, we use it as the drug of choice for short-term therapy of prostatitis. The best results have been obtained with 400–1200 mg daily, taken after meals every 12 h for 10 days.

Cinnarizine (Mitronal, Searle), has evoked our interest as a potential agent in the treatment of male adnexitis. Cinnarizine has a broad anti-inflammatory spectrum having, in addition to antihistaminic and antiserotonin effects, an antikinin activity (Di Perri and Auteri 1971), and a capacity to inhibit the complement system, especially by blocking the activation of C_4 (Di Perri 1973). The high tolerance to this drug may enhance its use during prolonged anti-inflammatory therapy. The achievement of an effective concentration of cinnarizine in male genital secretions needs to be investigated.

The administration of prostaglandin synthesis inhibitors, like anti-inflammatory drugs, may result in a decrease of seminal prostaglandin E (PGE) and prostaglandin F (PGF) concentrations (Collier and Flower 1971). Byjdeman et al. (1970), Collier et al. (1975) and Howkins (1968) claim that there is a correlation between low seminal levels and unexplained infertility. Isidori et al. (1980) have reported disturbed sperm concentration and motility associated both with high to low levels of PG-E or 19-OH PG-E in semen. Eliasson (1959) and Eliasson et al. (1968) found no change in sperm motility of washed spermatozoa when suspended in PG-

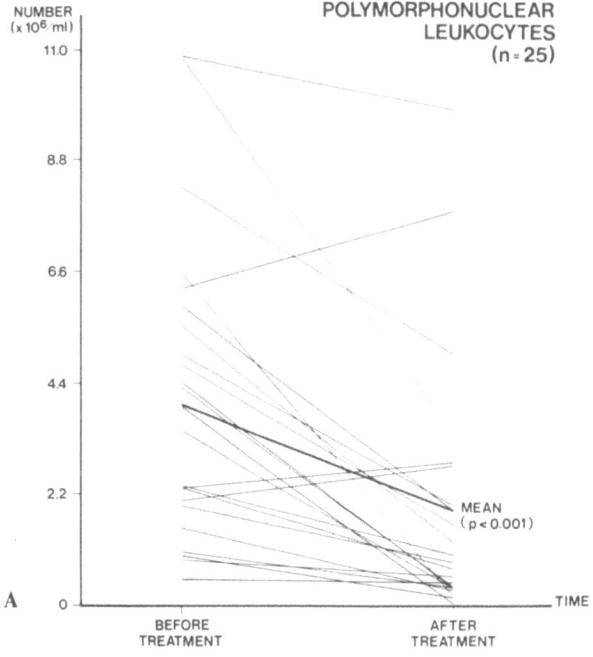

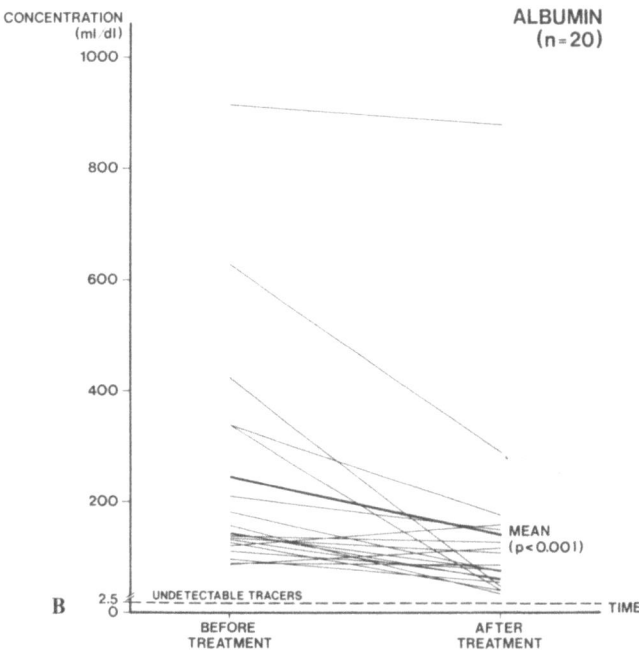

Fig. 5. A–D. The effects of a 30-day established treatment upon the seminal concentration of leukocytes **A**, albumin **B**, IgG **C**, and α_1-AG **D**. These figures seem to indicate that IgG and albumin levels are as useful as leukocyte counting in the laboratory follow-up of male adnexitis. Unexpectedly, α_1-AG has a variable response which remains to be clarified

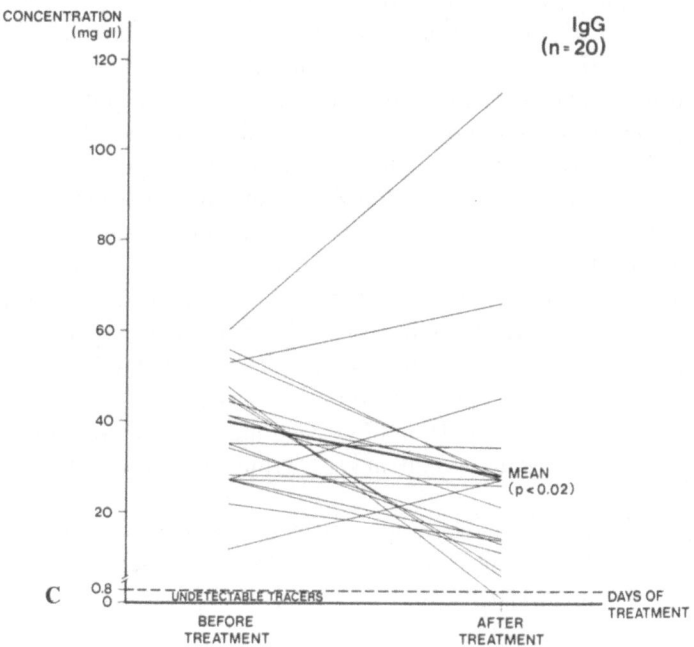

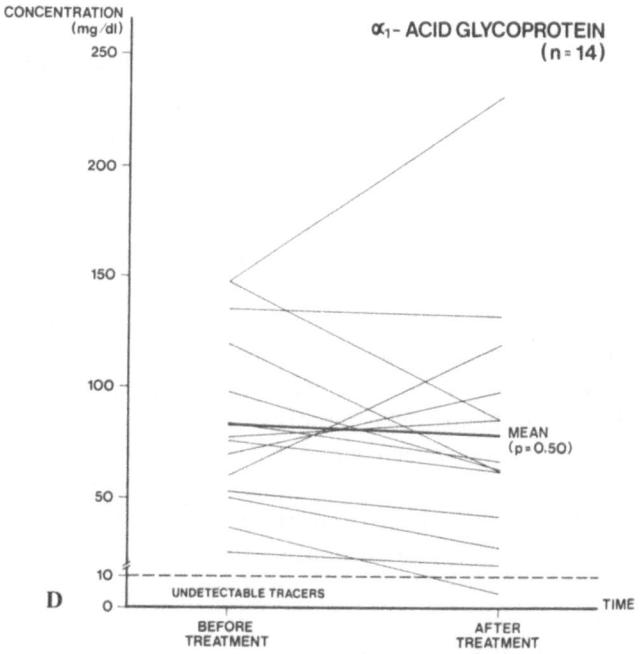

Fig. 5 C, D

containing solutions, but Didolkar and Roychowdhury (1980) have found that the addition of PG-E$\overset{2}{2}$ to human semen enhances sperm motility. Meiosis (Dellow and Miles 1975) and the fertilizing ability of spermatozoa are both prostaglandin-dependent phenomena in male adult rats (Chatterjee and Rej 1978). Badr (1976) reported the existence of a reciprocal relationship between androgen level and prostaglandin concentration in testicular tissue. Joseph and Bartke (1979) demonstrated that the intratesticular administration of indomethacin in adult male rats can interfere with the stimulation of testicular testosterone production by LH. Aspirin and indomethacin have pronounced antigonadal effects in adult male rats: These drugs directly inhibit Leydig's cell function, alter Sertoli's cell morphology, reduce accessory gland weight, and depress the spermatocyte-spermatid conversion process (Biswas et al. 1978; Sanyal et al. 1980; Tierney et al. 1979). Administration of LH in indomethacin-treated rats restores accessory gland weight. However, only the simultaneous injection of LH and PGE 2 to these animals was able to fully restore both sex accessory gland weight and sperm number to the level of controls (Biswas et al. 1978).

These marked effects upon rat gonads remain to be demonstrated in humans, but these observations mitigate against the indiscriminate use of anti-inflammatory drugs in infertile patients.

1.4.3 Follow-Up

There are several claims that treatment of genital tract inflammation and/or infection improves semen quality and fertility (Baker et al. 1979; Comhaire et al. 1977; Derrick and Dahlberg 1976; Quesada et al. 1968; Ulstein et al. 1976). Increased sperm motility and viability, reduced spontaneous agglutination (Derrick and Dahlberg 1976), restoration of prostatic secretory function (Eliasson 1976 b), and improved sperm count and morphology (Ulstein et al. 1976) are all benefits attributed to treatments in infertile patients with male adnexitis. However, there continues to be inadequate evidence for the true efficacy of anti-inflammatory and antimicrobial therapy under such conditions. Prospective studies of this subject are still needed.

The most acceptable criteria of cure in the follow-up of these patients are eradication of pathogenic microorganisms from genital secretions, a return to normal exfoliative cytology, and restoration of accessory gland secretory function: Other criteria include the number of neutrophils per volume of semen and PVF and the seminal concentration of some molecular tracers of the inflammatory process. Figure 5 illustrates the effect of therapy upon such parameters. Duration of treatment must be individualized for each patient. Therapy should be stopped only after normalization of seminal or PVF parameters.

1.5 Gaps in Our Knowledge

The real meaning, as well as the diagnosis and management of the inflammatory state of male accessory genital organs (ISMAGO) are still a matter of controversy. Concepts will continue to change. Some fundamental questions in this field can be asked:

(1) What is the real incidence of male adnexitis as a causative factor of male infertility? (2) What is the true incidence of seminal vesicular inflammation with or without prostatitis in fertile man? (3) What is the relationship between epididymitis and male infertility? (4) What is the real meaning of microorganisms like viruses, Trichomonas, chlamydia, and mycoplasma in inflammatory male infertility? (5) What are the mechanisms through which bacteria and/or substances released during the inflammatory reaction could affect sperm function? (6) Are there noninfectious accessory gland inflammations responsible for male infertility? (7) To what extent would therapeutic measures really improve seminal quality and pregnancy rates? (8) What are the best schemes for treating patients with inflammatory disease of the genital tract? (9) Are there significant harmful side effects of established therapy upon fertility? (10) The inflammatory response is a beneficial process. At what moment does the inflammatory reaction interfere with sperm function? Must all types and degrees of male accessory gland inflammation be treated?

The role of inflammation in the development of male infertility still remains to be clarified. As our diagnostic ability improves, so will our understanding of the cause and effect relationship between inflammation and decreased fertility. A consequence of this understanding will be new and improved therapeutic regimens intended to restore normalcy in the male reproductive tract and a return to the fertile state.

Acknowledgments. The suggestions of Drs. Rune Eliasson and Elisabeth Johanisson are gratefully acknowledged. The author is also grateful to Dr. Francisco Rodrigues Freire for his help in the revision of the manuscript. The author wishes to thank Dr. Denize Cardozo, Drs. José Augusto Soares Pantaleao and Roberto Paulo Dias Burlamaqui, Mr. Emerson Rocha Gonçalves, Mrs. Carla Hejstron Naritomi for their technical assistance and Miss Augusta R. Guimarães for her secretarial help. This work was partially supported by research grants from the Grupo de Estudos de Fertilidade e Esterilidade do Rio de Janeiro-GEFERJ.

1.6 References

Albert PS, Salerno RG, Kapoor SN, Davis IE (1975) The nitrofurans as sperm-immobilizing agents. J Urol 113:69–70

Apffel CA, Peters IH (1969) Tumors and serum glycoproteins. The "Symbodies". Progr Exp Tumor Res 12:1–54

Badr FM (1976) Effect of sexual maturation and androgens on prostaglandin levels in tissues of male reproductive system in mice. Endocrinology 98:1523–1527

Baker HWG, Straffon WGE, Murphy G, Davidson A, Burger HG, Kretser DM (1979) Prostatitis and male infertility: a pilot study. Possible increase in sperm motility with antibacterial chemotherapy. Int J Androl 2:193–201

Bedford IM (1975) Maturation, transport, and fate of spermatozoa in the epididymis. In: Greep RO, Astwood EB, Hamilton DW, Geiger SR (eds) Handbook of physiology: a critical, comprehensive presentation of physiological knowledge and concepts. American Physiological Society, Washington, D.C., pp 303–317

Bedford IM, Calvin HC, Cooper GW (1973) The maturation of spermatozoa in the human epididymis. J Reprod Fertil [Suppl] 18:199–213

Berger RE, Alexander ER, Monda GD, Ansell J, McCormick G, Holmes KK (1978) Chlamydia trachomatis as a cause of acute "idiopathic" epididymitis. N Eng J Med 298:301–304

Bianchi C (1972) Survey of the biological properties of 4-prenyl-1,2-diphenyl-3,5-py-razolidinedione, a novel agent in the class of anti-inflammatory drugs. Arzneim Forsch (Drug Res) 22:249–252

Biswas NM, Sanyal S, Patra PB (1978) Antispermatogenic effect of aspirin and its prevention by prostaglandin E_2. Andrologia 10:137–141

Blenk H, Hofstetter A, Böwering R, Buttler R, Hartmann M, Marx FI (1974) Im-munelektrophorese des Ejakulats. Möglichkeiten der Differentialdiagnose zwischen entzündlichen und nicht entzündlichen Adnexerkrankungen. Muench Med Wochenschr 116:35–38

Bracci U, di Silverio F, Alei G (1978) Antiandrogen management of prostatitis. In: Fabbrini A, Steinberger E (eds) Recent progress in andrology. Academic Press, New York, pp 447–451

Bygdeman M, Fredricsson B, Svanborg K, Samuelsson B (1970) The relation between fertility and prostaglandin content of seminal fluid in man. Fertil Steril 21:622–629

Chatterjee A, Rej SK (1978) The possible mode of action of prostaglandins. XV. Study of the effect of prostaglandin E_1, E_2 or E_{2a} in limiting the fertilizing capacity of epididymal sper-matozoa in rats. Int J Androl 1:563–569

Chernov A (1978) The occurrence of simple and mixed fungal infections in patients at the De-partment of Andrology. Hamburg (1972–1976). Andrologia 10:385–389

Chvapil M (1976) Effect of zinc on cells and biomembranes. Symposium on Trace Elements. Med Clin N Am 60:799–812

Chvapil M, Weldy PL, Stankova L (1975) Inhibitory effect of zinc ions on platelet aggregation and serotonin release reaction. Life Sci 16:1345–1362

Colleen S, Mårdh P-A (1975a) Studies on nonacute prostatitis. Clinical and laboratory find-ings in patients with symptoms of nonacute prostatitis. In: Danielsson D, Juhlin L, Mårdh P-A (eds) Genital infections and their complications. Almquist & Wiksell, Stockholm, pp 121–131

Colleen S, Mårdh P-A (1975b) Effect of metacycline treatment of nonacute prostatitis. Scand J Urol Nephrol 9:198–204

Colleen S, Mårdh P-A, Schytz A (1975) Magnesium and zinc in seminal fluid of healthy males and patients with nonacute prostatitis with and without gonorrhaea. Scand J Urol Nephrol 9:192–197

Collier IG, Flower RI (1971) Effect of aspirin on human seminal plasma prostaglandins. Lan-cet 2:852–853

Collier IG, Flower RL, Stanton SL (1975) Seminal prostaglandins in infertile men. Fertil Steril 26:868–871

Comhaire F, Carlier A, Verschraegen G, Vermeulen L (1977) Spermogramme et infection génitale. In: Suchet-Henry J, Steg A, Constatin A (eds) Infection et fécondité. Masson, Paris, pp 59–65

Comhaire F, Verschraegen G, Vermeulen L (1980) Diagnosis of accessory gland infection and its possible role in male infertility. Int J Androl 3:32–45

Couture M, Ulstein M, Leonard J, Paulsen CA (1976) Improved staining method for dif-ferentiating immature germ cells from white blood cells in human seminal fluid. Andro-logia 8:61–66

Dalet F, Marina S, Gimeno E, Pomerol J (1978) Cephalexin concentration in the human ejaculate following oral and parenteral administration. Andrologia 10:142–148

Dellow PG, Miles TS (1975) Meiosis, a prostaglandin response that is not inhibited by aspirin. Br J Pharmacol 55:157–159

Derrick FC jr (1977) Bacteriological examination of the ejaculate. In: Hafez ESE (ed) Tech-niques of human andrology. Elsevier/North-Holland Biomedical Press, Amsterdam, pp 311–320

Derrick FC jr, Dahlberg B (1976) Male genital tract infections and sperm viability. In: Hafez ESE (ed) Human semen and fertility regulation in men. Mosby, St. Louis, pp 389–397

Didolkar AK, Roychowdhury D (1980) Effects of prostaglandins E-1, E-2, F-1a and F-2a on human sperm motility. Andrologia 12:135–140

Di Perri T (1973) Anticomplementary properties of cinnarizine. Arch Int Pharmacodyn Ther 203:23–29

Di Perri T, Auteri A (1971) Action of cinnarizine on the immunohaemolytic system. Arch Int Pharmacodyn Ther 193:304–306

Eliasson R (1959) Studies on prostaglandins. Acta Physiol Scand [Suppl 158] 46:1–73

Eliasson R (1975) Analysis of semen. In: Behrman SI, Kistner RW (eds) Progress in infertility, 2nd edn. Little, Brown & Co., Boston, pp 691–713

Eliasson R (1976) Seminal plasma accessory genital glands and infertility. In: Cockett ATK, Urry RL (eds) Male infertility. Work-up, treatment and research. Grune & Stratton, New York, pp 189–204

Eliasson R, Dornbusch K (1977) Levels of trimethoprim and sulfamethoxazole in human seminal plasma. Andrologia 9:195–202

Eliasson R, Dornbusch K (1980) Secretion of metronidazole into the human semen. Int J Androl 3:236–242

Eliasson R, Johannisson E (1978) Cytological studies of prostatic fluids from men with and without abnormal palpatory findings of the prostate II. Clinical application. Int J Androl 1:582–588

Eliasson R, Kvist U (1976) Importance of seminal plasma components on the structural stability of human spermatozoa. Andrologia [Suppl 1] 8:119–120

Eliasson R, Fredrickson B, Johannisson E, Leander G (1966) Biochemical and morphological changes in semen from men with diseases in the accessory genital glands. Excerpta Med Int Congr Ser 133:625–627

Eliasson R, Murdoch RN, White IG (1968) The metabolism of human spermatozoa in presence of PGE 1. Acta Physiol Scand 73:379–382

Eliasson R, Molin L, Rajka G (1970) Involvement of the prostate and seminal vesicles in urethritis with special reference to semen analysis. Andrologia 2:179–182

Eliasson R, Johnsen O, Lindholmer C (1971) Effect of zinc on human sperm respiration. Life Sci 10:1317–1320

Endtz AW (1972) Een methode om het vochtipe urinesediment en het vochtipe menselijke sperma rechtstreeks te kleuren. Ned Tijdschr Geneesk D 116:681–685

Fari A, Trévoux R, Vergès J, Belaisch I, Latarge I (1977) Incidence des états inflammatoires ou infectieux des glandes génitales annexes sur le sperme. In: Henry-Suchet I. Steg A. Constantin A (eds) Infection et fécondité. Masson, Paris, pp 43–58

Ferreira SH, Vane IR (1974) New aspects of the mode of action of nonsteroid anti-inflammatory drugs. Annu Rev Pharmacol 14:57–73

Fink E, Klein G, Hammer F, Müller-Bardorff G, Fritz H (1971) Protein proteinase inhibitors in male sex glands. In: Fritz H, Tschesche H (eds) Proc Int Res Conf Proteinase Inhibitors, Munich 1970. De Gruyter, Berlin New York, pp 225–235

Fowlkes DM, MacLeod J, O'Leary WM (1975) T mycoplasmas and human infertility: correlation of infection with alterations in seminal parameters. Fertil Steril 26:1212–1218

Friberg J (1974) Sperm-agglutinating antibodies and immunoglobulins G and A in stored human seminal fluid. Acta Obstet Gynecol Scand [Suppl] 36:59–63

Frick J (1976) Exploration and treatment of obstructions and infections in the seminal duct and accessory genital glands. Treatment of infections. I. International Congress of Andrology. ECO, Barcelona, pp 81–85

Fritjoffsson A, Kihl B, Danielsson D (1973) Chronic prostatovesiculitis. Incidence and significance of bacterial findings. Scand J Urol Nephrol 8:173–178

Fritz H, Förg-Brey B, Fink E, Meier M, Schiessler H, Schirren C (1972) Humana Krosin: Gewinnung und Eigenschaften. Hoppe-Seyler's Z Physiol Chem 353:1943–1949

Fritz H, Schiessler H, Schill W-B, Tschesche H, Heimburger N, Wallner O (1975) Proteases and biological control. In: Reich E, Rifkin D-B, Shaw E (eds) Cold Spring Harbor symposium. Cold Spring Harbor, New York, pp 737–766

Gaddum P (1968) Sperm maturation in the male reproductive tract: Development of motility. Anat Rec 161:471–482

Gnarpe H, Friberg J (1973) T mycoplasmas on spermatozoa and infertility. Nature 245:97–98

Gomes WR (1970) Chemical agents affecting testicular function and male fertility. In: Johnson AD, Gomes WR, Vandemark NL (eds) The testis. Influencing factors, vol III. Academic Press, New York, pp 483–554

Grayhack JT (1980) Prostatic fluid in diagnosis of prostatic cancer. Prostatic Cancer Newsletter, Summer 7:1

Hensle TW, Prout GR, Griffin P (1977) Minocycline diffusion into benign prostatic hyperplasia. J Urol 118:609–611

Herrmann WP, Hermann G (1969) Immunoelectrophonetic and chromatographic demonstration of IgG, IgA and fragments of γ-globulin in the human seminal fluid. Int J Fertil 14:211–215

Hoare R, Delory GE, Penner DW (1956) Zinc and acid phosphatase in the human prostate. Cancer 9:721–726

Hofstetter A, Schill W-B, Wolff HH, David R (1978) Inhibition of spermotility by genital mycoplasma strains (in German). Therapiewoche 28:1923–1930

Homonnai TZ, Sasson S, Paz G, Kraicer PF (1975) Improvement of fertility and semen quality in men treated with a combination of anticongestive and antibiotic drugs. Int J Fertil 20:45–49

Homonnai ZT, Fainman N, Paz G, Kraicer PF (1979) The effect of a combination of prostatic massage and antibiotic plus anticongestive drugs and human semen quality and fertility. Andrologia 11:71–76

Howkins DF (1968) Relevance of prostaglandins to problems of human subfertility. In: Ramwell PW, Shaw IE (eds) Prostaglandins. Symposium of the Worcester Foundation for Experimental Biology. Interscience, New York, pp 1–36

Isidori A, Conte D, Laguzz G, Gionenco P, Dondero F (1980) Role of seminal prostaglandins in male fertility. I. Relationship of prostaglandin E and 19-OH prostaglandin E with seminal parameters. J Endocrinol Invest 3:1–4

Jayle MF, Janiaud P, Engler R, Degrelle H, Marcais I (1971) Incorporation of the APR sialoglycoproteins in granulomatous tissues. In: Peeters H (ed) Protides of the biological fluids. Pergamon, Oxford, pp 159–167

Jecht E, Haneke E (1978) Levamisole in the treatment of chronic urogenital infections. Andrologia 10:325–326

Johannisson E (1976) Cytological and biochemical evaluation of the male reproductive tract. Exfoliative cytology. I. International Congress of Andrology. ECO, Barcelona, pp 14–18

Johannisson E, Eliasson R (1978) Cytological studies of prostatic fluids from men with and without abnormal palpatory findings of the prostate. I. Methodological aspects. Int J Androl 1:201–212

Joseph MM, Bartke A (1979) Effects of prostaglandins and indomethacin on the response of rat testis to LH in vivo. Int J Androl 2:250–256

Kazimierczak W, Maslinski C (1974) The mechanism of the inhibitory action of zinc on histamine release from mast cells by compound 48/80. Agents Actions 4:203–204

Kerr WK, Keresteci AG, Mayoh H (1960) The distribution of zinc in the human prostate. Cancer 13:550–554

Kobelev AA (1971) Treatment of chronic prostatitis. Urol Nephrol 2:65–71

Koj A (1974) Biological functions of acute-phase reactants. In: Allison AC (ed) Structure and functions of plasma proteins. Plenum, London, pp 113–124

Li TS, Shulman S (1971) Immunoelectrophoretic analysis of human seminal plasma fractions after fractionation by various methods. Int J Fertil 16:87–100

Lillie RD, Fullmer HM (1976) Smear preparations, bacteria, protozoa, and other parasites. In: Lillie RD, Fullmer HM (eds) Histopathologic technique and practical histochemistry, 4th edn. McGraw-Hill, New York, pp 719–763

Lindholmer C (1974) Studies on the effects of human seminal plasma on sperm motility and survival. PhD dissertation. Stockholm University

Lindholmer C, Carlström A, Eliasson R (1974) Occurrence and origin of proteins in human seminal plasma with special reference to albumin. Andrologia 6:181–196

Mackenzie AR, Hall T, Whitmore WF (1962) Zinc content of expressed human prostatic fluid. Nature 193:72–73

Malmborg AS, Dornbusch K, Eliasson R, Lindholmer C (1975) Concentrations of various antibacterials in human seminal plasma. In: Danielsson D, Juhlin L, Mårdh P-A (eds) Genital infections and their complications. Almqvist & Wiksell, Stockholm, pp 307–312

Mårdh P-A, Colleen S (1975a) Search for urogenital tract pathogens in patients with symptoms of prostatitis. Scand J Urol Nephrol 9:8–16

Mårdh P-A, Colleen S (1975b) Antibacterial activity of human seminal fluid. Scand J Urol Nephrol 9:17–23

Mårdh P-A, Colleen S, Holmqvist B (1972) Chlamydia in chronic prostatitis. Br Med J 4:361–363

Mathur U, Data SL, Mathur BBL (1977) The effect of aminopterin-induced folic acid deficiency on spermatogenesis. Fertil Steril 28:1356–1360

Mears EM jr (1973) Bacterial prostatitis versus "prostatosis": A clinical and bacteriological study. JAMA 224:1372–1375

Moberg PJ, Eneroth P, Ljung A, Nord CE (1979) Bacterial growth in samples from cervix and semen from infertile couples. Int J Fertil 24:157–163

Moberg PJ, Eneroth P, Ljung A, Nord CE (1980) Bacterial flora in semen before and after doxyciline treatment of infertile couples. Int J Androl 3:46–58

Moller BR, Mårdh P-A (1980) Experimental epididymitis and urethritis in grivet monkeys provoked by chlamydia trachomatis. Fertil Steril 34:275–279

Nahoum CRD, Cardozo D (1980) Staining for volumetric count of leukocytes in semen and prostate-vesicular fluid. Fertil Steril 34:68–69

Naib ZM (1970) Exfoliative cytopathology. In: Naib ZM (ed) Exfoliation cytopathology. 2nd edn. Little, Brown & Co., Boston, pp 1–5

Nikkanen V, Grönroos M, Suominen J, Multamäki S (1979) Silent infection in male accessory genital organs and male infertility. Andrologia 11:236–241

O'Leary WM, Frick J (1975) The correlation of human male infertility with the presence of mycoplasma T-strain. Andrologia 7:309–316

Oosterlinck W, Wallijn E, Wijndaele JJ (1976) The concentration of doxycycline in human prostate gland and its role in the treatment of prostatitis. Scand J Infect Dis [Suppl] 9:85–88

Paulson JD, Polakoski KL (1977) Isolation of a spermatozoal immobilization factor from Escherichia coli filtrates. Fertil Steril 28:182–185

Plomp TA, Mattelaer JJ, Maes RAA (1978) The concentration of thiamphenicol in ejaculate and prostatic tissue. J Antimicrob Chemother 4:65–71

Polakoski KL, Zaneveld LJD (1976) Proteinases and proteinase inhibitors in andrology. In: Hafez ESE (ed) Human semen and fertility regulation in men. Mosby, St. Louis, pp 563–569

Pomerol JM (1978) Obstructions of the seminal duct. Int J Androl [Suppl 1] 50–52

Quesada EM, Dukes CD, Deem GH, Franklin PR (1968) Genital infections and sperm-agglutinating antibodies in infertile men. J Urol 99:106–108

Quinlivan GWL, Sullivan H (1972) The identity and origin of antigens in human semen. Fertil Steril 23:873–878

Quinlivan GWL, Sullivan H (1976) Antispermatozoal effects of human seminal plasma: an immunologic phenomenon. Fertil Steril 27:1194–1198

Rönnberg L, Ylostalo P, Jouppila P (1978) Estimation of the size of the seminal vesicles by means of ultrasonic β-scanning: a preliminary report. Fertil Steril 30:474–475

Rümke P (1974) The origin of immunoglobulins in semen. Clin Exp Immunol 17:287–297

Sanyal S, Patra PB, Nay S, Biswas NM (1980) Augmentation of luteinizing hormone action by prostaglandin E_2 in the prevention of antispermatogenic effect of indomethacin. Andrologia 12:179–185

Schill W-B (1976) Quantitative determination of high molecular weight serum proteinase inhibitors in human semen. Andrologia 8:359–364

Schirren C, Schaller D (1971) Nachweis der Kombination Trimethoprim/Sulfamethoxazol im menschlichen Spermaplasma. Andrologie 3:23–24

Schoysman R, Strosberg AD, Hoebeke J (1978) Viscosity of semen: a multifactorial problem. In: Fabbrini A, Steinberger E (eds) Recent progress in andrology. Academic Press, New York, pp 221–227

Stankova L, Drach GW, Hicks T, Zuroski CF, Chvapil M (1976) Regulation of some functions of granulocytes by zinc of the prostatic fluid and prostate tissue. J Lab Clin Med 88:640–648

Swenson ChE, Toth A, Toth Cl, Wolfgruber L, O'Leary WM (1980) Asymptomatic bacteriospermia in infertile men. Andrologia 12:7–11

Symes JM, Jarvis JD, Tresider GC (1974) An appraisal of cephalexin monohydrate levels in semen and prostatic tissue. Chemotherapy 20:257–262

Symoens J, Rosenthal M (1977) Levamisole in the modulation of the immune response: the current experimental and clinical state. J Reticuloendothel Soc 21:175–220

Taylor-Robinson D, Manchee RJ (1967) Spermadsorption and spermagglutination by mycoplasmas. Nature 215:484–487

Teague NS, Boyarsky S, Glenn JF (1971) Interference of human spermatozoa motility by E. coli. Fertil Steril 22:281–285

Tierney WJ, Daly IW, Abbatielo ER (1979) The effect of prostaglandins PGE 2 and PGF 2A on spermatogenesis in adult male Sprague-Dawley rats. Int J Fertil 24:206–209

Turner TF (1960) Fluorescence photomicrography of acridine orange-stained exfoliative cytologic preparations. J Biol Photogr Assoc 58:9–10

Ulstein M, Capell P, Holmes KK, Paulsen CA (1976) Nonsymptomatic genital tract infection and male infertility. In: Hafez ESE (ed) Human semen and fertility regulation in men. Mosby, St. Louis, pp 355–362

Weinstein L (1975) Antimicrobial agents. In: Goodman S, Gilman A (eds) The pharmacological basis of therapeutics. Macmillan, New York, pp 1090–1112

Woodbury DM, Fingl E (1975) Analgesic-antipyretics, anti-inflammatory agents and drugs employed in the therapy of gout. In: Goodman S, Gilman A (eds) The pharmacological basis of therapeutics. Macmillan, New York, pp 325–358

Woolf N (1977) Acute inflammation. In: Cell, tissue and disease. The basis of pathology. Baillière Tindall, London, pp 18–49

Wu DH (1957) Bacteriological studies on the semen, and experimental studies on the influences of antibiotics, crystalline penicillin potassium, dihydrostreptomycin sulfate and terramycin hydrochloride upon the semen. Keio J Med 34:508–527

Wybran J (1976) Experimental aspects of immunotherapy. In: Fuddenberg HH, Stites DP, Caldwell JL, Webbs JV (eds) Basic and clinical immunology. Lange Medical Publications, Los Altos, Cal, pp 606–611

Yunda IF (1972) Alteration of genital hormone excretion and possibilities of hormonotherapy in some urologic diseases. In: Actual problems of physiology, biochemistry and pathology of endocrine system. Moscow, pp 161–195

Yunda IF, Imshinetskaya LP (1977) Testosterone excretion in chronic prostatitis. Andrologia 9:89–94

Zaneveld LJD, Polakoski KL, Robertson RF, Williams WL (1971) Trypsin inhibitors and fertilization. In: Fritz H, Tschesche H (eds) Proc Int Res Conf Proteinase Inhibitors Munich 1970. De Gruyter, Berlin New York, pp 236–244

Zeineh RA, Kukral JC (1970) The turnover rate of orosomucoid in burned patients. J Trauma 10:493–498

2 Clomiphene Citrate in the Treatment of Male Infertility

A. M. C. M. Schellen

Clomiphene citrate (Clomid, Merrell Touraude) is a synthetic analog of chloro-trianisene (TACE), a nonsteroidal estrogen. TACE in turn is closely related to stil-bestrol (Fig. 1). Clomiphene citrate which stimulates ovulation in anovulatory women (Holtkamp et al. 1961) exists in two forms, the cis- and trans-isomers, which are both present in Clomid.

The cis compound is much more effective in stimulating ovulation (Wieland et al. 1972; Reyes and Faiman 1974). The cis form has two identical chemical groups on the same side of the double bond, while the trans form shows these groups lo-calized on different sides (Fig. 2). Greenblatt (1961) described the clomiphene ovu-lation-inducing effect, while Jungck (1964) was first to describe its effect on sper-matogenesis. Clomiphene binds competitively to steroid receptors in the hypothala-mus, thus inhibiting the negative feedback exerted by circulating steroids like 17β-estradiol. This results in an increase of LHRH and consequently of LH and FSH (Franchimont 1973). These effects of Clomid on the hypothalamic-pituitary level have made it possible to use Clomid in the dynamic evaluation of the hypothalamic-pituitary-gonadal axis in both females (Emperaire et al. 1979).

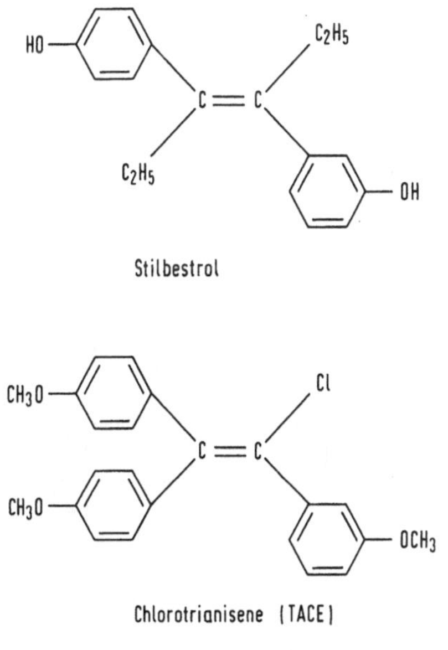

Stilbestrol

Chlorotrianisene (TACE)

Fig. 1. Structure of stilbestrol and chlorotriani-sene (TACE)

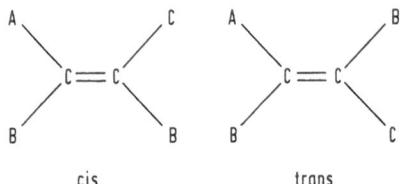

Clomiphene citrate

Fig. 2. Structure of Clomiphene citrate and its two isomers

cis   trans

2.1 Testicular Control and Function

The gonadotropic hormones of the pituitary gland, LH and FSH, stimulate testicular function. They, in turn, are stimulated by the neurohypophyseal factor LHRH, which is modulated by gonadal steroids through both positive and negative feed-

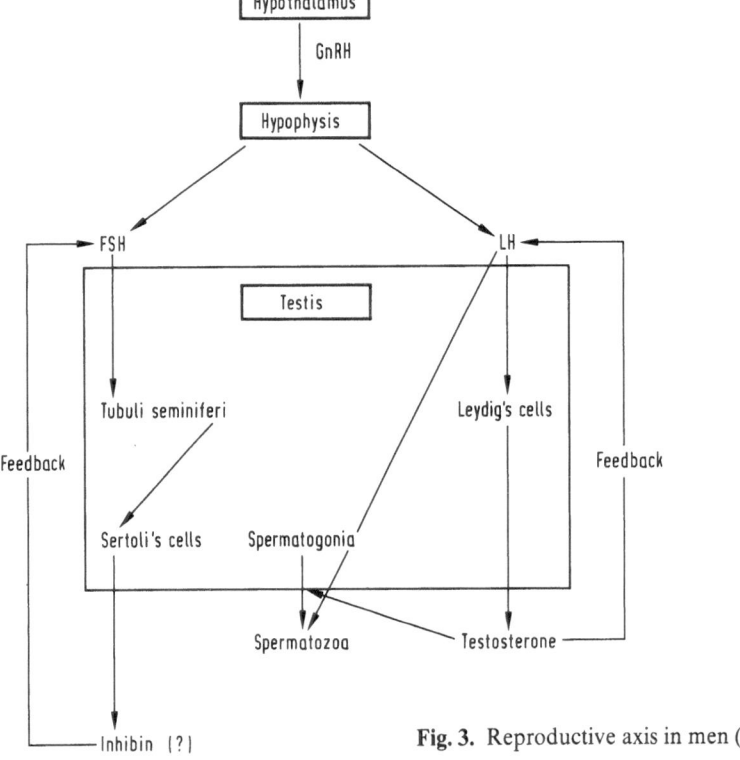

Fig. 3. Reproductive axis in men (Espinasse 1977)

Table 1. Factors involved in control mechanisms of testicular function

Site	Factors
Brain	Exteroceptive influences
	Stress
Hypothalamus	Monoamines (dopamine, norepinephrine)
	Releasing hormones
Pituitary	Gonadatropins (FSH, LH)
	Growth hormone
	Prolactin
	Others?
Testis	Androgens
	Estrogens
	Other steroids?
	Binding proteins (circulating, intratesticular)

back mechanisms (Martini 1970). These feedback mechanisms appear to take place at three levels: (1) a "long" feedback system, in which the inhibiting messages are mainly the gonadal steroids; (2) a "short" feedback system in which the inhibiting messages are represented by the gonadotropic hormones, which thus affect their own secretion; (3) an "ultrashort" feedback system in which the releasing hormones can have direct control on their rate of production.

Functional changes in the hypothalamus, anterior pituitary gland, or gonads significantly affect the entire reproduction axis (Fig. 3). The factors influencing the endocrinous functioning of the testis have been summarized by Burger et al. (1976) (Table 1). The total duration of spermatogenesis in humans is a biological constant which takes 74 days (Clermont 1970), while maturation of spermatozoa in the epididymis and deferential transport occur over a period of 16 days (Heller and Clermont 1964). Because of these time periods, therapy of male infertility promoting spermatogenesis must be maintained for at least 3 months.

2.2 The Clomiphene Test

The clomiphene test can be used to evaluate the integrity of the hypothalamic-hypophyseal-gonadal axis and to examine the secretory function of the hypophysis. There are several ways of using the test and eliciting different reactions (Bardin et al. 1967; Geller and Scholler 1971; Geller et al. 1977). In ten normal males who received 200 mg clomiphene citrate for 7 days, Franchimont et al. (1975) could show a significant rise of serum FSH and LH on day 4 (Fig. 4). The finding that the rise of LH precedes the rise in plasma testosterone by at least 2 days demonstrates that clomiphene citrate acts on the hypothalamic-pituitary axis to release gonadotropins, which in turn stimulate the testis.

Emperaire et al. (1979) used the clomiphene test in infertile patients and normal males to establish the hormonal response to clomiphene, to outline the positive and negative response in the individual subject, and finally to correlate the endocrine

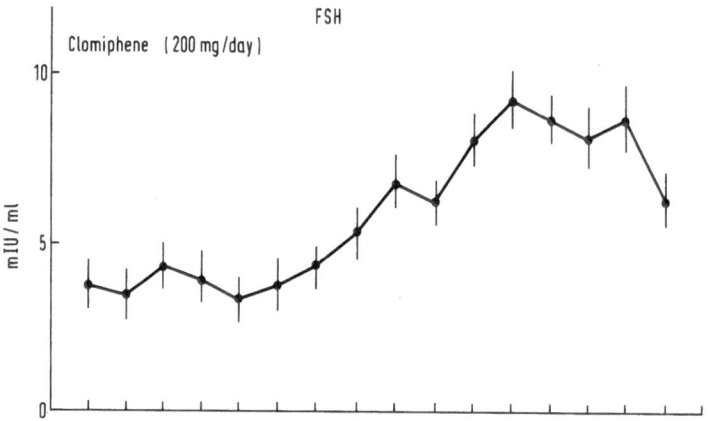

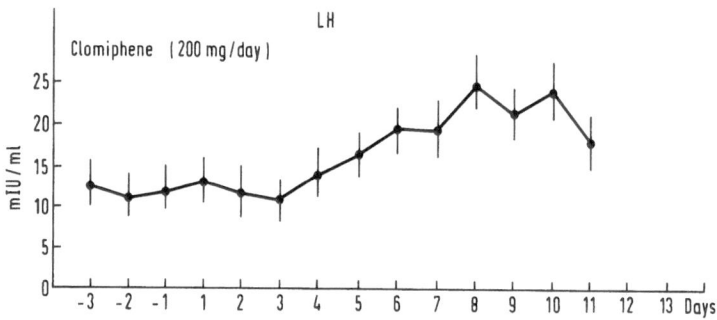

Fig. 4. Endocrine function of the testis: influence of Clomiphene citrate on FSH and LH in ten normal male subjects (mean±I SD)

with the semen response in the treated patients. They found that the infertile male population responded normally to Clomid administration. Three types of individual responses were observed (Table 2): a complete positive response, with elevation of all three hormones (LH, FSH, testosterone); a dissociated positive response, with increases in only one or two hormones; a negative response, with no increase in any hormone.

Table 2. Three types of individual response to Clomid (Emperaire et al. 1979)

Response	Hormones		
	FSH	LH	Testosterone
Complete	+	+	+
Dissociated FSH-LH	±	∓	
LH-Testosterone		±	∓
No response	–	–	–

The study of the correlations between hormone and semen responses showed that a complete or dissociated endocrine response was not an accurate predictor of a possible semen amelioration; on the other hand, the semen did not improve in patients without a positive hormonal response, particularly in those whose testosterone levels did not rise.

2.3 Clomiphene Citrate in Male Infertility

2.3.1 Clomiphene Citrate Therapy

Teoh (1972) described one of the first pregnancies apparently resulting from treatment of the male with clomiphene, and experience with clomiphene in male infertility has increased since then. The patients most likely to respond are those in whom gonadotropin secretion is low (Schellen and Beek 1974). Heller et al. (1969) studied the influence of Clomid on number and morphology of spermatozoa using several dosages (50, 100–200, and 400 mg/day) for 2–12 months: They found that a high dose of Clomid was associated with a decrease of sperm count, a low dose with an increase of sperm count, and intermediate doses with variable results. Although no consensus exists regarding dose and time period (Foss et al. 1973; Epstein 1977; Paulson 1977), we have found that a dose of 50 mg/day for a minimum of 6 weeks, but preferably 3 months is favored. In this respect, the only controlled double-blind crossover study (Rönnberg 1980) also found highly increased sperm count in patients with a FSH level below the mean value of the normal range and stressed the use of 50 mg daily for 3 months. Heller et al. (1969) found the morphology either unchanged or improved in subjects whose sperm counts were increased or not affected, while the number of abnormal forms increased as the sperm count decreased. Where sperm count decreased, testis biopsy showed a slight hyalinization of the tubular membranes, as well as a reduction of the tubular lumina. Following discontinuation of Clomid, histology of the germinal epithelium returned to normal. After studying the testicular biopsies before and after treatment, they concluded that clomiphene citrate has two effects on germinal epithelium; a stimulating effect resulting in an increased sperm count and an inhibiting effect, mainly with high dosages, resulting in an abundance of abnormal spermatids and a decrease of sperm concentration in the ejaculate.

2.3.2 Material and Methods

Although numerous reports on the effect of Clomid on hormone secretion are available, only a very few are devoted to the action of the drug on spermatogenesis and the spermiogram and these few show widely divergent results. It is obviously necessary to select the patients according to certain criteria and to maintain more uniformity with respect to the dosage and length of therapy. Nankin et al. (1971) showed that Clomid is only effective in the sense of increasing gonadotropins and testosterone levels, after maturation of the hypothalamic-pituitary centers. Kulin et al. (1976) showed that sexual maturation was a "conditio sine qua non" for the liberation of the gonadotropins by Clomid.

Table 3. Clomiphene citrate in azoospermic men

Reference	Number of treated patients	Sperm count (No. of patients)		Dosage (mg/day)	Duration of treatment
		Increased	No influence		
Jungck et al. (1964)	1	–	1	25	4–5 weeks
Mellinger et al. (1966)	5	–	5	Unknown	
Foss et al. (1967)	1	1	–	50–100	5–17 weeks
Potts (1968)	20	13	7	Unknown	
Orsola-Marti (1971)	Many	Clearly positive	?	Unknown	
Schellen et al. (1972)	17	2	15	50	40–90 days

Table 4. Clomiphene citrate in oligozoospermic men

Reference	Number of treated patients	Sperm count (No. of patients)			Dosage (mg/day)	Duration of treatment
		In-creased	De-creased	No influence		
Jungck et al. (1964)	28	17	6	5	25–50	4–5 weeks
Mellinger et al. (1966)	13	10	3	–	Unknown	
Conill et al. (1966)	4	2	–	2	100	10 days
Mroueh et al. (1967)	15	1	?	?	50	6 weeks
Pelligrini et al. (1967)	3	2	?	?	50	6 weeks
Schirren (1968)	20	10	?	?	Unknown	
Arrata et al. (1969)	Some	–	1	Some	Various	
Palti et al. (1970)	69	8	21	40	12.5–100	3–8 weeks
Lorenz (1971)	20	3	?	?	100	10 days
Mor (1971)	27	10	9	8	5–50	90–120 days
Orsola-Marti (1971)	Many	Clearly positive	?	?	Unknown	
Schellen et al. (1972)	84	59	–	25	50	40–90 days

Table 5. The use of Clomid in male infertility: a review (Espinasse 1977)

Reference	Number of patients	Dosage (mg/day)	Months of treatment	Improvement	Pregnancies
Jungck et al. (1964)	20	50	2	13	0
	8	25	2	4	0
Mellinger et al. (1966)	18	?	?	10	0
Mroueh et al. (1967)	15	50	1.5	1	0
Potts et al. (1968)	20	50	3	13	1
Principi et al. (1969)	6	100	3	6	0
Palti et al. (1970)	69	12.5–100	1–2	33	4
Ansari et al. (1972)	12	?	?	6	3
Wieland et al. (1972)	11	5–10	2	3	0
Kalin et al. (1973)	25	50	2	11	0
Schellen et al. (1974)	101	50	1–3	61	19
Paulson et al. (1975)	22	25	6	18	2
(1976)	35	25	?	31	8
Emperaire et al. (1976)	54	50	3–3.5	16	4
Jerome et al. (1977)	10	25	3–6	7	9
Jeanne et al. (1977)	16	100	4	10	5

Therapy can only be useful if increased FSH and LH values are expected: Thus, individuals with increased basal serum gonadotropins and azoospermia would not be expected to respond. Clomid therapy should be limited to cases of oligozoospermia, i.e., less than 20 million spermatozoa/ml, with low or normal FSH and LH levels. However, it is necessary that the pituitary is responsive, since an increase of FSH and LH is a proof of the integrity of the hypothalamus-pituitary-gonadal axis. In cases where no increase of FSH and LH is seen, a LHRH test will differentiate between hypothalamic and a hypophyseal insufficiency.

When no results can be obtained with Clomid, an explanation could be a disturbance of the FSH/LH ratio, since LH values can especially show disproportionate increases (Lunenfeld and Katz 1972).

Table 6. Clomid treatment in male infertility

Reference	Number of patients	Dosage (mg/day)	Duration of treatment	Improvement	Pregnancies
Da Rugna et al. (1974)	33	50	60 days	5	0
Sas et al. (1976)	21	50	3 months	15	3
Espinasse (1977)	37	25–50	3 months	16	3
Paulson (1977)	57	25	6 months	45	20
Meili et al. (1977)	37	50	3–6 months	19	5
Epstein (1977)	16	50	4 months or more	10	5
Paulson et al. (1977)	32	25	6–12 months	?	13
Check et al. (1977)	10	25	7 months or more	7	9
Emperaire et al. (1979)	54	50	100 days	11	0
Chiorboli et al. (1979)	24	25	3–8 months	?	6
Rönnberg et al. (1979)	46	50	3 months	33	?
Homonnai et al. (1979)	60	25–50	35–60 days	28	2

2.3.3 Review of Results Obtained with Clomid

Three major reasons for results with Clomid to differ so dramatically among various authors are patient selection, dosage, and duration of treatment.

Although considerable research has investigated the effect of Clomid on gonadotropins and steroidogenesis, little has been done to study the effect of Clomid on spermatogenesis. The results of Clomid therapy in male infertility or subfertility have been extensively reviewed for azoospermic and oligozoospermic patients (Schellen 1975), and no beneficial effect was found in treating azoospermic individuals (Table 3): The results in oligzoospermic men are shown in Table 4.

Espinasse (1977) reviewed the role of Clomid in male infertility (Table 5) and found that, in 422 patients who were not uniformly selected, improved sperm parameters were seen in 243 cases (55%) which resulted in 54 pregnancies (12%).

Table 6 summarizes our most recent review of the literature. Of these 427 cases, 189 (44%) showed an improvement in sperm parameters, and in 66 cases (16%) a pregnancy resulted.

From Tables 4, 5, and 6 one must conclude that optimal results can be obtained with a dose of 50 mg/day given continuously for at least 3 months. A dose of 25 mg/day for 25 days with a 5-day drug-free interval gives similar results, but therapy should be continued for at least 6 months.

2.4 Side and Secondary Effects of Clomiphene Citrate

The most popular dose of 25–100 mg/day clomiphene citrate does not cause important side effects or deviations of kidney function, hemopoiesis, thyroid function, and serum cholesterol values (Espinasse 1977). However, the following side effects have been observed in males (Mauss et al. 1974; Da Rugna et al. 1974; Espinasse 1977): aggressive behavior; slight depression; visual complaints (scotoma scintillans, blurry vision); nausea; dizziness or equilibrium disturbances; allergic dermatitis; hair loss. These side effects disappear rapidly after termination of therapy, though there is seldom a need to stop therapy.

Continuous administration of Clomid can interfere with cholesterol synthesis resulting in an increase of desmosterol levels (Espinasse 1977). In a small group an increase in bromsulphalein (BSP) retention was observed, while other liver tests were normal (Schreiber et al. 1966). Therefore, the use of Clomid is contraindicated only in patients with a history of serious liver disease.

After 4–6 months of cis-clomiphene treatment, one study found that testicular size definitely tended to increase bilaterally, commonly accompanied by a sensation of heavier testicles (Reyes and Faiman 1974). Some patients also observed an increased libido. In one patient the cis-clomiphene was stopped due to an enlargement of his underdeveloped gonad. An orchidectomy in this patient revealed a testicular tumor (adult teratoma) with seminoma of an unusual pattern. Although available evidence does not support a relationship between cis-clomiphene treatment and the appearance of testicular tumor, in patients undergoing treatment with any agent that stimulates the germinal epithelium, testicular size should be carefully measured.

2.5 Discussion

The influence of sex steroids on the secretion of LH and FSH may be both inhibitory and stimulatory, i.e., feedback may be positive or negative. Steroids exert their effect upon the hypothalamus or pituitary, or both.

Clomiphene, a synthetic monosteroid triarylethylene derivate, causes the release of LH and FSH by a direct action on the hypothalamus. Clomid may have a stimulating effect on the hypophysis as a result of direct action on the diencephalon or even the pituitary gland itself (Greenblatt 1961).

The success obtained with Clomid in the induction of ovulation (Holtkamp et al. 1961) lead to its use in certain cases of subfertility in males. The problem of achieving maximal therapeutic effect seems to lie in the difficulties associated with finding criteria for the appropriate selection of patients, an optimal dosage, an appropriate dose schedule for inducing a testicular response, and the best duration of treatment required for a response.

Absence of increased LH and FSH response in the clomiphene test points towards hypophyseal insufficiency or deficient gonadotropic function. Only among those patients in whom FSH is low or normal can positive results be expected. Patients with increased FSH secretion should not receive Clomid, since an elevated FSH level indicates severe testicular degeneration, and positive results from this therapy can not be expected.

In the literature and in our own experience we found encouraging results after proper selection of the patients, i.e., patients with low or normal FSH and LH levels and a functioning pituitary. In these cases, the resultant pregnancies are seen as a result of treatment and not a placebo effect. Although it is the experience of most workers in this field that about 20% of all oligozoospermic men will be responsible for a pregancy spontaneously with no drug therapy (almost the same result as with Clomid), it has to be stressed that success was obtained in well-selected patients and pregnancies occurred after many years of involuntary infertility and after other unsuccessful therapies. A dose of 50 mg/day for at least 90 days is favored over a cyclic therapy of 25 mg/day for 25 days with a 5-day drug-free interval because there is no rationale for cyclic therapy in men and effective administration of the drug can be limited to 3 months if given continuously.

Patients with azoospermia should be excluded from Clomid therapy unless there is evidence of spermatogenesis in the testicular biopsy. Although the results obtained with Clomid are controversial, the experience obtained with this drug appears to show sufficient effectiveness in some oligozoospermic men without producing undesireable side effects.

2.6 References

Ansari AH, Wieland RG, Klein DE (1972) Cis-clomiphene citrate in the management of oligospermia. J Urol 108:131
Arrata WSM (1969) The subfertile male. Fertil Steril 20:460
Bardin CW, Ross GT, Lipsett MB (1967) Site of action of clomiphene citrate in men: a study of the pituitary Leydig cell axis. J Clin Endocrinol 27:1558–1564
Burger HG, De Kretzer DM, Hudson B (1976) Spermatogenesis and its endocrine control. In: Hafez ESE (ed) Human semen and fertility regulation in men. Mosby, St. Louis, pp 3–16
Check JH, Rakoff AE (1977) Improved fertility in oligospermic males treated with clomiphene citrate. Fertil Steril 28:746
Chiorboli E, Gomes de Silva LFA (1979) Long term use of Clomiphene in low dosage for subfertility. Proc First Panca congress. Caracas, p 162
Clermont Y (1970) Dynamics of human spermatogenesis. In: Rosemberg E, Paulsen CA (eds) The human testis. Plenum, New York London, pp 47–59
Conill et al. (1966) (cited by Espinasse)
Da Rugna D, Dedes M, Ghossein E (1974) Erfahrungen mit Humangonadotropinen und Clomiphenzitrat bei Fertilitätsstörungen des Mannes. Der Informierte Arzt 470–474
Emperaire JC et al. (1976) (cited by Espinasse)
Emperaire JC, Riviere J, Ruffie A, Audebert AJM (1979) Clomiphene test and clomiphene therapy in idiopathic male infertility. Arch Androl 2:223–231
Epstein JA (1977) Clomiphene treatment in oligospermic infertile males. Fertil Steril 28:741–745

Espinasse J (1977) Utilisation du citrate de clomiphène isolément ou en association avec les androgènes dans le traitement des hypofertilités masculines idiopathiques. A propos de 74 cas. PhD dissertation, University of Toulouse

Foss GL, Tindall VR, Birkett JP (1967) The effect of clomiphene on spermatogenesis and hormone excretion in a patient with Klinefelter's syndrome. J Reprod Fertil 13:315

Foss GL, Tindall VR, Birkett JP (1973) The treatment of subfertile men with clomiphene citrate. J Reprod Fertil 32:167–170

Franchimont P (1973) Human gonadotropin secretion in male subjects. In: James VHT, Serio M, Martina L (eds) The endocrine function of the human testis, vol I. Academic Press, New York London, pp 445–458

Franchimont P, Legros JJ, Demoulin A, Bourguignon (1975) Investigations of gonadotrophin secretion in normal and pathological conditions. In: Schellen AM (ed) Releasing factors and gonadotropic hormones in male and female sterility. European Press, Ghent, pp 12–24

Geller S, Scholler R (1971) Potentialisation par le clomiphène de la réponse testiculaire à la stimulation gonadotrophique. Ann Endocrinol 32:6

Geller S, Dajoux R, Armoghathe JF, Scholler R (1977) Une nouvelle épreuve d'exploration de la fonction testiculaire: l'épreuve combinée clomiphene-HCG-Dexamethasone. Cah Sexuol Clin 17:475–486

Greenblatt RB (1961) Induction of ovulation with MRL-41. JAMA 178:101–104

Heller CG, Clermont Y (1964) Kinetics of the germinal epithelium in man. Recent Progr Horm Res 20:545–558

Heller CG, Rowley MJ, Heller GV (1969) Clomiphene citrate: a correlation of its effect on sperm concentration and morphology, total gonadotropins. ICSH, estrogen and testosterone excretion and testicular cytology in normal men. J Clin Endocrinol Metab 29:638–649

Holtkamp DE, Davis RH, Rhoads JE (1961) Effect of chloramiphene on fertility and ovulation. Fed Proc 20:419–423

Homonnai ZT, Peled M, Paz GF (1979) Changes in semen quality and fertility in response to endocrine treatment of subfertile men. Gyn Obstet Inv 9:244

Jeanne A, Epstein MD (1977) Clomiphene treatment in oligospermic infertile males. Fertil Steril 28:741

Jerome H, Check MD, Abraham E, Rakoff MD (1977) Improved fertility in oligospermic males treated with clomiphene citrate. Fertil Steril 28:746

Jungck EC, Roy S, Greenblatt RB, Matesh VB (1964) Effect of clomiphene citrate on spermatogenesis in the human. A preliminary report. Fertil Steril 15:40–43

Kalin et al. (1973) (cited by Espinasse)

Kulin HE, Reiter EO, Brindson WE (1976) Pubertal maturation of the gonadotrophin-stimulatory response to clomiphene: Case report. J Clin Endocrinol Metab 43:182–186

Lorenz E (1971) Medikamentöse Therapie männlicher Fertilitätsstörungen. Inaugural-Dissertation, Berlin

Lunenfeld B, Katz M (1972) Traitement de l'infertilité masculine par les gonadotrophines et le clomiphène. In: Masson (ed) Fécondité et sterilité du male. Masson, Paris, pp 135–152

Martini L (1970) Hypothalamic control of gonadotropin secretion in the male. In: Rosemberg E, Paulsen CA (eds) The human testis. Plenum, New York London, pp 187–204

Mauss J, Mohnfeld G, Börsch G (1974) Synthetic LH-releasing factor and clomiphene stimulation in oligospermic males with normal FSH excretion. J Reprod Fertil 40:171–175

Meili HU, Bandauer K (1977) Erfahrungen mit der kombinierten Mesterolon-Clomipheen-Citrat-Therapie bei Oligospermien. Helv Chir Acta 44:373

Mellinger RC, Thompson RJ (1966) The effects of clomiphene citrate in male infertility. Fertil Steril 17:94

Mor A (1971) The use of clomiphene citrate in male infertility. Fortsch Androl 2:100

Mroueh A, Lytton B, Kase N (1967) Effect of clomiphene citrate on oligospermia. Am J Obstet Gynecol 98:1033

Nankin HR, Yanaihara T, Troen P (1971) Response of gonadotrophins and testosterone to clomiphene stimulation in a pubertal boy. J Clin Endocrinol 33:360–363

Orsola-Marti (1971) Alterations in spermatogenesis. Sixth World Congr Fertil and Steril Tel Aviv 1968 (Abstracts) 104

Palti Z (1970) Clomiphene therapy in defective spermatogenesis. Fertil Steril 21:838

Paulson DF (1977) Clomiphene citrate in the management of male hypofertility: Predictors for treatment selection. Fertil Steril 28:1226–1229

Paulson DF, de Vere White R (1977) Staging profile of hypofertile males. J Urol 116:83

Paulson DF, Wacksman J (1976) Clomiphene citrate therapy in the management of male infertility. J Urol 115:73

Paulson DF, Wacksman J, Hammond CB, Wiebe HR (1975) Hypofertility and clomiphene citrate therapy. Fertil Steril 26:892

Pellegrini G, Piotti LE (1967) Bilan thérapeutique des insuffisances testiculaires dit secondaires. Actual Endocrinol (Paris) 8:191

Potts JF (1968) A clinical evaluation of two types of therapy for male infertility. Med J Aust 17:707

Principi ME et al. (1969) Experienceias del uso del citrato de clomifen en la esterilidad masculina. Rev Argentina Urol 38:265

Reyes FJ, Faiman C (1974) Long-term therapy with low-dose cisclomiphene in male infertility: effects on semen, serum FSH, LH, testosterone and estradiol, and carbohydrate tolerance. Int J Fertil 19:49–55

Rönnberg L (1980) The effect of clomiphene citrate on different sperm parameters and serum hormone levels in preselected infertile men: a controlled double-blind crossover study. Int J Androl 3:479–486

Rönneberg L, Tuimala R (1979) Treatment of oligozoospermia with clomiphene: Choice of patients on the basis of FSH values. Infertility 2:247

Sas M, Szöllösi J, Falkay G (1976) Traitement par clomiphène de la subfertilité de l'homme. Therapia Hungarica 3:127

Schellen AM (1975) Effects of gonadotropic hormones, clomiphene and releasing factors on human spermatogenesis. In: Beric BM, Lunenfeld B, Kovác T, Prudan R (eds) Gonadotropins in Modern Therapy (Serbo-Croatian). Novi Sad, pp 66–83

Schellen AM, Beek JJ (1972) Clomiphene in male sterility. J Gynecol Obstet Reprod 1:190

Schellen AM, Beek JJ (1974) The use of clomiphene treatment for male sterility. Fertil Steril 25:407–410

Schirren C (1968) Die konservative Therapie von Fertilitätstörungen des Mannes. Der Urologe 17:179

Schreiber E et al. (1966) Studies with ^{14}C-labeled clomiphene citrate. Clin Res 14:287–292

Teoh ES (1972) Pregnancy following the use of clomiphene citrate in male infertility. Ann Acad Med (Singapore) 1:43–45

Wieland RG, Ansari AH, Klein DE, Doshi NS, Hallberg MC, Chen JC (1972) Idiopathic oligospermia: Control observations to cisclomiphene. Fertil Steril 23:471–475

3 Tamoxifen

F. H. Comhaire

Management of patients with oligozoospermia should focus on the detection of treatable causes. If these have been excluded or if poor semen quality persists after adequate treatment of such causes, nonspecific modes of treatment can be considered. One theoretical approach is to stimulate the Leydig cell function and increase intratesticular testosterone concentration by interference with hypothalamo-pituitary feedback using antiestrogens (Bardin et al. 1967; Santen et al. 1971; Schill 1979).

In the past, several studies have been performed with clomiphene citrate, a drug which displays weak intrinsic estrogenic activity (Self et al. 1967; Charles et al. 1969; Barbosa et al. 1973; Richards and Griffith 1974; Lunan and Klopper 1975). The estrogenic activity of clomiphene may explain some adverse effects observed during the intake of high doses (Heller et al. 1968).

Tamoxifen is an antiestrogen structurally similar to clomiphene citrate. Whereas clomiphene citrate is a racemic mixture of equal parts of the trans and cis isomers, tamoxifen, due to its chemical structure, only contains one isomer. Tamoxifen has a much weaker intrinsic estrogenic activity than clomiphene and treatment with this drug, in a dose of 20 mg/day, does not increase the concentration of estrogen-sensitive binding proteins in the blood plasma. Hence, tamoxifen might be expected to be more suitable for treatment of males (Hemworth 1975). The use of tamoxifen in a total of 203 subfertile men has been reported by four groups (Comhaire 1976; Vermeulen and Comhaire 1978; Bartsch and Scheiber, to be published; Buvat et al., to be published; Schill and Landthaler 1980). The results of these studies should be interpreted cautiously, since none used appropriate (i.e., placebo-treated) controls.

3.1 Mode of Action

The mode of action of tamoxifen is relatively well known from studies in the treatment of female breast cancer. The drug competes with estrogens for the receptors in the tissues, to which it binds. The tamoxifen receptor complex is transported into the cell nucleus where it stimulates estrogen-dependent protein synthesis. Unlike estrogens, tamoxifen does not dissociate from the nuclear acceptors and, thus, blocks further effects of estrogens on the cell.

In the male, the biological consequence of this antiestrogenic activity is particularly remarkable at the hypothalamic level, where the feedback inhibition of GnRH secretion is greatly inhibited, and possibly also at the intratesticular level where estrogen receptors on Leydig cells are occupied. Through this action, hypothalamo-pituitary-testicular function is activated in the presence of a functionally normal hypothalamus.

3.2 Patients

Patients selected for treatment with tamoxifen fulfilled the following criteria: being the male partner of an infertile relationship at least 12 months in duration; presenting at least two semen samples with clearly abnormal characteristics; presenting no evident cause for poor semen quality; having been treated for either male adnexitis

Table 1. Semen characteristics of 15 oligozoospermic patients before and during treatment with tamoxifen (Comhaire 1976)

	Units	Before	During	Significance
Semen volume	ml	3.9	3.9	NS
Semen pH		7.7	7.7	NS
Semen fructose	mg/ml	3.0	2.6	<0.02
	mg/ejaculate	11.7	10.3	<0.05
Semen acid phosphatase	KAU[1]/ml	2 437	2 925	<0.1
	KAU[1]/ejaculate	9 180	11 680	NS
Sperm concentration	million/ml	12.7	28.3	<0.01
Sperm production	million/ejaculate	55.6	89.5	<0.02
Motile spermatozoa	%	36.4	33.5	NS
Production of motile spermatozoa	million/ejaculate	21.9	35.7	<0.05
Living spermatozoa	%	74	74	NS

[1] King-Armstrong Units

or varicocele more than 12 months before, without significant improvement of semen quality. Patients were referred by gynecologists who had performed necessary investigations in the female partner without detecting any significant abnormalities. All patients treated were normogonadotropic and had a normal testosterone concentration in peripheral blood.

We have studied two series of patients of 15 cases (Comhaire 1976) and 21 cases (Vermeulen and Comhaire 1978), respectively. Semen characteristics of these cases are listed in Table 1. Treatment consisted of 20 mg (two tablets) tamoxifen per day for 2–24 months. In order to control for the integrity of the hypothalamo-pituitary-testicular axis, the hormonal response was evaluated after 1 month of tamoxifen treatment. Only one case showed no testosterone concentration increase, and further endocrinologic investigation in this patient showed hypothalamic disorder.

Two to eight semen samples were analyzed before starting treatment and, during treatment, control semen analyses were performed every 3 months. Semen analysis included:

– measurement of the ejaculate volume and pH,
– estimation of ejaculate viscosity after liquefaction,

– semiquantitative measurement of sperm motility,
– estimation of sperm density in the hemocytometer,
– detailed light-microscopic examination of sperm morphology,
– estimation of the number of round cells in the ejaculate and differential staining between peroxidase-positive neutrophil leukocytes and peroxidase-negative spermatogenic cells,
– measurement of the concentration of fructose and acid phosphatase in the seminal plasma, and
– culture of the semen plasma for aerobic and anaerobic strains.

Plasma testosterone and estradiol levels were measured by well-established radioiummunological techniques. LH and FSH levels were measured by a double antibody method using the commercial CEA-IRE-SORIN kits (Cis, Bif-sur-Yvette, France). Statistical analysis was by Student's t-test or Wilcoxon's signed rank test for paired replicates where indicated.

3.3 Results

3.3.1 Plasma Hormone Levels

3.3.1.1 Testosterone

On day 5 of drug intake, testosterone concentration was significantly increased in all normal volunteers as well as in patients with oligozoospermia (Fig. 1). During long-term treatment (up to 1 year), these elevated testosterone concentrations were maintained at a constant level between 83% (Bartsch and Scheiber, to be published) and approximately 100% (Comhaire 1976; Vermeulen and Comhaire 1978) above basal levels.

3.3.1.2 Estradiol

Peripheral estradiol concentration increased roughly parallel to testosterone. The mean concentration before treatment was 37 pg/ml, it equaled 57 pg/ml during treatment. Estrogen-sensitive plasma transport proteins, such as transferrin, trans-

Table 2. Concentrations of steroids and binding proteins before and during treatment with tamoxifen in subfertile males (Comhaire and Dhont 1975)

	Units	Before	During	Significance
Plasma testosterone	ng/ml	4.7	10.0	<0.01
Plasma estradiol	pg/ml	37	57	<0.05
Total serum protein	g/dl	7.2	7.4	NS
Total iron binding capacity	µg/dl	373	356	NS
T3 uptake	%	108	105	NS
Total thyroxine	µg/dl	7.5	7.5	NS
Cortisol binding capacity	$10^6 \, \text{M}^{-1}$	1.0	1.5	NS
Testosterone binding capacity	$10^8 \, \text{M}^{-1}$	5.5	4.2	NS

cortin, thyroxine-binding globulin, and sex hormone-binding globulin, remained unchanged (Table 2).

3.3.1.3 Gonadotropins (LH and FSH)

Serum gonadotropin levels (particularly the concentration of LH) increased significantly and remained elevated during continuation of drug intake (Comhaire and

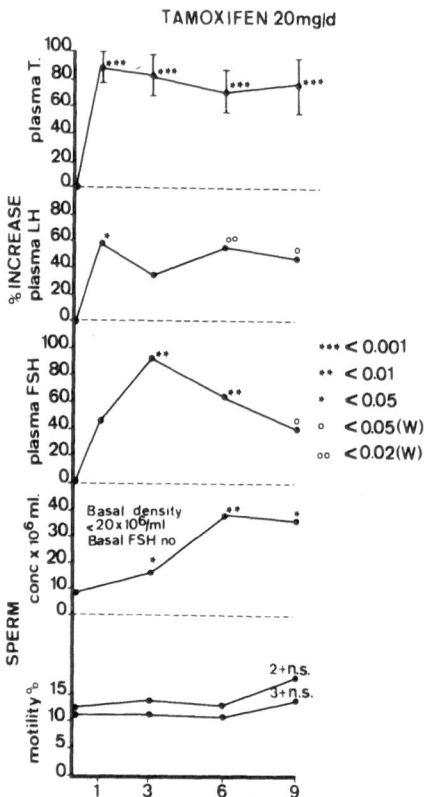

Fig. 1. Influence of tamoxifen treatment on serum concentrations of testosterone, LH, and FSH (expressed as percent increase compared to basal value), and on concentration and motility of spermatozoa in patients with oligozoospermia of less than 20 million/ml (Vermeulen and Comhaire 1978). The *abscissa* indicates the duration of treatment in months. Motility is subdivided into rapidly progressive (3+) and sluggishly progressive (2+). Student's *t*-test for paired observations (*stars*) and Wilcoxon's signed rank test for paired replicates (*W*) were used for analyses

Dhont 1975; Vermeulen and Comhaire 1978; Bartsch and Scheiber, to be published) (Fig. 1). This finding contradicts the results reported by Willis et al. (1977). In our patients the FSH increase was most pronounced after 3 months of treatment and tended to decrease after 6 months or more, nevertheless remaining significantly higher than basal levels (Fig. 1).

The stimulation of the hypothalamo-pituitary function was further documented by the increased LH and FSH response to exogenous GnRH stimulation observed during tamoxifen treatment (Dhont et al. 1976). Both the amplitude of the response (peak level after stimulation minus basal level) and the total gonadotropin release were clearly increased (Comhaire and Dhont 1975; Vermeulen and Comhaire 1978).

3.3.2 Sperm Characteristics

3.3.2.1 Sperm Concentration

Important effects were registered in the sperm concentration and sperm output per ejaculate. Indeed, 55% (Schill and Landthaler 1980) to 70% (Bartsch and Scheiber, to be published) or 80% (Comhaire 1976) of oligozoospermic patients with normal

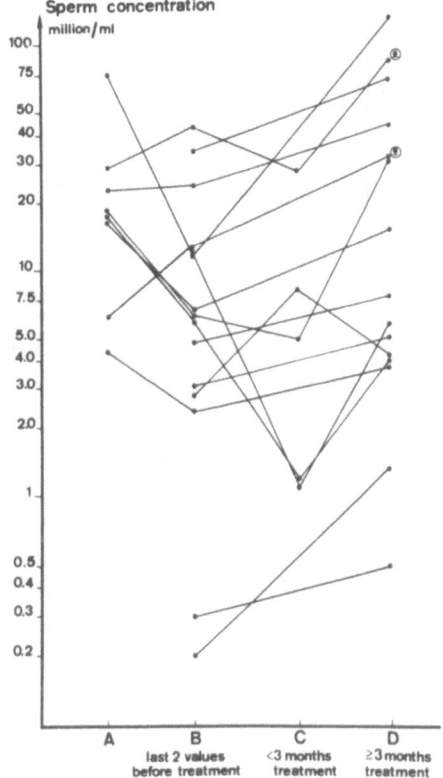

Fig. 2. Variations in sperm concentration in 15 subfertile patients treated more than 3 months with tamoxifen (note logarithmic scale!) (Comhaire 1976): *A* mean sperm concentration in the semen analyses preceding the last two pretreatment values; *B* mean sperm concentration in the two semen analyses obtained before starting tamoxifen treatment; *C* mean sperm concentration after less than 3 months treatment; *D* mean sperm concentration in semen analyses performed after tamoxifen treatment of 3 months or longer

basal FSH level responded to tamoxifen with a significant increase in sperm production, sperm concentration and sperm output increasing to values two- to threefold the basal value (Table 1, Fig. 2). Although this increase may be apparent by 3 months, further improvement generally occurs after 6 and 9 months of treatment (Comhaire 1976; Vermeulen and Comhaire 1978). If however, no increase in sperm count has occurred after 6 months, no effect can be expected by further treatment.

Cases responding to treatment by increases in sperm concentration present a correlation between the sperm density before and during treatment (Comhaire 1976), (Fig. 3). The best results were registered in patients with sperm concentrations below 20 million/ml (Vermeulen and Comhaire 1978).

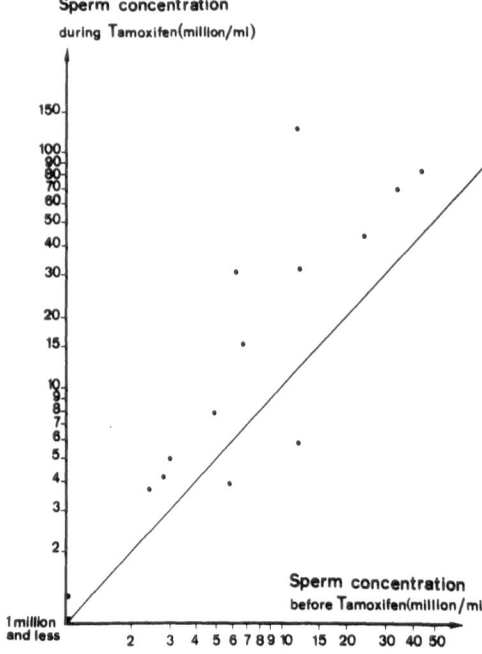

Fig. 3. Correlation between mean sperm concentration in semen analyses before tamoxifen treatment (*abscissa*) and semen analyses after 3 or more months of treatment (*ordinate*). Please note logarithmic scales. The line represents the bisectrix (Comhaire 1976)

3.3.2.2 Sperm Motility

The overall percent sperm motility remained virtually unchanged in the two studies (Comhaire 1976; Vermeulen and Comhaire 1978). Schill and Landthaler (1980) and Bartsch and Scheiber (to be published), however, demonstrated a significant improvement in percent sperm motility in those patients whose sperm concentrations also increased. In all four studies the number of spermatozoa with progressive motility per ml (so-called motile sperm count) and per ejaculate was significantly increased.

3.3.2.3 Sperm Morphology

Therapy with tamoxifen has not been found to influence sperm morphology. Schill and Landthaler (1980) and Buvat et al. (to be published) have reported results of tamoxifen treatment in 113 cases of males with infertility and oligozoospermia. These authors describe results identical to those reported in our studies. Thus, tamoxifen treatment generally results in improvement of the sperm concentration and sperm output per ejaculate, but probably does not significantly improve the quality of the spermatozoa as appreciated in sperm motility and sperm morphology. Nevertheless, the total production of "normal" spermatozoa per ejaculate clearly increases.

3.3.3 Biochemical Composition of Seminal Plasma

The volume and pH of the ejaculate are not significantly influenced by tamoxifen treatment. There are conflicting reports regarding fructose concentration and content per ejaculate. Comhaire (1976) found a significant decrease whereas Schill and Landthaler (1980) and Bartsch and Scheiber (to be published) reported no significant changes. The concentration and output of the prostatic markers, such as acid phosphatase (Comhaire, Vermeulen 1978) and citric acid (Bartsch and Scheiber, to be published), were not significantly changed. The effect of tamoxifen treatment on the secretory function of the accessory sex gland seems, therefore, to be negligible (Table 1).

3.3.4 Pregnancy

Not all of the studies reported sufficient data regarding the fertility status of the female partner. Our groups included male partners of infertile relationships, in which the female had always been examined clinically by a gynecologist. All females had a biphasic basal body temperature curve: when performed, hysterosalpingography was normal. Certainly, all the females were not fully explored endocrinologically, whereas laparascopy was only performed in exceptional cases. Since the duration of treatment was not clearly standardized, results in terms of pregnancies should be evaluated with care.

Comhaire (1976) reported five pregnancies in the first series of 15 cases, however, two of these ended in early abortion. Bartsch and Scheiber (to be published) recorded 19 pregnancies which all occurred in the group of patients who responded to tamoxifen treatment by an increased sperm concentration and no pregnancy occurred in the nonresponding group. No data are available on the outcome of the latter pregnancies.

Schill and Landthaler (1981) obtained a conception rate of 38% within an observation period of 1 year after 5 month's of tamoxifen treatment and Buvat et al. (to be published) reported a 30% pregnancy rate occurring after a mean duration of 3.5 months treatment. Careful examination of the children born after tamoxifen treatment in our study group revealed no abnormalities. In all our cases the placenta was found to be normal.

We know from placebo-controlled studies that spontaneous pregnancy rates in the population of males seen in our department is 8% within 1 year. The pregnancy rate of roughly 33% in our study groups treated with tamoxifen, therefore, favorably contrasts against the placebo-treated controls.

3.3.5 Side Effects

During treatment with tamoxifen no side effects were noticed in any of the patients. Symptoms such as scintillating scotoma, reported to occur during clomiphene treatment, were not registered in our cases. The treatment had, if anything, a positive influence on sexual life by increasing libido and orgasm in some of the cases. Gynecomastia never occurred in our patients: on the contrary, if initially present, gynecomastia regressed during treatment.

Some patients reported an increase in testicular volume during treatment and this was confirmed by orchidometry. A few patients noticed increased body hair growth. Systematic control determinations of blood concentrations of transaminases, alkaline and acid phosphatase, serum lipids, as well as of red and white blood cells, revealed no alterations in the several hundreds of patients so far treated in our department. In addition, Schill and Landthaler (1981) found no alterations of the number of thrombocytes and the serum calcium concentration.

3.4 Conclusions

Tamoxifen stimulates the hypothalamo-pituitary-testicular axis, resulting in increased testosterone secretion and a two- to threefold increase of sperm density in 75% of the patients. Since the proportion of motile and morphologically normal spermatozoa remains unaffected, the total output of "normal" spermatozoa per ejaculate increases. Related to the improved sperm production, a pregnancy rate of about 30% is obtained.

The treatment is easy, devoid of side effects, and well tolerated. The treatment can be administered to patients with either idiopathic oligozoospermia or persistent oligozoospermia after adequate treatment of varicocele or of male adnexitis. Patients with extreme astheno- or, particularly, teratozoopsermia (less than 10% sperm with ideal morphology) will probably not benefit from this treatment. The treatment is currently reserved for normogonadotropic individuals.

If the testicular hormonal response is satisfactory, tamoxifen treatment should be continued for at least 6 months. If semen quality improves, treatment can be continued for longer periods up to 2 years. If, however, no improvement occurs within 6 months of treatment, the drug should be discontinued since there is almost no chance of success in such cases. The results of our own studies and those reported by others suggest that tamoxifen is a valuable drug in the treatment of male infertility. Double-blind control trials are needed to further validate this impression.

3.5 References

Babosa J, Seal US, Doe RP (1973) Anti-estrogens and plasma proteins. I. Clomiphene and isomers, ethamoxytriphetol U-11, 100A and U-11, 555A. J Clin Endocrinol Metab 36:666–677

Bardin W, Ross GT, Lipsett M (1967) Site of action of clomiphene citrate in men: a study of the pituitary Leydig cell axis. J Clin Endocrinol Metab 27:1558–1564

Bartsch G, Scheiber K (to be published) Tamoxifen treatment in oligospermic males. Int J Urol

Buvat J, Ardaens K, Gauthier A, Buvat-Herbaut M, Lemaire A (1981) Treatment of 80 cases of hypospermia by tamoxifen. Proceedings of the II. International Congress of Andrology, Tel Aviv. Isr J Med Sci 57

Charles D, Klein T, Lunn SF, Loraine JA (1969) Clinical and endocrinological studies with the isomeric components of clomiphene citrate. J Obstet Gynaecol Br Commonwealth 76:1100–1110

Comhaire F (1976) Treatment of oligospermia with tamoxifen. Int J Fertil 21:232–238

Comhaire F, Dhont M (1975) Influence of current modes of treatment in male infertility on the hypothalamo-pituitary testicular function. In: Schellen T (ed) Releasing factors and gonadotropic hormones in male and female sterility. European Press Medicon, Ghent, pp 117–132

Comhaire F, Vermeulen A (1978) Treatment of oligozoospermia with tamoxifen (Abstract). Int J Androl [Suppl] 1:165

Dhont M, De Gezelle H, Vandekerkhove D (1976) Modulation of pituitary responsiveness to exogenous LHRH by an oestrogenic and an anti-oestrogenic compound in the normal male. Clin Endocrinol 5:175–180

Heller CG, Rowley MJ, Heller GV (1968) Clomiphene citrate: a correlation of its effect on sperm concentration and morphology, total gonadotrophins, ICSH, estrogen and testosterone excretion and testicular cytology in normal men. J Clin Endocrinol Metab 29:638–649

Hemworth BM (1975) Effect of the anti-cancer drug tamoxifen on spermatogenesis. IRCS Med Sci Libr Compend 3:627

Lunan CB, Klopper A (1975) Anti-estrogens: a review. Clin Endocrinol 4:551–572

Richards JF, Griffith DR (1974) Effects of cis- and trans-clomiphene on mammary gland development in the rat. Fertil Steril 25:74–78

Santen RJ, Leonard JM, Sherins RJ, Gandy HM, Paulsen CA (1971) Short- and long-term effects of clomiphene citrate on the pituitary-testicular axis. J Clin Endocrinol Metab 33:970–979

Schill WB (1979) Recent progress in pharmacological therapy of male subfertility: a review. Andrologia 11:77–107

Schill WB, Landthaler M (1980) Tamoxifen treatment of oligozoospermia. Andrologia 12:546–548

Schill WB, Landthaler M (1981) Erfahrungen mit dem Antiöstrogen Tamoxifen zur Therapie des Oligozoospermie. Hautarzt 32:306–308

Self LW, Holtkamp DE, Kuhn WL (1967) Pituitary-gonad related effects of isomers of clomiphene citrate. Fed Proc 26:534

Vermeulen A, Comhaire F (1978) Hormonal effects of an antiestrogen, tamoxifen, in normal and oligospermic men. Fertil Steril 29:320–327

Willis KS, London DR, Bevis BA, Butt WR, Lynch SS, Holder G (1977) Hormonal effects of tamoxifen in oligospermic men. J Endocrinol 73:171–173

4 LHRH and Its Analogs in the Treatment of Idiopathic Normogonadotropic Oligozoospermia

L. Schwarzstein and N. Aparicio

4.1 General Considerations

4.1.1 Hypothalamic Hormones

The isolation and synthesis of the hypothalamic hormone which stimulates the synthesis and release of both gonadotropins was a major and decisive step in confirming the hypothalamic control of pituitary function (Schally et al. 1971 a; Matsuo et al. 1971). It also created the possibility of using this hormone to perform physiological and clinical studies in the diagnosis and treatment of several entities involving the hypothalamic-pituitary-gonadal axis. This factor is called LH- and FSH-releasing hormone, abbreviated to LHRH/FSHRH or simply LHRH or gonadotropin releasing hormone (GnRH) (Schally et al. 1973).

LHRH is a polypeptide composed of ten amino acids. Its sequence was obtained after several steps of purification of sheep and pigs hypothalami and is similar in both species. Some of these amino acids are responsible for the physiological action of the compound, while the remaining ones are responsible for the affinity with the receptors and, thus, are related to the pharmacokinetic characteristics of the hormone (Spona 1975): LHRH was synthesized on the basis of the previous elucidated amino acid sequence and the synthetic preparation showed properties similar to the natural purified hormone. These properties were observed not only in sheep and pigs, but in many other species including humans (Schally et al. 1973).

The evidence to date suggests that LHRH is the only hormone responsible for the stimulation of the synthesis and release of LH and FSH. The release of both gonadotropins is also regulated by the levels of gonadal steroids (Schally et al. 1971 b). Synthetic LHRH can be administered intravenously, intramuscularly, or intranasally. Intestinal absorption is poor, hence the oral route cannot be used. Also, the short half-life of LHRH determines a brief duration of effect.

For these reasons, it was thought that the practical perspectives for the use of this hormone could be improved if it were possible to obtain a long-lasting vehicle or LHRH-related compounds with structural modifications and/or substitution of amino acids able to maintain a longer half-life and/or higher gonadotropin-releasing potency. In the few years following the isolation of LHRH and the determination of its structure and synthesis, an estimated 1000 analogs of LHRH have been synthesized (Schally et al. 1980).

These studies have led to the availability of different synthetic LHRH analogs, some with higher potency and long-lasting effect (Table 1) and others with the capacity to block the LHRH effect and, thus, to inhibit the pituitary gonadotropic function.

Hyperpotent analogs of LHRH are obtained by the substitution of glycine in position 6. Moreover, the incorporation of ethylamide in position 10 increases the potency and the duration of effect (Vilchez-Martínez et al. 1974). Up to now, LHRH

Table 1. Some of the stimulatory analogs under investigation

Analog	Potency in comparison to LHRH
D-Ala^6-LHRH	6–7-times (Monahan et al. 1973)
D-Leu^6-LHRH	5–9-times (Vilchez-Martínez et al. 1974)
D-Phe^6-LHRH	10–13-times (Coy et al. 1975)
D-Trp^6-LHRH	50–100-times (Coy et al. 1975)
D-Ser-(Bu^t)^6-LHRH-EA (Hoe 766)	30–100-times (Sandow et al. 1976)
D-Leu^6-LHRH-EA	50–60-times (Vilchez-Martínez et al. 1974)
D-Ala^6-LHRH-EA	30-times (de la Cruz et al. 1975)

and some analogs have been used therapeutically in the male, namely in the treatment of hypogonadotropic hypogonadism (Mortimer et al. 1974; Mortimer 1977; Happ et al. 1975, 1978 a; Vilchez-Martínez et al. 1979; Tharandt et al. 1977).

4.1.2 Male Infertility

The pathophysiology and etiology of male infertility are poorly understood and largely unknown. Therefore, specific therapy has eluded us and we have had to content ourselves with empiric forms of treatment.

It is well known that the majority of infertile males have normal basal levels of LH, FSH, and testosterone. In spite of this, treatment with gonadotropins, testosterone, and clomiphene citrate, was based on the assumption that an overstimulation of the testes could lead to improved spermatogenesis.

However, the evaluation of results of such studies faced several difficulties, such as spontaneous variations of the parameters of the spermiogram and even spontaneous pregnancies without treatment. As these studies were performed on small numbers of patients and seldom with double-blind methodology, the results should be interpreted with great caution. Moreover, certain causes of male infertility, such as genetic or immunological problems, were not taken into consideration in most of these studies. This fact suggests that the population under study was not homogeneous enough to guarantee a correct evaluation of results.

4.2 Experience with LHRH and Its Analogs

4.2.1 Selection of Patients

When we began our experiences with LHRH and, later with the analogs, these drugs had never been used in the treatment of the infertile or subfertile man. Contemporary to our first experiences, Zárate et al. (1973) treated a small group of infertile patients with LHRH. A total of ten patients, four of them azoospermic, were treated with 500 µg LHRH twice daily intramuscularly for a period of 6 months applying neither a clear selection of patients or criteria for evaluation of therapeutic results. Moreover, some patients experienced an increased spermatic output. It was, thus, necessary to design a trial protocol trying to select a homogeneous population according to the following criteria:

1. Only patients with no less than 3 years of infertility were incorporated.
2. Patients had idiopathic normogonadotropic oligoasthenozoospermia and normal androgenic function.
3. Oligoasthenozoospermia was diagnosed by at least three sperm counts performed during 3 months immediately preceding the inclusion of the patient into the study. Subjects with counts above 20×10^6 spermatozoa/ml were not included.
4. Selected clinical, roentgenologic, urologic, vascular, endocrinologic, and laboratory studies were performed in all patients. All these studies were within normal limits to consider the patients as having "idiopathic oligoasthenozoospermia".
5. In all patients, plasma circulating levels of LH, FSH, and testosterone were repeatedly determined by radioimmunoassay. The levels of the three hormones fell within the normal ranges of the assay methods.
6. Each patient underwent bilateral testicular biopsy, with ample testicular exposure at least 60 days before starting treatment. Patients selected for the study were those who showed no macroscopic alteration on the usual examination of the testes and epididymis. According to the type of light-microscopic histologic involvement, patients were classified as follows: quantitative alterations of spermatogenesis with foci of arrest at the spermatid stage (group 1) and patients with more severely altered spermatogenesis (group 2).

This classification was based on the results of previous experiences (Schwarzstein 1974; Meinhard et al. 1973; Aafjes and Van der Vijver 1974) which showed the best therapeutic results with human menopausal gonadotropin (HMG) and other agents in patients of group 1.

4.2.2 Evaluation of Results

Quantitative results were evaluated by means of variance analyses involving the concentration of spermatozoa/ml, the percentage of live and motile spermatozoa, and the percentage of spermatozoa with forward progression. The percentage of live spermatozoa was determined by substracting the percentage of eosin-positive spermatozoa from the total number of spermatozoa.

Results were also evaluated qualitatively. For this purpose, *frank improvement* was arbitrarily defined as the achievement of at least twice the initial values and

Table 2. Classification of qualitative evaluation (see text)

	Spermatozoa/ml	Percent and live motile spermatozoa	Percent spermatozoa with forward progression
Positive	Frank improvement	Frank improvement	Frank improvement
Doubtful	Improvement	Improvement or frank improvement	Improvement or frank improvement
Negative	No change	Improvement or no change	Improvement or no change

sperm count of more than 30×10^6 spermatozoa/ml, 40% live and motile spermatozoa, and 30% spermatozoa with forward progression. *Improvement* implied the achievement of at least twice the initial values without surpassing the figures mentioned for the previous category. "No change" meant that the patient had not achieved twice the initial values.

According to these arbitrary definitions, results were classified as shown in Table 2.

4.2.3 Experience with LHRH

Twenty-one patients were selected, who were considered to have idiopathic normogonadotropic oligozoospermia. Of these patients, 14 were classified according to testicular histology as group 1 and seven as group 2. The number of spermatozoa/ml was significantly lower in patients of group 2, while the percent live and motile sperm and percent spermatozoa with forward progression were similar in both groups (Table 3).

Five patients of group 1 and five of group 2 were treated once daily with intramuscular injections of LHRH for 60–135 days (long-term therapy): Three subjects of group 1 and one of group 2 underwent two courses of this regimen with a treatment-free interval of 3 months, the remaining patients receiving only one course of this treatment regimen. Nine patients of group 1 and two of group 2 received 30–45-day courses of treatment separated by a 1-month treatment-free interval (short-term therapy).

Most patients were treated with 100–200 µg/injection LHRH. Two patients, at the beginning of the study, were treated with 500 µg/injection. The dose was modi-

Table 3. Sperm count, percentage of live and motile spermatozoa and percentage of spermatozoa with forward-progressive motility in groups 1 and 2 prior to treatment with LHRH. Values are means ± SE of at least three sperm counts

Group	n	Sperm count $\times 10^6$/ml Mean ± SE (range)	Percent live and motile spermatozoa	Percent forward-progressive spermatozoa
1	14	7.9±1.5 (1.5–17.0)	31.7±4.3	12.5±3.4
2	7	3.5±0.9 (0.5–7.5)	34.4±7.1	13.2±4.1

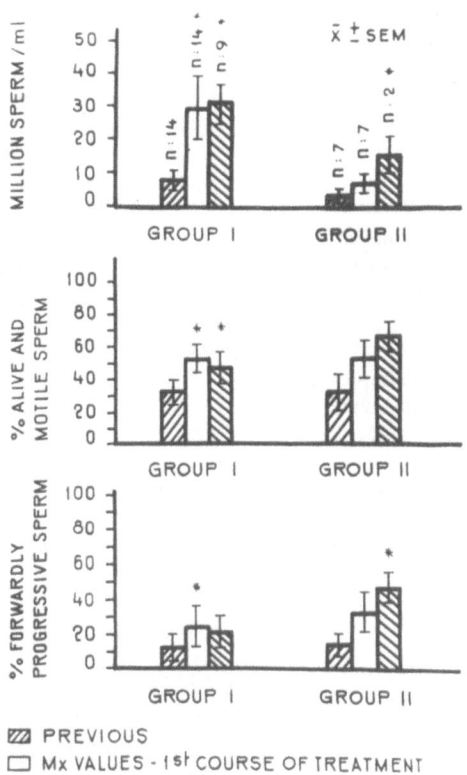

Fig. 1. Sperm counts, percentage of live and motile spermatozoa, and percentages of spermatozoa with forward progression in both groups before and after treatment with LHRH. The asterisks indicate values that are significantly different ($p < 0.05$) from pretreatment values

fied after a dose-response study (Turner et al. 1975), which showed that doses higher than 200–250 µg did not improve LH and FSH response. All the patients underwent control spermiograms every 20–30 days during the course of treatment and up to 45 days after withdrawal of medication. Spermiograms were obtained for 13 patients (seven of group 1, six of group 2) for up to 90–150 days after the end of the treatment, at 20–30-day intervals.

Figure 1 shows the evaluation of the parameters studied before and after treatment with LHRH, results in both groups given separately. Significant rises in all three parameters occurred in group 1 during treatment, mostly in the number spermatozoa/ml. Group 2 showed a rising trend, but significance was not reached after the first course of treatment. The patients in group 2 who received two courses of treatment experienced significant qualitative and quantitative improvement.

Table 4 summarizes the qualitative assessment of the results obtained in both groups. The proportion of *frank improvement* was similar in both groups as far as the parameters of vitality and motility are concerned. The proportion showing *frank improvement* in sperm concentration was significantly higher in group 1. Of the 21 patients studied, six obtained the maximal sperm concentration 30 or more days after treatment was discontinued. In the same period, ten subjects obtained the maximal percentage of live and motile spermatozoa and 15 the maximal percent forward-progressive spermatozoa.

Table 4. Qualitative assessment of sperm count, percentage of live and motile spermatozoa and percentage of forward progressive spermatozoa in groups 1 and 2 after treatment with LHRH

Parameter	Group 1 (n = 14) No. patients (%)	Group 2 (n = 7) No. patients (%)
Sperm count		
Frank improvement	7 (50.0)	0 (0.0)
Improvement	3 (21.4)	4 (57.1)
No change	4 (28.6)	3 (42.8)
Percent live and motile spermatozoa		
Frank improvement	7 (50.0)	4 (57.1)
Improvement	4 (28.6)	0 (0.0)
No change	3 (21.4)	3 (42.8)
Percent forward progressive spermatozoa		
Frank improvement	7 (50.0)	4 (57.1)
Improvement	4 (28.6)	0 (0.0)
No change	3 (21.4)	3 (42.8)

Six of seven patients in group 1 followed-up for 90–150 days after withdrawal of treatment retained the sperm count values above the initial number, whereas this occurred in only one of six patients in group 2.

Table 5 contains the overall results of treatment classified according to the severity of testicular involvement and type of treatment applied. Four of five group 1 patients receiving *long-term treatment* obtained *positive* results, and three of them were able to impregnate their wives. The same regimen in group 2 resulted in one pregnancy. With the *short-term regimen* in group 1 only one positive case with impregnation occurred. The significance of the difference between both treatment regimens was $P < 0.05$. No side effects were observed in any case. Fifteen patients spontaneously reported increased libido and sexual potency after the first follow-up 20–30 days from the start of treatment.

Under the conditions of this study, LHRH treatment resulted in qualitative and quantitative improvement in semen parameters in patients with idiopathic normogonadotropic oligozoospermia. Patients with the best prognosis were those with less severe spermatogenetic disorders, although improvement was also achieved in some subjects with more severe disorders of spermatogenesis.

Table 5. Overall results of treatment with LHRH, classified according to testicular biopsy and type of treatment

Group	Long-term treatment			Short-term treatment		
	Positive	Doubtful	Negative	Positive	Doubtful	Negative
1	4	1	0	1	4	4
2	1	3	1	0	1	1

Hypothetically, the therapeutic action of LHRH might result from two mechanisms; direct gonadotropin release or restoration of normal pituitary gonadotropin reserve (Yoshimoto et al. 1975). This may account for the amelioration seen after withdrawal of treatment. Although spontaneous variations in the number of spermatozoa, tubular and/or ductal patency and/or adnexal gland function cannot be ruled out, the fact that the above results occurred during or immediately after treatment with LHRH suggests that improvement can be ascribed to the treatment.

The increase in libido and sexual potency reported by the patients occurred 20–30 days after initiation of treatment. It has been suggested that this effect might be related to a central action of LHRH, in addition to stimulation of the pituitary-gonadal axis (Mortimer et al. 1974), although the possibility of placebo effect has yet to be evaluated.

It must also be stated that, since LHRH is a small peptide which is rapidly disintegrated in vivo, it rarely becomes immunogenic. Therefore, the possible incidence of antibody formation during or after a prolonged treatment of patients with LHRH is extremely low (Schally et al. 1980; Sandow et al. 1978).

There is only one report of secondary drug failure because of antibody formation in one hypogonadal patient treated for more than 1 year with LHRH (Van Loon and Brown 1975). In conclusion, LHRH may be useful in the treatment of subfertile men. Further experiences with a larger number of patients are needed to confirm its efficacy.

4.2.4 D-Leucine[6]-LHRH-Ethylamide

It was thought that an analog of LHRH with increased potency and longer duration of action would combine a more intense and prolonged releasing effect with the restoration of pituitary functional reserve.

D-leu[6]-LHRH-EA releases 50–60-times as much LH and 15-times as much FSH as do similar doses of LHRH, when administered to immature male rats over a 6-h period (Arimura et al. 1974; Vilchez-Martínez et al. 1974). D-leu[6]-LHRH-EA, given systemically, raises LH and FSH blood levels in men and women for as long as 24 h (de Medeiros-Comaru et al. 1976; Soria et al. 1975). This analog has also been found to be active when administered intranasally to normal men (González-Barcena et al. 1976; Happ et al. 1978 c). It is also effective when given intravaginally or rectally (Saito et al. 1977). Our own dose-response study using intramuscular injections of D-leu[6]-LHRH-EA in oligozoospermic men showed significant increases of LH and FSH for 6 and even 12 h after the injection. Peak levels were obtained between 4 and 6 h (Turner et al. 1976). We tested the therapeutic action of this analog in 17 patients (ages 19–42 years old) with idiopathic normogonadotropic oligozoospermia. The criteria of selection were the same as the one used for LHRH treatment.

According to histologic study of their testes, all patients had hypospermatogenesis with foci of alterations at the spermatid stage (group 1), with the exception of two subjects who had more severe alterations in some tubules (group 2).

The patients were treated for 90 days with intramuscular injections of D-leu[6]-LHRH-EA at doses of 5 µg daily (four patients), 10 µg daily (four patients), 20 µg daily (five patients), and 200 µg daily (four patients). All patients underwent control spermiograms every 30 days during the course of treatment and 90 days after withdrawal of medication. Results were evaluated as previously stated.

Table 6 shows data obtained before treatment in the four groups. Figure 2 shows average values for all the parameters considered before treatment and the maximal values during and after treatment. No significant changes were observed, with the exception of patients treated with 20 µg analog, who experienced significant increases in the percentage of live and motile spermatozoa and in the percentage of spermatozoa with forward-progressive motility. Table 7 summarizes the qualitative assessment of the results obtained in the four groups. No frank improvement in sperm count was obtained. Only few patients experienced frank improvement in vitality and motility without correlation to dosage. Table 8 shows overall results of treatment. No positive results were observed and results were not dose-dependent.

Table 6. Data before treatment with D-Leu[6]-LHRH-EA

Dose per day	No. of sub-jects	No. spermatozoa/ml		Percent live and motile spermatozoa		Percent forward-progressive spermatozoa	
		Mean ±SE	Range	Mean±SE	Range	Mean±SE	Range
5 µg	4	1.9±0.6	1.0 – 4.0	33.6±8.2	18.0±61.0	19.4±7.5	1.7 – 38.0
10 µg	4	5.7±1.0[a]	3.1 – 8.5	47.3±5.3	33.0 – 62.0	26.5±1.1	23.0 – 29.0
20 µg	5	3.1±1.4	0.5 – 9.0	45.0±5.8	29.0 – 60.0	10.4±3.7[b]	0.0 – 25.0
200 µg	4	4.2±0.7	1.0 – 8.0	30.5±4.1	10.0 – 56.0	11.8±3.3[b]	0.0 – 32.0

[a] Compared to 5 µg, $P < 0.05$
[b] Compared to 10 µg, $P < 0.05$

Table 7. Qualitative assessment of results with D-leu[6]-LHRH-EA

Parameter	Group 5 µg No. of patients (%)		Group 10 µg No. of patients (%)		Group 20 µg No. of patients (%)		Group 200 µg No. of patients (%)	
Sperm count								
Frank improvement	0	(0.0)	0	(0.0)	0	(0.0)	0	(0.0)
Improvement	1	(25.0)	1	(25.0)	4	(80.0)	0	(0.0)
No change	3	(75.0)	3	(75.0)	1	(20.0)	4	(10.0)
Percent live and motile spermatozoa								
Frank improvement	1	(25.0)	0	(0.0)	0	(0.0)	0	(0.0)
Improvement	0	(0.0)	0	(0.0)	1	(20.0)	0	(0.0)
No change	3	(75.0)	4	(100.0)	4	(80.0)	4	(10.0)
Percent forward-progressive spermatozoa								
Frank improvement	0	(0.0)	2	(50.0)	3	(60.0)	0	(0.0)
Improvement	0	(0.0)	0	(0.0)	2	(40.0)	0	(0.0)
No change	4	(100.0)	2	(50.0)	0	(0.0)	4	(10.0)

D-LEU-6-LH/RH-EA
SPERM EVOLUTION

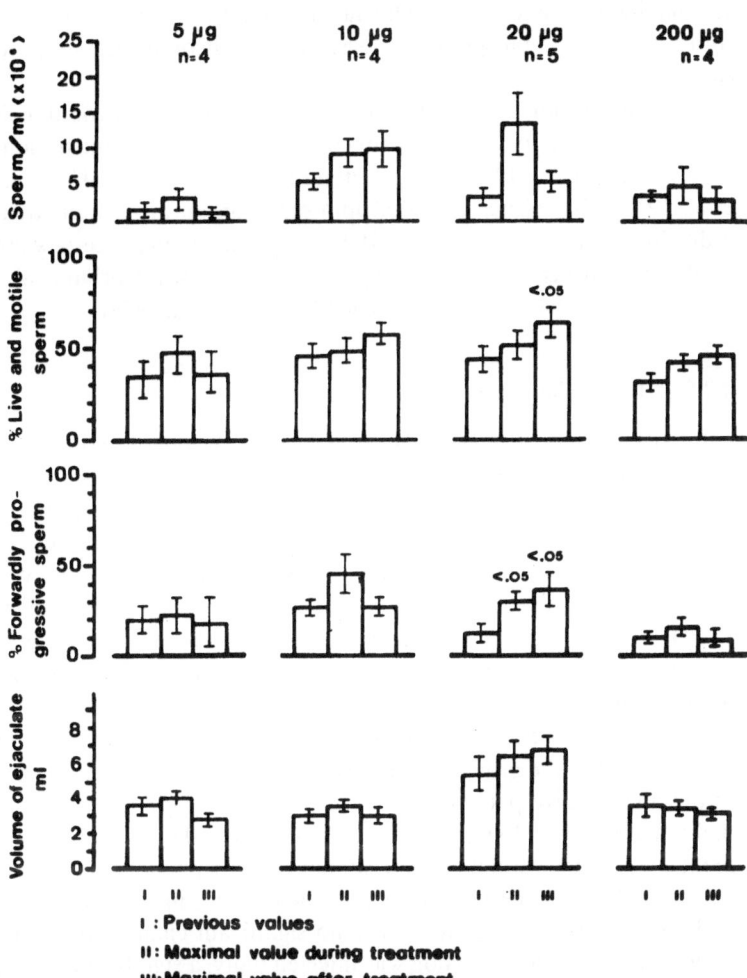

Fig. 2. Sperm counts, percentage of live and motile spermatozoa, percentage of spermatozoa with forward progression, and volume of ejaculate before treatment and maximal values during and after treatment with D-leu⁶-LHRH-EA

Table 8. Overall results of treatment with D-leu⁶-LHRH-EA

Group	Positive No. of patients (%)	Douptful No. of patients (%)	Negative No. of patients (%)
5 μg	0 (0.0)	0 (0.0)	4 (100.0)
10 μg	0 (0.0)	0 (0.0)	4 (100.0)
20 μg	0 (0.0)	3 (60.0)	2 (40.0)
200 μg	0 (0.0)	0 (0.0)	4 (100.0)

Results were doubtful in three patients of the group treated with 20 µg, whereas in the remaining patients the results were considered negative.

The results showed no significant improvement from either the quantitative or the qualitative point of view. This fact is even more significant because, for the majority of patients, the prognosis was at least theoretically good according to the histologic study.

Possible explanations of the lack of therapeutic benefit could include an exhaustion of the pituitary after prolonged and repeated administration of the analog (Schwarzstein et al. 1977) or inhibition of the testicular LH-HCG receptor (Auclair et al. 1977). Diminished gonadotropin secretion during chronic treatment due to a reduction in the number of LHRH receptors in the pituitary and paradoxical antifertility effects of several analogs have been shown (Corbin et al. 1977; Labrie et al. 1978; Bergquist et al. 1979; Vilchez-Martínez et al. 1979).

4.2.5 D-Tryptophan⁶-LHRH

D-trp[6]-LHRH, recently synthesized, is 13–21-times more potent than LHRH in releasing LH and FSH in rats (Coy et al. 1976). Given intravenously or intramuscularly it raises serum LH, FSH, testosterone, and 17-β-estradiol levels for a period of at least 6 h (Jaramillo et al. 1977). When administered intranasally in doses of 500 µg, it elevates LH and FSH levels for up to 24 h (Wass et al. 1979). Chronic treatment of men with hypogonadotropic hypogonadism with D-trp[6]-LHRH improves their testicular function (Jaramillo et al. 1978). It is also useful for women with hypothalamic-pituitary dysfunction (A. Zañartu 1980, personal communication).

Eighteen infertile patients with idiopathic normogonadotropic oligozoospermia, all belonging to the group 1 biopsy type, were treated with intramuscular injections of this analog. Five patients received 5 µg every 2 days, three patients received 5 µg daily, five received 10 µg every 2 days, and five 10 µg daily. The schemes of treatment control and evaluation were similar to those previously described.

Table 9 shows sperm count values before, during, and after treatment. With 5 and 10 µg every 2 days, there were no significant changes in the number of spermatozoa/ml. When the analog was injected daily, a significant decrease in the number of spermatozoa/ml was observed, and four patients, two treated with 5 µg and two with 10 µg, became azoospermic. They recovered during the following 60 days. Only one patient, treated with 10 µg each 2 days, showed improved sperm count with a slight improvement of motility.

Table 10 shows the qualitative evaluation. The negative results observed could be attributed to the large dosage utilized. There is no experience with dose regimens for this hormone. Recent studies with D-trp[6]-LHRH showed decrease in pituitary function and depletion of pituitary LH, as well as some extrapituitary gonadal inhibitory effects of high doses (Vilchez-Martínez et al. 1979). Daily administration of D-trp[6]-LHRH to male rats caused a reduction in testicular tubules, loss of LH receptor sites in the testes, and decreased plasma testosterone levels. All these effects disappeared 4 weeks after cessation of treatment (Schally et al. 1978).

These results suggest that the paradoxical antifertility effects of LHRH analogs on the gonad result, at least in part, from a direct action that leads to the reduction

Table 9. Data before, during and after treatment with D-trp[6]-LHRH. The abbreviation % FPS indicates percent forward-progressive spermatozoa

	5 μg every 2 days		5 μg daily		10 μg every 2 days		10 μg daily	
	No. spermatozoa/ml	% FPS	No. spermatozoa/ml	% FPS	No. spermatozoa/ml	% FPS	No. spermatozoa/ml	% FPS
Pretreatment	9.32±1.42	6.8±1.3	8.4±1.9	5.7±1.9	8.9±1.3	2.6±0.9	5.7±1.3	3.5±1.1
Maximal values during treatment	10.25±1.29	10.0±2.2	1.4±0.9	2.2±2.2	8.4±2.9	3.7±1.2	3.9±1.1	1.6±0.9
Maximal values after treatment	7.36±1.31	9.3±3.3	0.6±0.4	0	6.3±1.5	1.7±1.4	3 ±1.1	0

Table 10. Qualitative assessment of results obtained with D-trp⁶-LHRH

Parameter	5 µg every 2 days		5 µg daily		10 µg every 2 days		10 µg daily	
	No. of patients	(%)	No. of patients	(%)	No. of patients	(%)	No. of patients	(%)
Sperm count								
Frank improvement	0	(0)	0	(0)	0	(0)	0	(0)
Improvement	0	(0)	0	(0)	1	(20)	0	(0)
No change	5	(100)	3	(100)	4	(80)	5	(100)
Percent forward-progressive spermatozoa								
Frank improvement	0	(0)	0	(0)	1	(20)	0	(0)
Improvement	1	(20)	0	(0)	0	(0)	0	(0)
No change	4	(80)	3	(100)	4	(80)	5	(100)

of LH/HCG receptors (Arimura et al. 1979). On the contrary, smaller doses, such as a daily injection of 1 µg D-trp⁶-LHRH increases LH/HCG receptors three- to five-fold by a direct effect (Schally et al. 1980).

A number of recent studies demonstrate antifertility effects of large doses of LHRH and some long-acting analogs. Prolonged treatment with these compounds causes impairment of reproductive functions. In view of these paradoxical antifertility effects of relatively large pharmacological doses of LHRH and some stimulatory analogs, the doses of analogs should be limited. We still lack a suitable clinical regimen for parenteral or intranasal administration which could lead to increasingly successful use of these compounds in male infertiliy.

4.3 Conclusions

In spite of the great advance registered in recent years with the isolation, identification of the structure and synthesis of LHRH and, subsequently, of the so-called "superactive" stimulatory analogs, the usefulness of these agents in the treatment of male infertility still remains to be established. Synthetic LHRH seems promising in a limited and very selected group of patients, although further experiences with larger numbers of patients are needed to confirm its therapeutic benefit.

At the same time, we should mention the fact that approaches based on LHRH may possibly lead to the development of birth control methods for the male. These methods could be based on the development and application of the paradoxical antifertility effects which occur when relatively large doses of the stimulatory analogs are employed or in the utilization of inhibitory analogs.

This last fact is based in the possibility of modifying the structure of the LHRH molecule, thus inhibiting biological activity without destroying binding affinity. These inhibitory analogs can complete with biologically active compounds for the same receptor sites.

The knowledge that relatively large doses of the stimulatory analogs have paradoxical antifertility effects should foster the development of more suitable clinical regimens for parenteral and intranasal application. This could lead to increasingly successful use of these compounds for the treatment of male infertility. Also, we need to establish better criteria for the selection of patients to be treated and to encourage laboratory and clinical research to determine whether the use of LHRH or its analogs offers future promise in the treatment of the subfertile male.

Acknowledgements. We are grateful to Mrs. María Luz Rueda and Mrs. Mónica González Sabathié for their invaluable secretarial assistance and to Mrs. Mabel Slulitell de Santos for her careful technical help.

4.4 References

Aafjes JH, Van der Vijver JCM (1974) A relationship between testicular biopsy score count and fertility of men treated for oligospermia. Fertil Steril 25:809–812

Arimura A, Vilchez-Martínez JA, Coy DH, Coy EJ, Hirotsu Y, Schally AV (1974) (D-ala[6]-Des-Gly-NH$_2$[10])-LH-RH-ethylamide: a new analogue with unusually high LH-RH/FSH-RH activity. Endocrinology 95:174–177

Arimura A, Serafini PC, Sonntag W (1979) Does LH-RH agonist decrease ovarian and testicular LH/HCG receptors by direct action? Program of the 61st Annual Meeting in the Endocrine Society, Anaheim, California (Abstract 433), Endocrine Society, p 181

Auclair C, Kelly PA, Coy DH, Schally AV, Labrie F (1977) Potent inhibitory activity of [D-Leu[6]-Des-Gly-NH$_2$[10]] LHRH ethylamide on LH/HCG and PRL testicular receptor levels in the rat. Endocrinology 101:1890–1893

Bergquist Ch, Nillius SJ, Bergh T, Skarin G, Wide L (1979) Inhibitory effects on gonadotrophin secretion and gonadal function in men during chronic treatment with a potent stimularory luteinizing hormone-releasing hormone analogue. Acta Endocrinol 91:601–608

Corbin A, Beattie CW, Rees R, Yardley J, Foell TJ, Chai SY, McGregor H, Sarantakis D, McKinley WA (1977) Postcoital contraceptive effects of agonist analogs of luteinizing hormone-releasing hormone. Fertil Steril 28:471–475

Coy DH, Schally AV, Vilchez-Martínez JA, Coy EJ, Arimura A (1975) Stimulatory and inhibitory analogs of LH-RH. In Motta M, Crosignani PG, Martini L (eds) Hypothalamic hormones. Chemistry, physiology, pharmacology and clinical uses. Academic Press, London New York San Francisco, pp 1–12

Coy DH, Vilchez-Martínez JA, Coy FJ, Schally AV (1976) Analogs of luteinizing hormone-releasing hormone with increased biological activity produced by D-amino acid substitutions in position 6. J Med Chem 19:423–425

de la Cruz A, de la Cruz KG, Arimura A, Coy DH, Vilchez-Martínez JA, Coy EJ, Schally AV (1975) Gonadotropin-releasing activity of two highly active and long-acting analogs of luteinizing hormone-releasing hormone after subcutaneous, intravaginal and oral administration. Fertil Steril 26:894–900

De Medeiros-Comaru AM, Rodriguez J, Povoa LC, Franco S, Dimetz T, Coy DH, Kastin AJ, Schally AV (1976) Clinical studies with long-acting superactive analogs of LH-RH in women with secondary amenorrhea. Int J Fertil 21:239–242

González-Barcena D, Kastin AJ, Schalch DS, Coy DH, Schally AV (1976) Prolonged elevation of LH after intranasal administration of an analogue of LH-RH. Fertil Steril 27:1246–1249

Happ J, Neubauer M, Egri A, Demisch K, Schoffling K, Beyer J (1975) GnRH therapy in males with hypogonadotrophic hypogonadism. Horm Metab Res 7:526–531

Happ J, Kollmann F, Krawelh C, Neubauer M, Kranse U, Demisch K, Sandow J, von Rechenberg W, Beyer J (1978a) Treatment of cryptorchidism with pernasal gonadotrophin-releasing hormone therapy. Fertil Steril 29:546–551

Happ J, Weber T, Callensee W, Ermet JA, Eshkol A, Beyer J (1978 b) Treatment of cryptorchidism with a potent analog of gonadotrophin-releasing hormone. Fertil Steril 29:552–556

Happ J, Hartmann U, Weber T, Crodes U, Beyer J (1978 c) Gonadotropin and testosterone secretion in normal human males after stimulation with gonadotropin-releasing hormone (GnRH) or potent GnRH analogs using different modes of application. Fertil Steril 30:666–673

Jaramillo CJ, Pérez-Infante V, Macía AL, Salgado AC, Coy DH, Schally AV (1977) Serum LH, FSH and testosterone response to the administration of a new LH-RH analog, D-trp[6]-LH-RH in normal men. Int J Fertil 22:77–84

Jaramillo CJ, Charro-Salgado AL, Pérez-Infante V, Bordiú Obanza E, Cano Iglesias F, Fernandez-Cruz A, Coy DH, Schally AV (1978) Clinical studies with D-trp[6]-luteinizing hormone-releasing hormone in men with hypogonadotropic hypogonadism. Fertil Steril 30:430–435

Labrie F, Auclair C, Cusan L, Kelly PA, Pelletier G, Ferland L (1978) Inhibitory effect of LH-RH and its agonists on testicular gonadotrophin receptors and spermatogenesis in the rat. Int J Androl [Suppl] 2:303–318

Matsuo H, Arimura A, Nair RMG, Schally AV (1971) The synthesis of proteine LH and FSH releasing hormone by the solid-phase method. Biochem Biophys Res Commun 45:822–827

Meinhard E, McRae CU, Chisholm GD (1973) Testicular biopsy in evaluation of male infertility. Br Med J 3:577–579

Monahan MW, Amoss MS, Anderson HA, Vale W (1973) Synthetic analogs of the hypothalamic luteinizing hormone releasing factor with increased agonist or antagonist properties. Biochemistry 12:4616–4620

Mortimer CH (1977) Clinical applications of the gonadotrophin releasing hormone. J Clin Endocrinol Metab 6:167–179

Mortimer LH, McNeilly AS, Fisher RA, Murray MAF, Besser GM (1974) Gonadotrophin releasing hormone therapy in hypogonadal males with hypothalamic or pituitary dysfunction. Br Med J 4:617–621

Saito M, Kamusaki T, Yaoi Y, Nishi N, Arimura A, Coy DH, Schally AV (1977) Stimulation of luteinizing hormone (LH) and follicle-stimulating hormone by (D-Leu[6],Des-Gly[10]-NH$_2$)-LH-releasing hormone ethylamide after subcutaneous, intravaginal and intrarectal administration to women. Fertil Steril 28:240–246

Sandow J, von Rechenberg W, Koenig W, Hahn M, Ierzabek G, Fraser H (1978) Physiological studies with highly active analogues of LH-RH. In: Gupta D, Voelter M (eds) Hypothalamic hormones – chemistry, physiology and clinical application. Edited by Chemie, Weinheim, p 307

Schally AV, Arimura A, Baba Y, Nair RMG, Matsuo H, Redding TW, Debeljuk L, White WF (1971 a) Isolation and properties of the FSH and LH releasing hormone. Biochem Biophys Res Commun 43:393–399

Schally AV, Kastin AJ, Arimura A (1971 b) Hypothalamic follicle-stimulating hormone (FSH) and luteinizing hormone (LH)-regulating hormone: Structure, physiology and clinical studies. Fertil Steril 22:703–721

Schally AV, Arimura A, Kastin AJ (1973) Hypothalamic regulatory hormones. Science 179:341–350

Schally AV, Arimura A, Coy DH (1980) Recent approaches to fertility control based on derivatives of LH-RH. In: Munson PL, Diczfalusy E, Glover J, Olson RE (eds) Vitamins and hormones. Academic Press, London, 38:258

Schwarzstein L (1974) Human menopausal gonadotropins in the treatment of patients with oligospermia. Fertil Steril 25:813–816

Schwarzstein L, Aparicio NJ, Turner D, Turner EA, Coy DH, Schally AV (1977) Luteinizing hormone (LH), follicle-stimulating hormone, and testosterone responses to consecutive injections of D-leucine[6]-LH-releasing hormone ethylamide in normal men. Fertil Steril 28:451–455

Soria J, Zárate A, Canales ES, Ayala A, Schally AV, Coy DH, Coy EJ, Kastin AJ (1975) Increased and prolonged LH-RH/FSH-RH activity of synthetic D-Ala[6],Des-Gly-NH$_2$[10]-LH-RH-ethylamide in normal women. Am J Obstet Gynecol 123:145–146

Spona J (1975) Some structural requirements for LH-RH actions. Endocrinol Exp 9:159–165

Tharandt L, Schulte H, Benker G, Hackenberg K, Reinwein D (1977) Treatment of isolated gonadotropin deficiency in men with synthetic LH-RH and a more potent analogue of LH-RH. Neuroendocrinology 24:195–207

Turner D, Turner EA, Schwarzstein L, Aparicio NJ (1975) Response of luteinizing hormone and follicle-stimulating hormone to different doses of synthetic luteinizing hormone-releasing hormone intramuscular administration in normal and oligospermic men: Preliminary report. Fertil Steril 26:337–339

Turner D, Turner EA, Aparicio NJ, Schwarzstein L (1976) Response of luteinizing hormone and follicle-stimulating hormone to different doses of D-leucine[6]-LH-RH-ethylamide in oligospermic patients. Fertil Steril 27:545–548

Van Loon GR, Brown GM (1975) Secondary drug failure occurring during chronic treatment with LH-RH: Appearance of an antibody. J Clin Endocrinol Metab 41:640–643

Vilchez-Martínez JA, Coy DH, Arimura A, Coy EJ, Hirotsu Y, Schally AV (1974) Synthesis and biological properties of (Leu-6)-LH-RH and (D-Leu,Des-Gly-NH_2[10]-LH-RH-ethylamide). Biochem Biophys Res Commun 59:1226–1232

Vilchez-Martínez JA, Pedroza E, Arimura A, Schally AV (1979) Paradoxical effects of D-Trp[6]-luteinizing hormone-releasing hormone on the hypothalamic-pituitary-gonadal axis in immature female rats. Fertil Steril 31:677–682

Wass JAH, Besser GM, Gómez Pan A, Scanlon MF, Hall R, Kastin AJ, Coy DH, Schally AV (1979) Comparison of long-acting analogues of luteinizing hormone-releasing hormone in man. Clin Endocrinol 10:419–425

Yoshimoto Y, Moridera K, Imura H (1975) Restoration of normal pituitary gonadotropin reserve by administration of luteinizing hormone-releasing hormone in patients with hypogonadotropic hypogonadism. N Engl J Med 292:242–245

Zárate A, Valdés-Vallina F, González A, Pérez-Ubierna C, Canales ES, Schally AV (1973) Therapeutic effect of synthetic luteinizing hormone-releasing hormone (LH-RH) in male infertility due to idiopathic azoospermia and oligospermia. Fertil Steril 24:485–486

5 Hyperprolactinemia in Male Infertility: Treatment with Bromocriptine

E. del Pozo

The importance of prolactin (PRL) as a lactogenic hormone and its role in the control of reproduction has long been recognized in the experimental animal. It is only recently that this hormone has been identified in humans as an entity separate from other lactogens and its biological properties investigated. Furthermore, its action in physiology and pathophysiology has been studied since specific PRL inhibitors were made available to experimental and clinical investigators.

The mechanisms of release and the biological effects of PRL in male subjects are presented here. The clinical role of this proteohormone in states of oversecretion and the response to bromocriptine treatment are reviewed.

5.1 Control of PRL Release: The Role of Dopamine and Estrogens

Findings of experimental and clinical studies indicate that the pituitary galactotropes are subjected to a predominantly inhibitory influence from the hypothalamus. Thus, it has been known that section of the pituitary stalk increases PRL secretion in experimental animals (Kanematsu and Sawyer 1973). This mechanism has also been confirmed in humans (Turkington et al. 1971), supporting the presence of a PRL-inhibiting factor (PIF). More insight into the mechanisms governing the secretion of PIF by the hypothalamus was obtained after the characterization of the tuberoinfundibular system (Halasz and Pupp 1965) and its identification as a part of complex mechanisms regulating the secretion of PRL by the anterior pituitary (Hökfelt and Fuxe 1972a). This system presumably acts at the level of the median eminence to release PIF, using dopamine (DA) as the neurotransmitter. Thus, any stimulation of the synthesis of DA, e.g., the administration of L-dopa, which is endogenously transformed into DA, would in turn increase PIF and subsequently reduce PRL secretion from the pituitary galactotropes. Mechanisms leading to the opposite effect (namely, a block in DA-PIF release) elevate serum PRL. By reason of its DA-dependency, this functional unit has been characterized as the tuberoinfundibular-dopaminergic (TIDA) system (Hökfelt and Fuxe 1972b). Although many researchers favor the idea that PIF may be identical with DA, an inhibitory effect on PRL release has been detected in brain extracts devoid of DA activity (Schally et al. 1976; Enjalbert et al. 1978). The influence of serotonergic, ad-

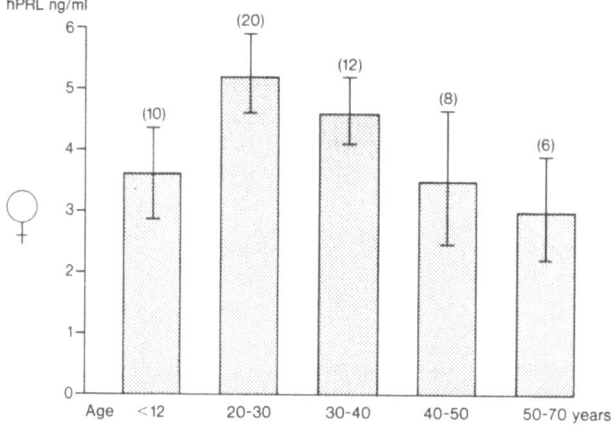

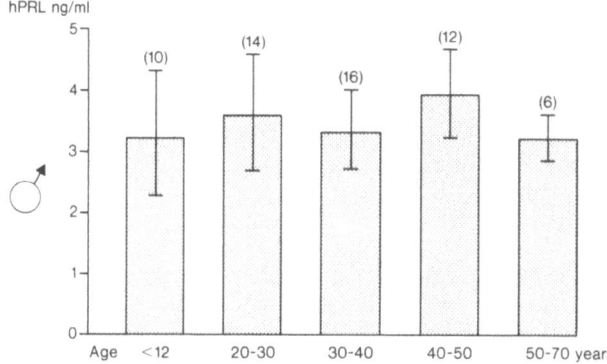

Fig. 1. PRL values during the human life cycle. There is an obvious dependency on ovarian activity in female subjects

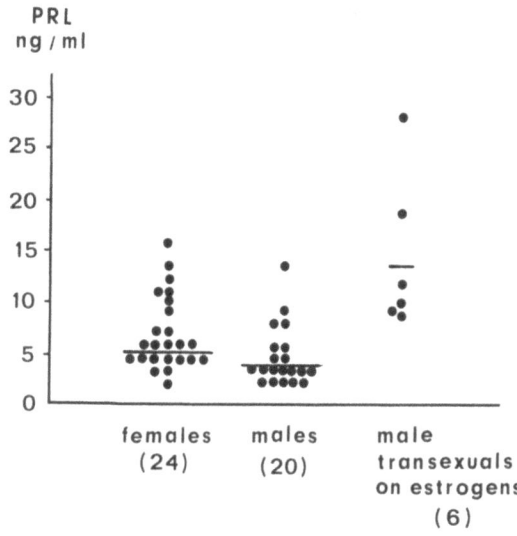

Fig. 2. Basal plasma PRL values in normal female and male subjects as compared with estrogen-treated men. Normal males exhibit values slightly lower than females because of lack of estrogen effect, whereas plasma PRL is elevated in men on sex steroid treatment

renergic, and cholinergic mechanisms in the control of PRL secretion has also been investigated, but their possible roles in humans remain without clinical relevance.

In humans, the relationship between sex steroids and PRL has been the subject of investigation. In males and hypogonadal women, PRL secretion has been augmented by estrogen (Frantz et al. 1972; Yen and Siler 1974). Throughout life, PRL follows different patterns in male and female subjects in relation to dependency upon estrogen production (Fig. 1). The stimulatory effect of sex steroids becomes manifest in male transsexuals on chronic estrogen intake. Figure 2 presents basal PRL levels in normal male and female individuals compared with a group of male subjects receiving variable amounts of estrogen.

5.2 Modification of PRL Secretion by Pharmacological Agents and Drug Interaction

A number of pharmacological agents, mainly neuroleptics (e.g., phenothiazine derivatives, sulpiride, and metoclopramide) elevate plasma PRL by altering brain DA turnover or by blocking specific DA receptors (Table 1). This property may also be inherent in compounds not known to act primarily as tranquilizers, but as depletors of central catecholamine (CA) stores (e.g., reserpine or α-methyldopa). Other sub-

Table 1. Drugs inducing hyperprolactinemia

Neuroleptics	*Hormones and antagonists*
Phenothiazines	TRH
Butyrophenones	Estrogens
Butyl-piperidine	Cyproterone acetate
Sulpiride	
Domperidone	*Opiates*
	Morphine
Antidepressants	Met-enkephaline
Dibenzazepine derivatives [a]	
	Others
Antihypertensives	Metoclopramide [b]
α-Methyldopa	Cimetidine
Reserpine	

[a] Imipramine, a weak PRL stimulator at doses of 25 and 50 mg
[b] Structurally related to sulpiride

Table 2. Prolactin inhibitors

Ergoline derivatives	3. Amino-ergolines
1. Clavines	Lisuride (Schering)
Metergoline (Farmitalia)	Sandoz CU 32-085
Pergolide (Elli-Lilly)	Nonergot drugs
2. Lysergic acid compounds	Apomorphine
Bromocriptine (Sandoz)	Piribedil (Eutherapie)
	Nomifensine (Hoechst)

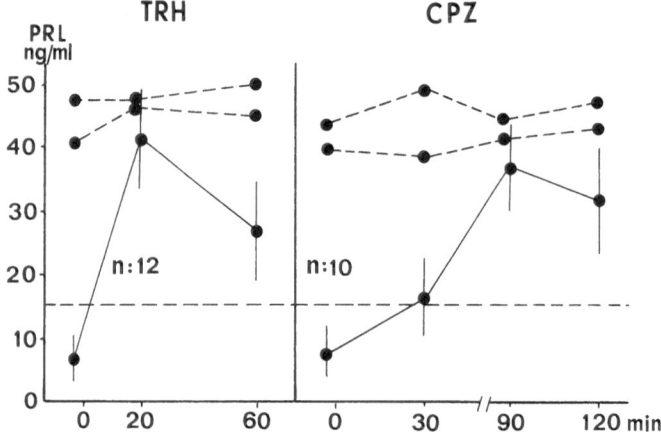

Fig. 3. PRL response to 100 µg TRH i.v. or 25 mg chlorpromazine (CPZ) i.m. in normal male volunteers as compared with two hyperprolactinemic subjects (*broken lines*). In these, the response to the stimulus is lessened or absent

stances can act via opiate receptors (enkephalins), probably linked to dopaminergic mechanisms. The mode of action of some drugs, such as cimetidine, a histamine$_2$-blocking agent, or the testosterone antagonist cyproterone acetate, remains uncertain.

Although TRH does not seem to play a physiologic role in the control of PRL (Gautvik et al. 1974), it stimulates the secretion of this lactogen strongly when administered intravenously in doses of 50–400 µg. Maximal PRL increments are recorded 15–20 min after injection. Figure 3 depicts this effect as compared with DA blockade with chlorpromazine (CPZ). It is interesting to note that, in pathological

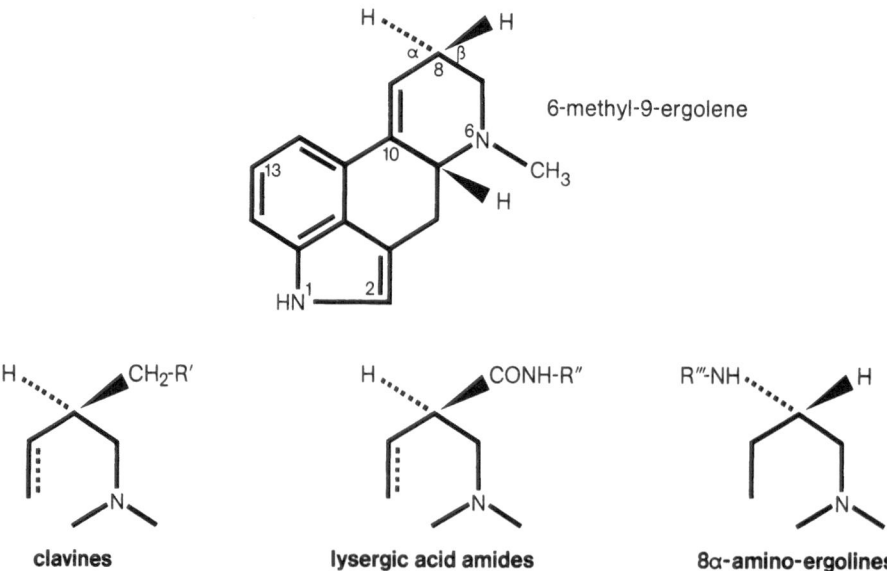

Fig. 4. Ergolene derivatives

hyperprolactinemia, the response to TRH and also to DA antagonists can be decreased. A number of drugs reduce PRL secretion by the pituitary (Table 2) and attention has been devoted to the agonistic effect of ergot compounds on the dopaminergic system. The endocrine profile of these drugs has been reviewed (Flückiger et al. 1978). They are made up of a 6-alkyl-ergolene or ergoline with different side-chains to position 8 of the tetracyclic moiety to form the three groups depicted in Fig. 4. Among them bromocriptine (2-Br-α-ergocriptine) was selected because of its strong PRL-inhibitory action (Flückiger 1972). This compound is a

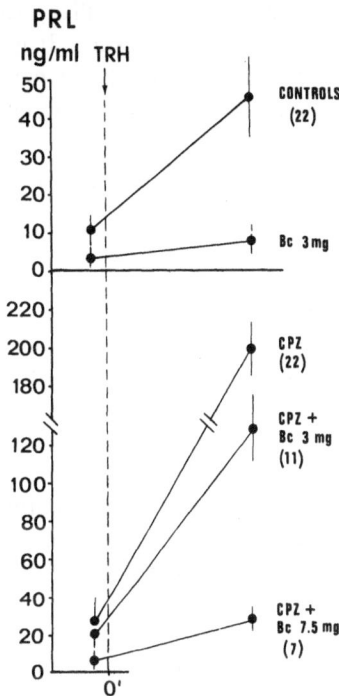

Fig. 5. Interaction between a DA-agonist drug (bromocriptine, Bc) and an antagonist (chlorpromazine, CPZ)

derivative of lysergic acid, but it is free of the hallucinogenic properties of LSD, a related substance also with strong PRL-inhibiting power. Bromocriptine lacks the uterotonic and vascular effects common to other ergots of the same group and its specificity as a DA agonist is supported by the strong competitive action with other substances exhibiting high affinity for DA receptors. Average daily dosages producing maximal PRL inhibition in humans are 3 to 5 mg, although in some cases dosage increases up to 10 mg or more can be required. Because of its marked dopaminergic effect (e.g., apomorphine) initial nausea and dizziness can be observed in some instances. These symptoms can be usually prevented by taking the drug after meals and starting with a low dosage, generally 1.25 mg, in the evening.

Flückiger and del Pozo (1978) reported that the inhibitory effect of bromocriptine on ovum implantation in the rat could be antagonized in a dose-dependent linear pattern by CPZ. In order to test a possible interaction between bromocriptine and neuroleptic drugs in the clinical situation, studies have been conducted in a group of psychiatric patients receiving 100 mg CPZ or more daily. Average basal

PRL levels were significantly (p < 0.001) elevated (28±2.6 ng/ml, mean ±SE), in comparison with normal male controls (11.1±1.3 ng/ml). The response to 100 µg TRH i.v. is depicted in Fig. 5. Psychiatric patients exhibited significantly (p < 0.001) higher peak PRL values (198±9.8 ng/ml) than the normal nontreated subjects (43.7±5.2 ng/ml). A gradual dosage increase of bromocriptine to 2.5 mg three times daily was necessary before plasma PRL was significantly (p < 0.01) lowered (7.3±1.8 ng/ml) and the peak response to TRH reduced to 20.4±3.4 ng/ml (p < 0.001). These results were interpreted as reflecting competitive drug antagonism. Thus, under these conditions a higher bromocriptine dosage can be required to fully normalize PRL secretion when dealing with patients subjected to dopaminergic blockade. It is noteworthy that treatment with bromocriptine for 4 weeks did not modify the neuroleptic effect of CPZ, indicating a duality of DA-mediated mechanisms at different brain levels.

5.3 Physiology and Physiopathology of PRL in Men

Although PRL circulates in male plasma in appreciable concentrations (2–15 ng/ml), its physiological role has not been clarified. Similar to women, male PRL secretion is subjected to a nyctohemeral rhythm, but oscillations seem of lower magnitude. The lack of lactational requirements does not preclude that with adequate priming the male mammary gland will respond to a PRL challenge with milk production. Thus, the mechanisms of the so-called witch's milk in the newborn can be explained by the same hormonal mechanisms responsible for lactogenesis in the mother, as shown by Hiba et al. (1977). Also, PRL stimulation with TRH induced milk secretion in a man pretreated with estrogens (Wyss and del Pozo, unpublished data).

More attention has been given to the effect of PRL on the male gonad. Initial reports on a possible correlation between the biological rhythms of PRL and testosterone have been contested (Jacobs et al. 1978; Seppälä et al. 1976). Furthermore, PRL suppression throughout pregnancy has failed to alter gonadal function in male fetuses, as demonstrated by the normal testosterone concentrations measured in cord blood of the neonates (Martin-Perez et al. 1979). However, there are data to support a role of PRL in the regulation of male gonadal function. In the experimental field, Aragona et al. (1977) demonstrated specific binding sites for PRL within the male reproductive system. The authors provided evidence in rats that this lactogen modulates LH binding to Leydig's cells, whereas FSH receptors are unaffected. Also radioiodinated PRL has been shown to bind specifically to Leydig's cells (Costlow and McGuire 1977) and testosterone secretion is enhanced by PRL in the hypogonadal hamster (Bex et al. 1978). Thus, this lactogen seems to act by sensitizing Leydig's cells to respond to LH stimulation.

Clinical work in humans presented by Magrini et al. (1976) suggests a modulating role for PRL in 5-α-reductase activity. Plasma elevations of this lactogen would accordingly impair dihydrotestosterone synthesis by specific tissues. A heterologous downward-regulating mechanism could explain this effect, in that a certain concentration of PRL would be required for normal androgen synthesis to occur. Exposure of androgenic receptors to a PRL excess would reduce the number of these, being reflected later in a decrease of androgen synthesis and, subsequently, in secondary hypogonadism and oligo- or azoospermia. Such a mechanism has been proven for other peripheral PRL receptors (Kelly et al. 1980).

A direct effect of PRL on spermatogenesis seems unlikely and limited experience by the author in male hyperprolactinemia indicates androgen-dependency in defective sperm maturation. There is no clear evidence for a role of PRL in oligozoospermia accompanied by normal testosterone and lactogen levels (Rjosk and Schill 1979). This is supported by the poor response following PRL inhibition (see Sect. 5.6).

Most male patients with hyperprolactinemia present normal basal plasma LH levels. It is interesting to note that Thorner and Besser (1977) found no changes in the LH fluctuating pattern of two hyperprolactinemic males after normalization of PRL secretion as compared with untreated control profiles. Similar to hyperprolactinemic women, the male PRL response to a TRH challenge or to dopaminergic blockade is lessened (see Fig. 3), probably due to a primary hypothalamic DA disturbance or by PRL itself via a short loop mechanism.

5.4 Incidence and Causes of Male Hyperprolactinemia

The criterion for the diagnosis of hyperprolactinemia is the persistence of plasma concentrations above 15 ng/ml in at least three basal resting samples. Hyperprolactinemia varies in incidence according to the selection procedure. Thus, this lactotrope has been found elevated in 2 of 68 hypogonadal males screened by the author. However, in cases of pituitary tumors the incidence can increase to 65% (Fossati et al. 1976; Franks et al. 1978; Carter et al. 1978; Nagulesparen et al. 1978). On the other hand, oligozoospermia in the absence of endocrine abnormality exhibits an extremely variable incidence of hyperprolactinemia between 3.6% (Da Rugna, unpublished data) 9% and 40% (Roulier et al. 1976; Boucher et al. 1977).

Renal and hepatic insufficiency are two conditions in which moderately elevated PRL is frequently seen (Nagel et al. 1973; Hagen et al. 1976; Wernze and Burghardt 1979). Whereas in the former no causative mechanism can be identified, a predominant estrogenic effect can be assumed in liver disease. This mechanism is further supported by the exaggerated PRL response to TRH found in some of these patients; a phenomenon characteristic of estrogenic dominance. It is interesting to note that the hyperprolactinemia of advanced renal insufficiency is not relieved by dialysis but by kidney graft, indicating that the causative factor originates in the renal parenchyma itself (Cowden et al. 1978; Lim et al. 1979). Certainly the chronic ingestion of DA antagonists may lead to sustained hyperprolactinemia (Falaschi et al. 1978) and the same effect can be expected in male subjects taking chronic estrogen treatment because of prostatic cancer or transsexuality (Frantz et al. 1972).

Processes involving basal brain areas can cause hyperprolactinemia, especially meningitis and meningoencephalitis, sarcoidosis, and tumors compressing the pituitary stalk. In some instances, the search for an ectopic source of PRL is necessary. Thus, lactogen-secreting cells have been localized in a hypernephroma and in lung cancer (Turkington 1971). A possible relationship between PRL and gynecomastia seems questionable. Normal plasma PRL has been found in this condition (Turkington 1972), and the self-limiting character of the disease makes the study of a causal relationship difficult. Finally, hyperprolactinemia may be associated with other endocrinopathies, such as acromegaly, hypothyroidism, and Cushing's disease.

5.5 Biological and Biochemical Effect of Excessive PRL Secretion in Men

Clinical and biological signs of excessive PRL production in the male are depicted in Table 3. They reflect a dual effect of this androgen; disturbance of control mechanisms at the CNS level and possible interference with gonadal receptors. The clinical expression of this phenomenon is the failure to enter puberty at preadolescent onset (Koenig et al. 1977) or the insiduous development of a syndrome of relative hypoandrogenism and defective sperm maturation. As in female subjects, the nyctohemeral rhythm of PRL is disturbed and the sleep-induced elevation is missing.

Biochemically, plasma PRL is elevated and testicular androgen synthesis reduced. The central inhibitory effect of PRL is localized at a suprasellar level since a positive LH response to exogenous LHRH occurs (Franks et al. 1978). As already mentioned, and similar to hyperprolactinemic women, the PRL response to a TRH or CPZ challenge is lessened, probably due to pre-existent decreased hypothalamic dopaminergic tone induced by PRL itself via a short loop mechanism or as a basic hypothalamic disturbance. A clear positive response to these stimulating agents is found in estrogen-induced hyperprolactinemia (see Sect. 5.1) (Fig. 6).

Despite experimental data (Magrini et al. 1976) for a direct action of PRL at the gonadal level, this effect has not been clearly demonstrated clinically. Hypogonadal

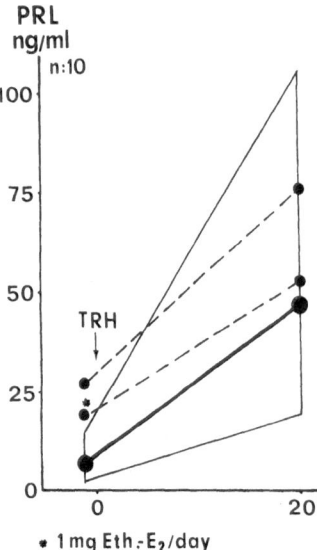

Fig. 6. Normal PRL response to 200 µg TRH in two estrogen-primed male subjects despite moderate elevation of basal lactogen. *Continuous lines* represent mean values and range recorded in ten normal men

Table 3. Effects of inappropriate prolactin (PRL) secretion in male subjects

Clinical	Biochemical
Failure to enter puberty	Elevated plasma PRL concentrations
Galactorrhea	Low androgen production
Oligoazoospermia	Absence of nocturnal PRL elevations
Signs of androgen failure	Positive pituitary and testicular response to exogenous stimulation
	Blunted response to TRH or DA blockade

Table 4. Incidence of clinical signs in male hyperprolactinemia

Signs	Incidence (%)	Range
Impotence	80	58 – 90
Hypoandrogenism and Hypospermatogenesis	65	45 – 100
Visual impairment	61	41 – 91
Headache	27	0 – 6
Gynecomastia	9.5	9 – 10
Galactorrhea	3	0 – 9

males with elevated plasma PRL usually exhibit adequate sex steroid responses to exogenous chorionic gonadotropin (CG) (Fossati et al. 1976; Franks et al. 1978). It can be speculated that the amounts of hCG administered pharmacologically may counteract the effect of PRL at receptor level.

Table 4 depicts the incidence of clinical signs and symptoms in male hyperprolactinemia taken from the author's files and from a review of the literature comprising 117 cases (Fossati et al. 1976; Franks et al. 1978; Carter et al. 1978; Nagulesparen et al. 1978). It is obvious that impotence and subfertility are the signs motivating the patients to seek medical advice. Because of the higher incidence of tumoral hyperprolactinemia in male subjects, visual impairment is a common finding, whereas the lack of female steroids prevents mammary tissue proliferation and incidence of galactorrhea is low.

5.6 Bromocriptine Treatment of Male Hypogonadism

The therapy of hyperprolactinemia is focused on the suppression of the abnormal secretion of pituitary lactogen by (1) discontinuation of medication enhancing PRL secretion, e.g., neuroleptics; (2) excision of a pituitary adenoma or ectopic source of PRL; (3) renal transplantation; and (4) medical inhibition with a DA receptor stimulator or pharmacological agent enhancing the synthesis of DA itself. In the past decade, broad experience has been gained with the use of bromocriptine. This compound is usually administered in doses of 1.25–2.5 mg two to three times daily. Under this schedule, plasma PRL is normalized within hours and there is a gradual recovery of signs of hypoandrogenism concomitant with improvement in sexual activity.

Some authors have investigated the effect of bromocriptine in prolactinoma cases. Carter et al. (1978), treating 11 of 22 such patients with bromocriptine, observed a major decline in plasma PRL and an improvement in potency. Plasma testosterone increased from a mean of 135 ng% to 396 ng%. It is interesting to note that in two subjects who remained impotent after testosterone replacement therapy, potency returned when hyperprolactinemia was reduced with bromocriptine. In another series of 29 patients, Franks et al. (1978) also noted a return of potency in subjects treated with bromocriptine. Similar results have been reported by Fossati et al.

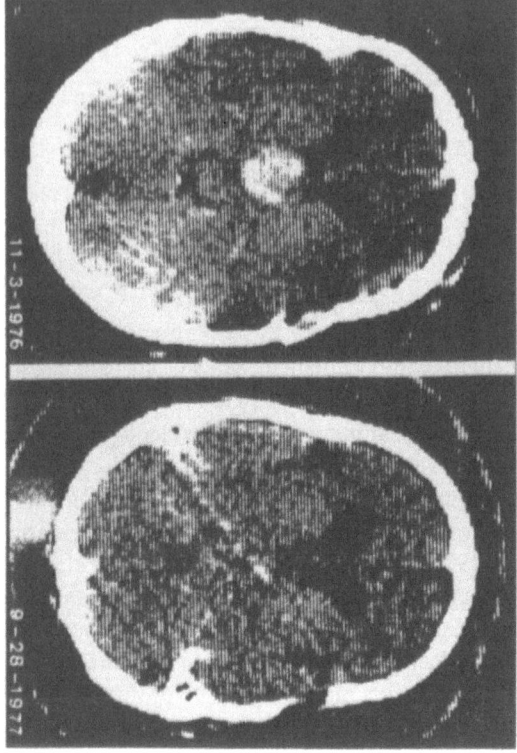

Fig. 7. Computerized tomographs of basal cranial sections in a male subject with a pituitary tumor (plasma PRL 620 ng/ml). There is complete disappearance of tumor shadow after 11 months of bromocriptine treatment (10 mg/day), and serum PRL had fallen below 2 ng/ml (courtesy of Dr. Landolt)

(1976). It is striking that, in males, pituitary lesions seem far more advanced and mean plasma PRL levels substantially higher than in hyperprolactinemic women. This is probably due to the absence of the alarming sign of cessation of cyclic activity in women which makes lesions clinically apparent at an earlier stage of development. As previously mentioned, bromocriptine treatment has induced sexual maturation in a subject with pubertal retardation and elevated plasma PRL (Koenig et al. 1977).

More difficult to assess is the relationship between oligozoospermia and PRL in normoprolactinemic individuals without other signs of endocrine abnormality. In a study of 18 oligozoospermic patients screened by the author, all had normal plasma PRL concentrations, but in another study (Roulier et al. 1976) elevated levels were found in 4 of 51 (8%) cases. More recently, Hovatta et al. (1979) treated 40 oligozoospermic low-androgen men with bromocriptine or placebo. While PRL levels (elevated in three men from each group) were normalized during bromocriptine treatment and plasma testosterone and dihydrotestosterone levels increased slightly in both groups, no significant difference in sperm counts between the two treatments was seen. Further reports appeared recently to confirm this lack of action of dopaminergic stimulation on defective spermatogenesis and sexual impotence (Ambrosi et al. 1977; Masala et al. 1979; Merino et al. 1980; Legros et al. 1980) despite isolated communications showing favorable results (Pierini and Nusimovich 1978).

A reduction of pituitary prolactinoma size during bromocriptine treatment with or without radiotherapy has recently been reported by a number of investigators (Corenblum et al. 1978; Sobrinho et al. 1978; Landolt et al. 1979; McGregor et al. 1979; Wass et al. 1979). In general, return of libido and sexual potency correlated with improvement in biochemical tests of pituitary function, visual field, and radiological findings. Figure 7 provides tomographic evidence of tumor regression following bromocriptine therapy in a male subject with hyperprolactinemia and a suprasellar mass. More recently, Thorner et al. (1980) reported very rapid reduction in basal PRL and in tumor size in two male subjects harboring very large suprasellar tumors under the same therapy. Doses given for this indication have ranged from 5 to 30 mg/day over 6–78 months.

Impairment of sexual function is a well-known accompaniment to hemodialysis in patients with renal insufficiency (Nagel et al. 1973; Levy and Wynbrandt 1975; Bommer et al. 1976), and elevated PRL levels and hypogonadism may also be associated with this condition (Nagel et al. 1973; Strickler et al. 1974; Geisthövel et al. 1976). Improvement of sexual performance in seven male hemodialysis patients has been observed following treatment with bromocriptine (2.5 mg twice daily) (Bommer et al. 1979). While there were no changes in basal and stimulated FSH and LH concentrations during the placebo-controlled trial, plasma PRL levels that were elevated before and during control treatment were reduced during therapy with bromocriptine.

5.7 Conclusions

The measurement of PRL has become clinically important not only in lactation, but also in the control of gonadal function. Elucidation of the secretory mechanism of PRL via modulation of the central dopaminergic system and its modification by drugs has provided new tools for the management of hyperprolactinemic conditions. In males, these are manifested by failure to enter puberty or by a syndrome of relative hypoandrogenism and defective sperm maturation. Its incidence is lower than in female populations and the lack of clinical signs during the early stages of development means that pituitary lesions leading to adenoma formation may be quite advanced by the time the diagnosis is established. Treatment with the dopaminergic drug bromocriptine rapidly normalizes PRL secretion and gonadal function in such patients. Moreover, clinical and radiological studies have shown that arrest of prolactinoma growth and reduction in tumor size are frequent findings in hyperprolactinemic subjects harboring such lesions. Thus, dopaminergic stimulation with bromocriptine seems to not only decrease PRL secretion, but also to limit the reproductive capacity of prolactinoma cells, offering a noninvasive way of treating these tumors.

5.8 References

Ambrosi B, Bara R, Travaglini P, Weber G, Beck Peccoz P, Rondena M, Elli R, Faglia G (1977) Study of the effects of bromocriptine on sexual impotence. Clin Endocrinol 7:417–421

Aragona C, Bohnet HG, Friesen HG (1977) Localization of prolactin binding in prostate and testis: The role of serum prolactin concentration on the testicular LH receptor. Acta Endocrinol 84:402–409

Bex F, Bartke A, Goldman BD, Dalterio S (1978) Luteinizing hormone receptors and seasonal changes in testicular activity in the golden hamster. Endocrinology 103:2069–2080

Bommer J, Tschöpe W, Ritz E, Andrassy K (1976) Sexual behaviour of hemodialysed patients. Clin Nephrol 6:315–318

Bommer J, Ritz E, del Pozo E, Bommer G (1979) Improved sexual function in male hemodialyses patients on bromocriptine. Lancet 2:496–497

Boucher D, Hermabessière J, Doly M (1977) Prolactin secretion in infertile men before and after treatment with bromocriptine. Ann Biol Anim Biochim Biophys 17:483–498

Carter JN, Tyson JE, Tolis G, Van Vliet S, Faiman C, Friesen HG (1978) Prolactin-secreting tumors and hypogonadism in 22 men. N Engl J Med 299:847–852

Corenblum B (1978) Bromocriptine in pituitary tumours. Lancet 2:786

Costlow ME, McGuire WL (1977) Autoradiographic localization of the binding of ^{125}I-labelled prolactin to rat tissue in vitro. J Endocrinol 75:221–226

Cowden EA, Ratcliffe WA, Ratcliffe JG, Dobbie JW, Kennedy AC (1978) Hyperprolactinemia in renal disease. Clin Endocrinol 9:241–248

Enjalbert A, Ruberg M, Kordon C (1978) Neuroendocrine control of prolactin secretion. In: Robyn C, Harter M (eds) Progress in prolactin physiology and pathology. Elsevier/North-Holland, New York Oxford, p 83

Falaschi P, Frajese G, Sciarra F, Rocco A, Conti C (1978) Influence of hyperprolactinaemia due to metoclopramide on gonadal function in men. Clin Endocrinol 8:427–433

Flückiger E (1972) Drugs and the control of prolactin secretion. In: Boyns AR, Griffith K (eds) Prolactin and carcinogenesis. Alpha Omega Alpha, Cardiff, p 162

Flückiger E, del Pozo E (1978) Influence on the endocrine system. In: Berde B, Schild HO (eds) Ergot alkaloids and similar compounds. Springer, Berlin Heidelberg New York (Handbook of experimental pharmacology, Vol. 49, p 616)

Flückiger E, Vigouret JM, Wagner HR (1978) Ergot compounds and prolactin. In: Robyn C, Harter M (eds) Progress in prolactin physiology and pathology. Elsevier/North-Holland Biomedical Press, Amsterdam Oxford New York, p 383

Fossati P, Strauch G, Tourniaire J (1976) Etude de l'activité de la bromocriptine dans les états d'hyperprolactinémie. Nouv Presse Med 5:1687–1690

Franks S, Jacobs HS, Martin N, Nabarro JDN (1978) Hyperprolactinemia and impotence. Clin Endocrinol 8:277–287

Frantz AG, Kleinberg DL, Noel GL (1972) Studies on prolactin in man. Recent Prog Horm Res 28:527–550

Gautvik KM, Tashjian AH, Kourides IA, Weintraub BD, Graeber CT, Maloof F, Suzuki K, Zuckerman JE (1974) Thyrotropin-releasing hormone is not the sole physiologic mediator of prolactin release during suckling. N Engl J Med 290:1162–1165

Geisthövel W, von zur Mühlen A, Bahlmann J (1976) Untersuchungen über die Hypophysen-Testes-Function bei chronisch nierenkranken Männern mit unterschiedlicher Glomerularfiltration. Klin Wochenschr 54:1027–1037

Hagen C, Ølgaard K, McNeilly AS, Rischer R (1976) Prolactin and the pituitary-gonadal axis in male uraemic patients on regular dialysis. Acta Endocrinol 82:29–38

Halasz B, Pupp L (1965) Hormone secretion of the anterior pituitary gland after physical interruption of all nervous pathways to the hypophysiotropic area. Endocrinology 77:553–562

Hiba J, del Pozo E, Genazzini A, Pusterla E, Lancranjan I, Sidiropoulos D, Gunti J (1977) Hormonal mechanism of milk secretion in the newborn. J Clin Endocrinol Metab 44:973–976

Hökfelt T, Fuxe K (1972a) On the morphology and the neuroendocrine role of the hypothalamic catecholamine neurons. In: Knigge KM, Scott DE, Weindl A (eds) Brain-endocrine interaction. Median eminence: structure and function. Karger, Basel, p 181

Hökfelt T, Fuxe K (1972b) Effects of prolactin and ergot alkaloids on the tubero-infundibular dopamine (DA) neurons. Neuroendocrinology 98:100–122

Hovatta O, Koskimies AI, Ranta T, Stenman UH, Seppälä M (1979) Bromocriptine treatment of oligospermia: a double-blind study. Clin Endocrinol 11:377–382

Jacobs LS, Mendelson WB, Rubin RT, Bauman JE (1978) Failure of nocturnal prolactin suppression by methysergide to entrain changes in testosterone in normal men. J Clin Endocrinol Metab 46:561–566

Kanematsu S, Sawyer CH (1973) Elevation of plasma prolactin after hypophyseal stalk section in the rat. Endocrinology 93:238–241

Kelly PA, Djiane J, de Léan A (1980) Interaction of prolactin with its receptor: dissociation and down regulation. In: MacLeod RM, Scapagnini U (eds) Central and peripheral regulation of prolactin function. Raven, New York, pp 173–188

Koenig MP, Zuppinger K, Liechti B (1977) Hyperprolactinemia as a cause of delayed puberty: Successful treatment with bromocriptine. J Clin Endocrinol 45:825–828

Landolt AM, Wüthrich R, Fellmann H (1979) Regression of pituitary prolactinoma after treatment with bromocriptine. Lancet 1:1082–1083

Legros JJ, Chiodera P, Mormont C, Servais J (1980) A psychoneuroendocrinological study of sexual impotence in patients with abnormal reaction to a glucose tolerance test. Adv Biol Psychiatry 5:117–124

Levy NB, Wynbrandt GD (1975) The quality of life on maintenance haemodialysis. Lancet 2:1328–1330

Lim VS, Kathpalia SC, Frohman LA (1979) Hyperprolactinemia and impaired pituitary response to suppression and stimulation in chronic renal failure: reversal after transplantation. J Clin Endocrinol Metab 48:101–107

Magrini G, Ebiner JR, Burckhardt P, Felber JP (1976) Study on the relationship between plasma prolactin levels and androgen metabolism in man. J Clin Endocrinol Metab 43:944–947

Martin-Perez J, del Pozo E, Clarenbach P, Brownell J, Derrer F (1979) Lack of dependency between androgen production and prolactin in man. Acta Endocrinol [Suppl] 225:174

Masala A, Delitala G, Alagna S, Devilla L, Rovasio PP (1979) Effects of long-term treatment with metergoline in patients with idiopathic oligospermia. Clin Endocrinol 11:349–352

McGregor AM, Scanlon MF, Hall K, Cook DB, Hall R (1979) Reduction in size of a pituitary tumor by bromocriptine therapy. N Engl J Med 300:291–293

Merino G, Canales ES, Vadillo ML, Forsbach G, Solis J, Zarate A (1980) Abnormal prolactin levels in serum and seminal plasma in infertile men. Arch Androl 4:353–355

Nagel TC, Freinkel N, Bell RH, Friesen H, Wilber JF, Metzger BW (1973) Gynecomastia, prolactin and other peptide hormones in patients undergoing chronic hemodialysis. J Clin Endocrinol Metab 36:428–432

Nagulesparen M, Ang V, Jenkins JS (1978) Bromocriptine treatment of males with pituitary tumours, hyperprolactinaemia, and hypogonadism. Clin Endocrinol 9:73–79

Pierini AA, Nusimovich B (1978) Bromocriptina y oligospermia. Sem Med 152:426–428

Rjosk HK, Schill WB (1979) Serumprolactin in male infertility. Andrologia 11:297–304

Roulier R, Mattei A, Reuter A, Franchimont P (1976) Taux de prolactine dans les stérilités et hypogonadismes masculines. Nouv Presse Med 5:1911

Schally AV, Dupont A, Arimura A, Takahara J, Redding TW, Clemens J, Shaar C (1976) Purification of a catecholamine-rich fraction with prolactin release-inhibiting factor (PIF) activity from porcine hypothalami. Acta Endocrinol 82:1–14

Seppälä M, Hirvonen E, Unnerus H-A, Ranta T, Laatikainen T (1976) Prolactin and testosterone: independent circulating levels in hyperprolactinemia prolactin suppression by bromocriptine. J Clin Endocrinol Metab 43:198–200

Sobrinho LG, Nunes MC, Santos MA, Mauricio JC (1978) Radiological evidence for regression of prolactinoma after treatment with bromocriptine. Lancet 2:257–258

Strickler RC, Woolever CA, Johnson M, Goldstein M, DeWeber G (1974) Serum gonadotropin patterns in patients with chronic renal failure on hemodialysis. Gynecol Invest 5:185–198

Thorner MO, Besser GM (1977) Hyperprolactinemia and gonadal function: results of bromocriptine treatment. In: Crosignani PG, Robyn C (eds) Prolactin in human reproduction. Academic Press, London, p 285

Thorner MO, Martin WH, Rogol AD, Morris JL, Perryman RL, Conway BP, Howards SS, Wolfman MG, MacLeod RM (1980) Rapid regression of pituitary prolactinomas during bromocriptine treatment. J Clin Endocrinol Metab 51:438–445

Turkington RW (1971) Ecotopic production of prolactin. N Engl J Med 285:1455–1458

Turkington RW (1972) Serum prolactin in patients with gynecomastia. J Clin Endocrinol 34:62–66

Turkington RW, Underwood LW, van Wyk JJ (1971) Elevated serum prolactin levels after pituitary-stalk section in man. N Engl J Med 285:707–710

Wass JAH, Moult PJA, Thorner MO, Dacie JE, Charlesworth M, Jones AE, Besser GM (1979) Reduction of pituitary tumor size in patients with prolactinomas and acromegaly treated with bromocriptine with or without radiotherapy. Lancet 2:66–69

Wernze H, Burghardt W (1979) Hyperprolactinemia bei Lebererkrankung. Med Klin 74:1615–1623

Yen SSC, Siler TM (1974) Augmentation of prolactin secretion by estrogen in hypogonadal women. J Clin Invest 53:652–655

6 Gonadotropin Therapy in Male Infertility

S. J. Winters and P. Troen

It is well established that the glycoprotein hormones LH and FSH are required for normal testicular function. Classical teaching is that the former stimulates testosterone production by Leydig cells, whereas FSH stimulates the tubules. This concept is supported by the presence of molecules which bind LH with high affinity on the cell membranes of Leydig cells (Catt and Dufau 1973), while FSH binding occurs on the surface of Sertoli cells (Means 1973). Following receptor binding, both gonadotropins work via adenyl cyclase-mediated systems.

The magnitude of the gonadotropin effect on the testis is primarily a function of the circulating hormone concentration. At least for LH, changes in receptor number also modulate the testicular response (Purvis and Hansson 1978). A reduction in LH receptors follows hypophysectomy in the rodent and results in decreased responsiveness of Leydig cells: treatment with small doses of LH increases the magnitude of the steroidogenic response. LH regulation of its receptor activity appears to be biphasic, however, in that treatment with large doses of LH/hCG results in desensitization of the Leydig cell. This has been correlated with a decrease in the numbers of LH receptors. Further, both prolactin (PRL) and FSH, and perhaps gonadotropin-releasing hormone (GnRH), affect LH receptor activity in some experimental systems.

The synthesis and secretion of both LH and FSH from pituitary gonadotrophs appears to be primarily regulated by the decapeptide GnRH. LH, but not FSH, is secreted into the blood in bursts; one occuring approximately every 2 h (Nankin and Troen 1971). The lack of discrete FSH pulses may relate to its longer half-life. Pulsatile administration of GnRH to prepubertal female rhesus monkeys produces elevations of both gonadotropins and induces regular ovulatory cycles (Wildt et al. 1980). Further, pubertal patterns of LH and FSH secretion can be induced by low-dose GnRH pulses in hypogonadotropic individuals (Jacobson et al. 1979). Lastly, rodents injected with anti-GnRH antiserum demonstrate a decrease in basal LH and FSH concentrations (Fraser et al. 1974) and both gonadotropins fail to rise in the serum after castration (Arimura et al. 1976).

Sex steroids regulate LH and FSH secretion as well, such that the castration response of increased serum gonadotropin levels is a classic example of negative feedback control. That testosterone administration results not only in suppression of serum LH levels, but also of FSH levels is not surprising when one considers that a single GnRH appears to control both LH and FSH, and both gonadotropins are thought to be secreted by the same cell. However, the failure of the nonaromatizable androgen dihydrotestosterone to suppress serum FSH levels significantly casts some doubt on the role of androgen in the regulation of FSH secretion (Stewart-Bently et al. 1974; Winters et al. 1979). Despite the suppression by testosterone of both LH and FSH, there is a large body of literature which suggests that a nonsteroidal factor of seminiferous tubular origin, inhibin, is also involved in the regulation of FSH (Baker et al. 1976; Franchimont et al. 1977). Biochemical characterization and elucidation of the true physiologic significance of this material is not yet available.

Estrogens also suppress gonadotropin concentrations in men (Loriaux et al. 1977). Studies of the pulsatile patterns of LH secretion reveal that nonaromatizable, as well as aromatizable androgen administration reduces the frequency of LH pulses whereas estradiol decreases the amplitude of the LH pulse (Santen 1975). These data suggest that different mechanisms are operative in the feedback control of LH by androgen and estrogen. Estradiol is produced by the testis in response to gonadotropin administration, yet the major fraction of circulating estradiol is derived from the peripheral aromatization of testosterone and androstenedione (MacDonald et al. 1979). This bioconversion is affected by age (Hemsell et al. 1974), body weight (MacDonald et al. 1978), thyroid hormone (Southren et al. 1974), and the presence of liver disease (Gordon et al. 1975) such that changes in circulating estradiol may influence gonadotropin secretion in these conditions. The reversible hypogonadotropic hypogonadism which characterizes Cushing's syndrome suggests that glucocorticoid may also affect LH and FSH secretion (Luton et al. 1977).

Although LH primarily affects Leydig cells and FSH affects Sertoli cells within tubules, the effects of these hormones are inter-related. Anatomically, this interaction is permitted by the close relationship of the two compartments within the testis, i.e., the interstitium and the tubules. Thus, both LH and FSH are needed to initiate spermatogenesis during pubertal maturation (Lee et al. 1975) and to reinitiate spermatogenesis in the hypophysectomized regressed rat (Steinberger 1971), FSH affects a permissive role on LH-stimulated testosterone secretion (Odell et al. 1973), and Sertoli cells may contribute to androgen production (Tcholakian and Steinberger 1978).

A series of studies has indicated that increased LH secretion is associated with an increase in the testosterone concentration within Leydig cells (Knorr et al. 1970) which may be, in turn, maintained by binding of testosterone to a high-affinity macromolecule whose synthesis is controlled by FSH, i.e., androgen-binding protein (ABP) (Ritzen et al. 1975). The ABP-androgen complex may be important in the transfer of androgen to the Sertoli cells and germinal epithelium to participate in the differentiation of germ cells (Steinberger et al. 1979). Once initiated, testosterone alone can maintain spermatogenesis in the hypophysectomized rodent (Steinberger 1971).

The demonstration of ABP in the human testis (Hsu and Troen 1978) and the recent finding that human ABP activity correlates with intratesticular testosterone levels in testes of elderly men (Lee et al. 1980) suggests that similar mechanisms to those of the rodent could be operative in humans. Therefore, the induction of spermatogenesis in hypogonadotropic men would be expected to require the presence of both LH and FSH, whereas spermatogenesis might be maintained without continuous FSH administration. The precise role for FSH in the initiation or maintenance of human spermatogenesis is not clear. Further understanding of the effects of gonadotropins on intratesticular steroids and proteins may provide some insight into the use of these agents in normogonadotropic oligozoospermia. A review of experience accrued in the treatment of hypospermatogenesis with gonadotropins is discussed here.

6.1 Gonadotropin Preparations

6.1.1 Pituitary Gonadotropins

Highly purified human pituitary gonadotropins have been prepared by various investigators for structural studies. Purification techniques are laborious, requiring, for example, molecular sieve chromatography, ion exchange chromatography, and preparative electrophoresis. The yields are small; in the range of 50 mg/1000 pituitaries. These limitations preclude the meaningful use of pituitary gonadotropins for clinical therapy at present.

6.1.2 hCG

hCG is a glycoprotein hormone containing approximately 30% carbohydrate. It resembles hLH both structurally and biologically. Like hLH, hCG is composed of two noncovalently bound subunits which have been designated α and β. Akin to LH, hCG interacts with membrane receptors on the surface of Leydig cells to stimulate testosterone secretion (Dufau et al. 1971; Hsu et al. 1978). Because it is purified from first trimester-pregnancy urine, hCG is a readily available product. One commercial preparation requires absorption on permutit, elution with ethanolic ammonium acetate and precipitation with alcohol. Potencies of commercial preparations are approximately 2000–4000 IU/mg (Second International Reference Preparation). Although hCG was previously thought to be present only during pregnancy and as a paraneoplastic hormone, it now appears that small amounts of hCG may normally be found in a wide variety of tissues, most notably the pituitary (Chen et al. 1976; Braunstein et al. 1979).

6.1.3 FSH

FSH is a glycoprotein hormone that, like LH, is composed of a nonspecific α subunit and a specific β subunit. Dissociation of FSH into its subunits can be accomplished by incubation with 8 M urea. The separate subunits are of minimal biologic activity.

FSH is extracted from the urine of postmenopausal women, hence, the designation human menopausal gonadotropins (hMG). Although this material also contains LH, the biological activity of the latter is small.

hMG is available as Pergonal (Serono Laboratories). The manufacturer's literature indicates that each ampule contains 75 IU FSH and 75 IU LH.

6.2 Hypogonadotropic Hypogonadism

Although they comprise a relatively small segment of the total population with hypospermatogenesis, men with hypogonadotropic hypogonadism are important beyond their numbers due to our knowledge of the pathogenesis of the disorder and because of the potential for successful therapy in these men. This syndrome is characterized by clinical hypogonadism with hypospermatogenesis and low serum testosterone levels associated with inappropriately low serum LH and FSH concentrations. The underlying cause may be within either the hypothalamus or pituitary. A differential diagnosis of hypogonadotropic hypogonadism is found in Table 1.

Panhypopituitarism in childhood is most often idiopathic, whereas in adults it usually results from an acquired lesion involving either the hypothalamus or pituitary. In addition to complete endocrine diagnostic testing, these patients require ophthalmologic evaluation and radiologic assessment including sellar tomography and cranial CT scans. Generally, mass lesions require neurosurgery and most patients become candidates for gonadotropin therapy. In subjects with PRL-producing tumors (Pont et al. 1979) and Cushing's syndrome (Bigos et al. 1980), removal of the adenoma may result in restoration of normal gonadal function.

Idiopathic hypogonadotropic hypogonadism (IHH) is thought to result from a deficiency in either the synthesis or secretion of GnRH. Associated pituitary and hypothalamic function is normal in these subjects (Boyar et al. 1973; Winters et al. 1978). Affected patients fail to enter puberty due to deficient gonadotropin secretion and may present associated midline defects which serve as clinical markers for their disease. The association of familial IHH with anosmia was first reported by Kallmann et al. in 1944, hence the designation Kallmann's syndrome.

Men with partial hypogonadotropism may present testes which are slightly enlarged when compared to those of prepubertal boys and with varying degrees of Leydig cell insufficiency. Although originally considered to have an isolated deficiency in LH secretion, some of these men have been found to have nocturnal increases in serum LH and testosterone levels similar to those of the pubertal boys

Table 1. Disorders associated with hypogonadotropic hypogonadism

Idiopathic hypogonadotropic hypogonadism and related syndromes	Hypothalamic tumors and cysts
	Dysgerminoma
Kallmann's syndrome	Craniopharyngioma
"Fertile eunuch" syndrome	
Prader-Willi syndrome	CNS infections
Lawrence-Moon-Biedl syndrome	Meningitis (bacterial and fungal)
Möbius' syndrome	Encephalitis
Idiopathic hypopituitarism (partial and complete)	Miscellaneous
	Head trauma
Pituitary adenomas	Sarcoidosis
	Hemochromatosis
Chromophobe adenomas	Histiocytosis
Prolactinomas	Pituitary irradiation
Cushing's syndrome	Anorexia nervosa
Acromegaly	

whom they resemble clinically (Boyar et al. 1976). Thus, they seem to lack the factor which permits the transition from sleep-related LH bursts to the adult pattern of continuous pulsatile LH secretion. Isolated FSH deficiency has been described in a woman with primary amenorrhea (Rabin et al. 1972), but no similar cases have been found in men.

6.2.1 Treatment of Hypogonadotropics with hCG

Leydig cell function can be studied by evaluating the response of serum testosterone levels to hCG administration. Both intravenous and intramuscular routes of administration have been used, although only the latter is approved in the United States. Intramuscular injections of 1500–5000 IU for 1–7 days produce a 100% increase in serum testosterone concentrations and in the blood production rate of testosterone. After 1500–4000 IU hCG i.m., serum testosterone concentrations remain elevated for 4–5 days, presumably due to the long biological half-life (30 h) of hCG. Single-dose administration and daily doses for 4 days have both been frequently employed as diagnostic protocols.

Recently, a two-component response of testosterone to single-dose hCG was noted with the first increment occurring 1–8 h after injection, whereas the second peak is observed 2–3 days after intramuscular administration (Saez and Forest 1979; Nankin et al. 1980). The physiological significance of these observations remains to be established. The repetitive administration of hCG has been found to result in refractoriness to acute hCG stimulation (Saez and Forest 1979). This may relate to both a loss of LH receptor activity and to a relative enzymatic defect in testosterone biosynthesis, perhaps at the 17–20 desmolase step (Cigorraga et al. 1978).

By current standards the clinical use of hCG as a stimulation test must be considered imprecise. The diagnosis of primary gonadal failure is now easily accomplished by the measurement of serum levels of LH and FSH by specific RIA. However, there continue to be some practical applications for hCG stimulation, e.g., the destinction between bilateral cryptorchidism and congenital anorchia (Aynsley-Green et al. 1976).

Santen and Paulsen (1973) reported testosterone responses to hCG administration in men with idiopathic hypogonadotropism. Although previous short-term studies had suggested a Leydig cell defect in these men, prolonged hCG administration produced serum testosterone levels similar to those of normal adults. The exception was in men with hypogonadotropism and concomitant bilateral cryptorchidism, who failed to respond to hCG.

Clinical androgenization can be successfully accomplished with hCG in hypogonadotropic men with scrotal testes. Several protocols have been suggested. We favor a dose of 1500–2000 IU every 5 days, as this generally maintains serum androgen concentrations within the adult male range yet minimizes the frequency of injections (Fig. 1). Further, it has recently been recognized that excessive hCG administration may result in refractoriness to the action of hCG (Saez and Forest 1979). Lastly, hCG treatment increases not only testosterone production, but also estradiol secreton by the testis (Kelch et al. 1972) and smaller, less frequent dosages may result in a lesser tendency for accompanying gynecomastia.

Alternatively, the patient can be masculinized with a long-acting testosterone ester, such as the enanthate. Doses of 200 mg i.m. every 3 weeks are most often satisfactory, but should be adjusted to the clinical needs of the patient. The suggestion that testosterone treatment could result in tubular fibrosis precluding the eventual induction of spermatogenesis by gonadotropins does not seem to be substantiated by the literature (see below). Dose-related side effects, such as priapism, acne, and prostatism, rarely occur but do require appropriate dose adjustments.

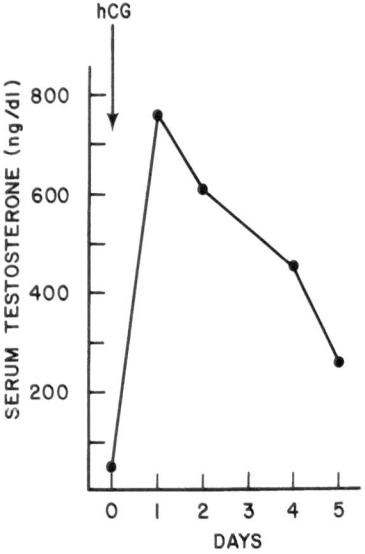

Fig. 1. Response of serum testosterone to a single injection of hCG (2000 IU i.m.) in a patient with idiopathic hypogonadotropic hypogonadism. The patient had received his last hCG dose 1 week prior to the study

In addition to stimulating testosterone secretion, hCG has been shown to influence tubules. Tubular growth, Sertoli cell maturation, and development of spermatocytes and spermatids were observed by Paulsen in two men with hypogonadotropic hypogonadism treated with 2000–5000 IU hCG three times weekly for 20–50 weeks, though azoospermia persisted (Paulsen 1965). Bergada and Mancini (1973), in their studies of cryptorchid children, found similar tubular growth using 28,000–30,000 IU hCG over 3–6 months. When FSH was added to these regimens, full complete spermatogenesis was observed.

hCG alone may result in sperm production in selected subjects with hypogonadotropic hypogonadism: in each responder it appears that some endogenous FSH secretion is present. It is less likely that this relates to the slight FSH activity of hCG, since hCG alone is ineffective in most hypogonadotropics. Del Pozo et al. (1975) reported a 23-year-old male with partial idiopathic hypogonadotropism who was clinically hypogonadal, but whose testicular volumes were 5.2 and 4.4 ml, slightly enlarged when compared to the prepubertal testis. Serum testosterone was 167 ng/dl. Testicular biopsy revealed normal size tubules (180 µ), but partially arrested spermatogenesis. After 4 months of therapy with 1000 IU i.m. hCG three times weekly, serum testosterone levels rose to 695 ng/dl and total sperm output rose from an initial 0.35 million hypomotile spermatozoa to 40 million spermatozoa with 50% normal motility. In a preliminary report, Sherins et al. (1977 a) documented the induction of spermatogenesis with hCG in two subjects with idiopathic hypogonadotropic hypogonadism in whom pretreatment testis size was prepubertal (4 ml), but in whom slight tubular stimulation was indicated by a somewhat increased tubular diameter (40–50 μ) compared to nonresponders (25–30 μ). Total sperm output increased to 6–7 million within 12 months and pregnancy occurred in one spouse. Luboshitsky et al. (1979) have recently reported gonadotropin treatment of two men with PRL-secreting pituitary adenomas and hypogonadism. hCG in doses of 5000 IU three times weekly for 4 months produced an increase in sperm output from 1.5 to 27 million/ml in one subject and from azoospermia to 20 million/ml in the second patient.

Therapy with hCG has maintained for more than 1 year spermatogenesis which was initiated with hCG-hMG (Johnsen 1978). This may be explained by endogenous secretion of small amounts of FSH or by the slight FSH activity of hCG. Alternatively, FSH may not be required in the maintenance of spermatogenesis. Instead, high concentrations of intratesticular testosterone, analogous to those which maintain spermatogenesis in newly hypophysectomized rats (Steinberger 1971), may be produced by hCG therapy and may be sufficient to sustain already existent, complete spermatogenesis.

6.2.2 Therapy with hMG

The administration of hMG alone to subjects with IHH (Paulsen 1965) or prepubertal children (Bergada and Mancini 1973) produced some increase in seminiferous tubular diameter, but failed to effect germ cell maturation. Further, there is no measurable effect of hMG on serum testosterone concentrations. Treatment with FSH alone has, therefore, not been pursued.

6.2.3 Therapy with hCG and hMG

The administration of hCG and hMG together to initiate spermatogenesis in well-defined hypogonadotropic hypogonadism is the clinical analogy of the studies by Greep in hypophysectomized rodents (Greep and Fevold 1937). Clinical experience began with the studies of Gemzell and Kjessler (1964) and MacLeod et al. (1964). These agents are generally effective in both IHH and acquired hypopituitarism but, because no large series have yet appeared in the literature, no precise success rates are available. Different investigators have used slightly different regimens, but most seem to give good results. It should be recognized that therapy designed to stimulate spermatogenesis remains both expensive and complex.

Generally therapy is begun with hCG alone. This results in stimulation of testosterone secretion, which produces an increase in libido and potency and increases intratesticular testosterone concentrations. Occasionally hCG alone may result in the appearance of spermatozoa in the ejaculate. Most investigators have continued hCG in doses of 3000 IU three times weekly for 6–12 months before adding hMG. The usual FSH dose is 75 IU three times weekly, although recent data suggest that the minimum FSH requirement may be less (Sherins et al. 1977 b). These observations are of practical importance when one considers the high cost of the FSH preparation.

Table 2. Published reports of pregnancies in the partners of men with hypogonadotropic hypgonadism treated with a combination of hCG and hMG

Author	Age	Dosages (IU)		Highest sperm concentration (million/ml)	Duration of therapy before pregnancy
		hCG	hMG		
Idiopathic hypogonadotropic hypogonadism					
Paulsen et al. (1970)	20	2000 × 3/week	64.5 – 74.3 daily	39	19 – 59 weeks[b]
Paulsen et al. (1970)	20	1000 – 5000 × 3/week	64.5 – 74.3 daily	71	15 weeks[b]
Mac Leod (1970)	25	4000 × 3/week	75 × 3/week	10	5 months
Spitz et al. (1978)	24	5000 × 2/week	75 × 2/week	16	9 months
Johnsen (1978)	31	3000 × 2/week	75 × 2/week	2[a]	10 months
Acquired hypogonadotropism					
Mac Leod (1970)	28 (PA[c])	4000 × 3/week	75 × 3/week	114	15 months[b]
Granville (1970)	29 (PA[c])	4000 × 2/week	75 weekly	50	18 months
Johnsen (1978)	32 (Crn[d])	3000 × 2/week	60 × 3/week	16[a]	6 months
Schroffner (1978)	25 (Crn[d])	3000 × 3/week	150 × 3/week	50	10 months

[a] Reported as total sperm output
[b] Precise duration of therapy prior to conception is unclear
[c] Pituitary adenoma
[d] Craniopharyngioma

Table 2 summarizes the experience of several centers which have reported successful pregnancies in the partners of hypogonadotropic men receiving hCG-hMG treatment. Of great interest is the relatively low sperm output associated with pregnancy. The light-microscopic morphology and the motility of these spermatozoa is usually normal. We are unaware of studies of the prevalence of congenital defects in children born to fathers in whom spermatogenesis was initiated with gonadotropins. Yet, because IHH is often familial and the mode of inheritance is presumably autosomally dominant, an increased frequency of this disorder is to be expected in the offspring of affected individuals. We are aware of only one such case, a 9-year-old boy with cryptorchidism and anosmia whose father had partial hypogonadotropic hypogonadism treated with hCG (Merriam et al. 1977).

In the treatment of patients with hypopituitarism acquired postpubertally, gonadotropins rather than testosterone are sometimes chosen as initial therapy even when androgenization rather than fertility is the clinical goal. This approach is based upon testicular biopsy data revealing maturation arrest, germ cell loss, and peritubular hyalinization in postpubertal hypopituitarism (Wong et al. 1974). It was suggested that, in the absence of gonadotropin, the seminiferous tubules could ultimately hyalinize and preclude the subsequent induction of spermatogenesis. On this basis, it has also been suggested that hCG rather than testosterone be used to androgenize subjects with idiopathic hypogonadotropic hypogonadism. Because of the greater cost and the more frequent injection schedule with gonadotropins, this hypothesis deserves more precise documentation. In fact, androgen therapy was given for 1 year by Johnsen (1978) to a 32-year-old patient with a craniopharyngioma and for 4 years by Schroffner (1978) to a 20-year-old with the same diagnosis and in neither case did it preclude a favorable response with ultimate pregnancy when therapy was changed to hCG-hMG. Further, Mancini et al. (1969) reported the restoration of spermatogenesis and the disappearance of peritubular hyalinization in a 32-year-old patient treated with hCG-hMG 10 years after hypophysectomy. Testosterone has been used for as long as 7 years in a subject with IHH without adversely affecting the subsequent response to hCG-hMG (Johnsen 1978).

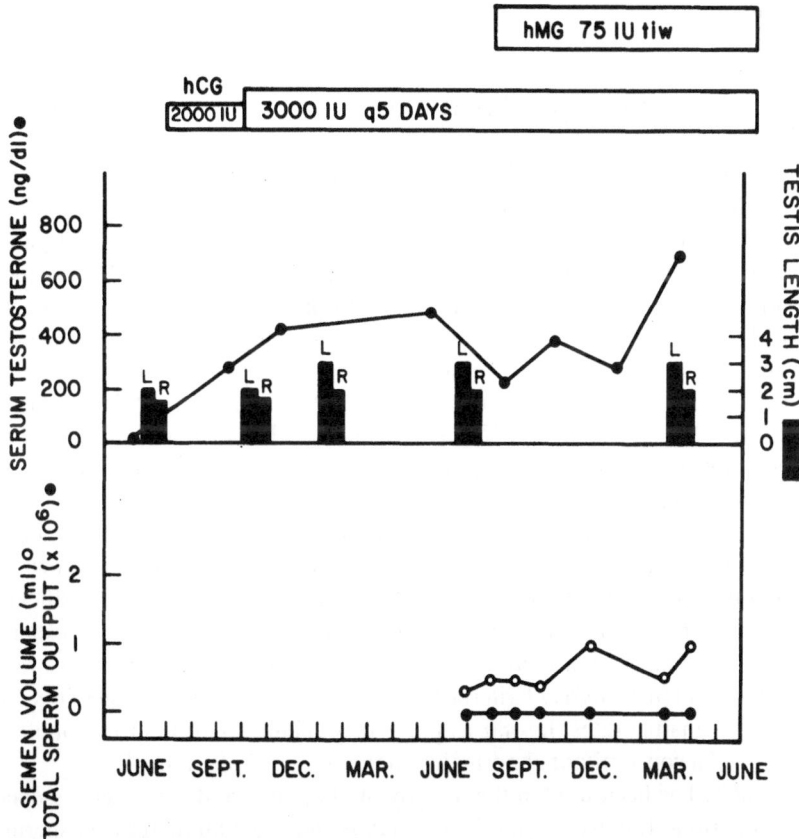

Fig. 2. Changes in serum testosterone, testes size, and sperm output in a 27-year-old man with IHH. Undescended testes were present at birth. At age 15 years, sexual infantilism lead to inhibition of hCG treatment. The left testis then descended spontaneously; right orchiopexy was performed at age 17 years. Only minimal testes growth occurred and azoospermia persisted during 10 months of treatment with hCG and hMG combined

It seems that patients with IHH and coexistent cryptorchidism may not be favorable candidates for gonadotropin therapy. Although the experience is small, patients who undergo orchiopexy in the early teen years have remained azoospermic when treated with the hCG-hMG combination (Fig. 2) (Sherins et al. 1977 b). Perhaps the current treatment of cryptorchidism in childhood will improve the fertility potential in these subjects with IHH.

It has recently been suggested that in some IHH patients with scrotal testes hCG-hMG may be ineffective in stimulating spermatogenesis (Check et al. 1979): The subject of this case report was a 26-year-old man with IHH in whom therapy was begun concomitantly with hCG 2000 IU and hMG 75 IU three times weekly. The serum testosterone level rose from 33 ng/dl to 1972 ng/dl. After 6 months, persistent azoospermia in a 1.5-ml ejaculate volume prompted an increase in the hMG dose to 150 IU. After a total 8 months of therapy, testis length had increased from 1.5–3.5 cm and a biopsy revealed incomplete spermatogenesis: treatment was abandoned. It should be noted that hCG pretreatment was not utilized prior to hMG. Further, the time needed to restore spermatogenesis has been noted to be 2–12 months. Thus, continued therapy in this subject might have produced positive results.

6.3 Gonadotropin Treatment in Idiopathic Oligozoospermia

The effectiveness of gonadotropins in the treatment of various anovulatory disorders prompted the extrapolation of this form of therapy to oligozoospermic men. Anovulation is characterized by a lack of the midcycle LH-FSH surge, a physiologic event which can be mimicked by drug therapy. In most idiopathic oligozoospermic men, however, no such deficiency in gonadotropin secretion is evident. Basal LH and FSH levels are either normal or elevated, and when testosterone concentrations are low they are associated with increased gonadotropin secretion that suggests a primary testicular defect (de Kretser et al. 1972; Purvis et al. 1975; Nankin and Troen 1976; Nankin et al. 1977). Nevertheless, the known stimulatory effects of gonadotropins on spermatogenesis serve as the incentive for their study in idiopathic oligozoospermia.

It is difficult to evaluate the efficacy of gonadotropin treatment in oligozoospermic men. Because the pathogenesis of this disorder is unknown, it is likely that the patient populations studied have been heterogeneous. Classifications based upon sperm output, motility, and morphologic abnormalities in testicular biopsy specimens have been used. Often, conclusions are based upon an insufficient number of semen analyses. Criteria for success include both changes in sperm output and pregnancy rates. Insofar as pregnancy relates to an infertile couple, the possibility of a concomitant abnormality in the spouse is often invoked.

hCG has been used in the therapy of idiopathic and varicocele-associated oligozoospermia. Futterweit and Sobrero (1968) reported an increase in sperm output in 15 of 27 patients and pregnancies in the spouses of ten of these men treated with hCG for 9 weeks. These changes occurred 4–8 months after completion of the treatment protocol. Recently, Cheval and Mehan (1979) reported improvement in 44 of 64 subfertile men: sperm density increased from 23 to 40.2 million/ml when spermiograms were analyzed 10 weeks after completing a 6-week course of hCG therapy. Twenty-three spouses (38%) became pregnant. These time relationships seem important in data analysis insofar as approximately 74 days are required for the formation of mature spermatozoa from spermatogonia. The results of other workers are very different; some finding changes in motility alone (Misurale et al. 1969) and others reporting pregnancy rates of 10% or less (Homonnai et al. 1978). It was suggested that large-dose hCG administration produced tubular sclerosis (Maddock and Nelson 1952), however, smaller doses of hCG which, in a carefully coordinated study, had no positive effects on sperm output, also had no deleterious effects (Sherins 1974). hCG administration does result in a fall in serum FSH concentrations, presumably due to feedback inhibition by the sex steroids produced (Reiter et al. 1972). LH production has not been evaluated because of the cross-reactivity between hLH and hCG in most assays.

Rosemberg (1976) summarized studies which evaluated the effects of hMG or hCG-hMG on hypospermatogenesis and divided the patients into two groups; those with severe (less than 10 million/ml) and those with moderate (11–20 million/ml)

Table 3. Effect of gonadotropin therapy in men with moderate idiopathic oligozoospermia (11 – 20 million/ml)

Authors	No. of subjects	No. improved (>30 million/ml)	No. pregnancies
Treatment with hMG			
Schoysman (1964)	4	2	2
Abelli and Falagario[a]	26	9	9
Lytton and Mroueh (1966)	10	6	2
Cittadini and Quartaravo[a]	2	1	0
Danezis and Batrinos (1967)	3	2	1
Debiasi and Misurale[a]	7	4	2
Lunenfeld et al. (1967)	24	13	0
Troen et al. (1970)	1	0	0
Schwarzstein (1964)	3	3	1
Rosemberg (1976)	1	1	0
	81	41 (51%)	17 (21%)
Treatment with hCG-hMG			
Mroueh et al. (1967)	4	2	0
Polishuk et al. (1967)	7	2	0
Anton et al. (1968)	3	0	0
Troen et al. (1970)	1	1	0
Sherins (1974)	2	0	0
Sina et al. (1974)	6	4	2
Rosemberg (1976)	3	2	0
Homonnai et al. (1978)	37	8	3
Schill (1979)	12	4	0
	75	22 (29%)	5 (7%)

[a] Quoted from Rosemberg (1976)

Table 4. Effects of gonadotropin therapy in men with severe idiopathic oligozoospermia (less than 10 million/ml)

Authors	No. of subjects	No. improved (million/ml)		Pregnancies
		10 – 30	> 30	
Treatment with hMG				
Abelli and Falagario[a]	6	1	1	0
Lytton and Mroueh (1966)	9	1	0	1
Danezis and Batrinos (1967)	8	3	1	1
Debiasi and Misurale[a]	8	1	0	0
Lunenfeld et al. (1967)	27	7	8	1
Troen et al. (1970)	6	1	0	0
Schwarzstein (1964)	9	0	2	1
Rosemberg (1976)	4	1	1	1
	77	15 (19%)	13 (17%)	5 (6%)
Treatment with hCG-hMG				
Cittadini and Quartaravo[a]	12	5	1	1
Polishuk et al. (1967)	7	3	0	1
Mroueh et al. (1967)	4	1	0	1
Anton et al. (1968)	16	0	0	0
DeKretscr et al. (1968)	3	1	0	0
Troen et al. (1970)	3	0	0	0
Pellegrini[a]	7	2	4	3
Sherins (1974)	5	0	0	0
Sina et al. (1974)	11	7	0	4
Schill (1979)	14	3	0	2
	122	22 (18%)	5 (4%)	12 (10%)

[a] Quoted from Rosemberg (1976)

oligozoospermia. These summary data have been recently extended by Schill (1979). Not unexpectedly, they find that moderate oligozoospermia responds more favorably than severe oligozoospermia, with a 16% pregnancy rate in the former and only 8.2% in the latter. Similarly, 35.5% of patients in the moderate oligozoospermia group achieved a sperm count of 30 million/ml, whereas only 19.8% reached these levels if their initial sperm concentration was less than 10 million/ml.

Some investigators who attempt to stimulate spermatogenesis with gonadotropins in idiopathic oligozoospermia favor the combination of hCG-hMG in dosages similar to those which are effective in hypogonadotropic subjects. Tables 3 and 4 contrast summary data from patients treated with hMG alone with those treated with the gonadotropin combination: for both moderate and severe oligozoospermia the results are strikingly similar, and dosages and frequencies of administration varied considerably among the different studies. Because of the current expense of FSH the dosages used were small if, in fact, the production rate of FSH in men approximates that calculated in women of 200 IU/day (Coble et al. 1969). No relationship between response rate and regimen used was apparent.

From our review of this literature we are impressed that summary data are drawn from very heterogeneous studies. From the 17 centers with data for moderate oligozoospermia, 22 pregnancies were seen in the spouses of 156 treated men (14%) (see Table 3). Nine centers reported no pregnancies in 60 couples, whereas the remaining eight enters report pregnancy rates of 23% in the 96 couples studied. It is safe to conclude that gonadotropins are not a uniformly successful therapy for all oligozoospermic men. The evaluation of therapeutic trials is also made more difficult by the variability of sperm density (Sherins et al. 1977 a), by the uncertainty of the relationship of sperm density to fertility, and by the difficulty of establishing proper controls (Smith and Steinberger 1977). Unfortunately, no parameters have yet been identified which will help predict who will respond to a given therapeutic regimen. Most authors do agree that patients with elevated gonadotropin concentrations are not good candidates for therapy.

The possibility that a subpopulation of idiopathic oligozoospermic men may suffer from an isolated deficiency of FSH secretion was raised recently by Maroulis et al. (1977). They reported two men with hypospermatogenesis, persistently low FSH concentrations, and normal LH and testosterone levels who responded to clomiphene administration with an increase in FSH secretion. No data on the effects of therapy on sperm production were included. Because basal serum FSH levels in normal men may occasionally be below the detection limits of conventional RIA, these data should be interpreted with caution. However, the repetitive measurement of basal and GnRH-stimulated serum FSH levels in sensitive immunoassays, perhaps in conjunction with measurement of intratesticular steroid concentrations, may uncover a subpopulation of apparently idiopathic oligozoospermic men who might respond to gonadotropin administration.

6.4 Conclusions

It is now over 15 years since gonadotropin treatment with FSH and hCG was introduced for hypospermatogenesis. This therapeutic combination clearly plays a successful role in ovulation induction in women and in the treatment of hypogonadotropic men. Many workers are of the opinion that in idiopathic oligozoospermia no effective treatment will evolve until the pathogenesis of the disorder is defined. Since a positive therapeutic response may lead to the elucidation of the etiology of a given disorder, clinical trials need not be abandoned. We believe that only a carefully controlled clinical study in which the patient population is clearly defined is likely to shed additional light on the use of gonadotropins in idiopathic oligozoospermia. Furthermore, although the success of gonadotropins as replacement therapy is established, the use of gonadotropins as pharmacologic agents in idiopathic oligozoospermia requires further study.

Acknowledgements. This work was supported in part by NIH grant 1-RO1-HD-11468.

6.5 References

Anton JP, Guéguen J, Genet P, Patoiseau JY (1968) Etude de 26 cas d'azoospermies et d'oligoasthénospermies traités par les gonadotrophines humaines extraites d'urines de femmes ménopausées (hMG). Gynecol Obstet 67:509–514

Arimura A, Shino M, De la Cruz KG, Rennels EG, Schally AV (1976) Effect of active and passive immunization with luteinizing hormone-releasing hormone on serum luteinizing hormone and follicle-stimulation hormone levels and the ultrastructure of pituitary gonadotrophs in castrated male rats. Endocrinology 99:291–303

Aynsley-Green A, Zachmann M, Illig R, Rampini S, Prader A (1976) Congenital bilateral anorchia in childhood. A clinical endocrine and therapeutic evaluation of twenty-one cases. Clin Endocrinol 5:381–391

Baker HWG, Bremner HG, Burger HG, de Kretser DM, Dulmanis A, Eddie LW, Hudson B, Keogh EJ, Lee VWK, Rennie GC (1976) Testicular control of follicle-stimulating hormone secretion. Recent Prog Horm Res 32:429–469

Bergada C, Mancini RE (1973) Effect of gonadotropins in the induction of spermatogenesis in human prepubertal testis. J Clin Endocrinol Metab 37:935–943

Bigos ST, Somma M, Rasio E, Eastman RC, Lanthier A, Johnston HH, Hardy J (1980) Cushing's disease: management by transsphenoidal pituitary microsurgery. J Clin Endocrinol Metab 50:348–354

Boyar RM, Finkelstein JW, Witkin M, Kapen S, Weitzman E, Hellman L (1973) Studies of endocrine function in "isolated gonadotropin deficiency". J Clin Endocrinol Metab 36:64–72

Boyar RM, Wu RHK, Kapen S, Hellman L, Weitzman ED, Finkelstein JW (1976) Clinical and laboratory heterogeneity in idiopathic hypogonadotropic hypogonadism. J Clin Endocrinol Metab 43:1268–1275

Braunstein GD, Kamdar V, Rasor J, Swaminathan N, Wade ME (1979) Widespread distribution of a chorionic gonadotropin-like substance in normal human tissues. J Clin Endocrinol Metab 49:917–925

Catt KJ, Dufau ML (1973) Interactions of LH and hCG with testicular gonadotropin receptors. In: O'Malley BW, Means AR (eds) Receptors for reproductive hormones. Plenum, New York pp 379–418

Check JH, Caro JF, Criden L, Meltz R, Brownstein K (1979) Leydig cell responsiveness with germinal cell resistance to gonadotropin therapy in Kallman's syndrome. Am J Med 67:495–497

Chen HC, Hodgen GD, Matsura S, Lin LJ, Gross E, Reichert LE jr, Birken S, Canfield RE, Ross GT (1976) Evidence for a gonadotropin from nonpregnant subjects that has physical, immunological, and biological similarities to human chorionic gonadotropin. Proc Natl Acad Sci 73:2885–2889

Cheval MJ, Mehan DJ (1979) Chorionic gonadotropins in the treatment of the subfertile male. Fertil Steril 31:666–668

Cigorraga SB, Dufau ML, Catt KJ (1978) Regulation of luteinizing hormone receptors and steroidogenesis in gonadotropin-desensitized Leydig cells. J Biol Chem 253:4297–4304

Coble YD jr, Kohler PO, Cargille CM, Ross GT (1969) Production rates and metabolic clearance rates of human follicle-stimulating hormone in premenopausal and postmenopausal women. J Clin Invest 48:359–363

Danezis JM, Batrinos ML (1967) The effect of human postmenopausal gonadotropins on infertile men with severe oligospermia. Fertil Steril 18:788–800

de Kretser DM, Taft HP, Brown JB, Evans JH, Hudson B (1968) Endocrine and histological studies on oligospermic men treated with human pituitary and chorionic gonadotrophin. J Endocrinol 40:107–115

de Kretser DM, Burger HG, Fortune D, Hudson B, Long AR, Paulsen CA, Taft HP (1972) Hormonal, histological and chromosomal studies in adult males with testicular disorders. J Clin Endocrinol Metab 35:392–401

Del Pozo E, Bolte E, Very M (1975) Suprasellar disturbance in the syndrome of fertile eunuchoidism: case report. Acta Endocrinol 80:165–170

Dufau ML, Catt KJ, Tsuruhara T (1971) Gonadotrophin stimulation of testosterone production by the rat testis in vitro. Biochim Biophys Acta 252:574–579

Franchimont P, Chari S, Hazee-Hagelstein MT, Debruche ML, Duraiswami S (1977) Evidence for the existence of inhibin. In: Troen P, Nankin HR (eds) The testis in normal and infertile men. Raven, New York, pp 253–270

Fraser HM, Gunn A, Jeffcoate SL, Holland DH (1974) Effect of active immunization to luteinizing hormone releasing hormone on serum and pituitary gonadotrophins, testes and accessory sex organs in the male rat. J Endocrinol 63:399–406

Futterweit W, Sobrero AJ (1968) Treatment of normogonadotropic oligospermia with large doses of chorionic gonadotropin. Fertil Steril 19:971–976

Gemzell C, Kjessler B (1964) Treatment of infertility after partial hypophysectomy with human gonadotrophins. Lancet 1:644

Gordon GG, Olivo J, Rafii F, Southren AL (1975) Conversion of androgens to estrogens in cirrhosis of the liver. J Clin Endocrinol Metab 40:1018–1026

Granville GE (1970) Successful gonadotropin therapy of infertility in a hypopituitary man. Arch Intern Med 125:1041–1044

Greep RO, Fevold H (1937) The spermatogenic and secretory function of the gonads of hypophysectomized adult rats treated with pituitary FSH and LH. Endocrinology 21:611–618

Hemsell DL, Grodin JM, Brenner PF, Siiteri PK, MacDonald PC (1974) Plasma precursors of estrogen. II. Correlation of the extent of conversion of plasma androstenedione to estrone with age. J Clin Endocrinol Metab 38:476–479

Homonnai ZT, Peled M, Paz GF (1978) Changes in semen quality and fertility in response to endocrine treatment of subfertile men. Gynecol Obstet Invest 99:244–255

Hsu AF, Troen P (1978) An androgen-binding protein in the testicular cytosol of human testis. Comparison with human plasma testosterone-estrogen binding globulin. J Clin Invest 61:1611–1619

Hsu AF, Stratico D, Hosaka M, Troen P (1978) Studies of the human testis. X. Properties of human chorionic gonadotropin receptor in adult testis and relation to intratesticular testosterone concentration. J Clin Endocrinol Metab 47:529–536

Jacobson RI, Seyler LE, Tamborlane WV jr, Gertner JM, Genel M (1979) Pulsatile subcutaneous nocturnal administration of GnRH by portable infusion pump in hypogonadotropic hypogonadism: Initiation of gonadotropin responsiveness. J Clin Endocrinol Metab 49:652–654

Johnsen SG (1978) Maintenance of spermatogenesis induced by hMG treatment by means of continuous hCG treatment in hypogonadotrophic men. Acta Endocrinol 89:763–769

Kallmann FJ, Schoenfeld WA, Barrera SE (1944) The genetic aspects of primary eunuchoidism. Am J Ment Defic 68:203–236

Kelch RP, Jenner MR, Weinstein RL, Kaplan SL, Grumbach MM (1972) Estradiol and testosterone secretion by human, simian, and canine testes, in males with hypogonadism and in male pseudohermaphrodites with the feminizing testes syndrome. J Clin Invest 51:824–830

Knorr DW, Vanha-Perttula T, Lipsett MB (1970) Structure and function of rat testis through pubescence. Endocrinology 86:1298–1304

Lee JA, Yoshida KI, Hosaka M, Stratico D, Hsu AF, Winters SJ, Oshima H, Troen P (1980) Studies of the human testis. XV. Androgen-binding protein and function of Leydig cells and tubules in aged men with prostatic carcinoma. J Clin Endocrinol Metab 50:1105–1110

Lee VWK, de Kretser DM, Hudson BH, Wang C (1975) Variations in serum FSH, LH and testosterone levels in male rats from birth to sexual maturity. J Reprod Fertil 42:121–126

Loriaux DL, Vigersky RA, Marynick SP, Janick JJ, Sherins RJ (1977) Androgen and estrogen effects in the regulation of LH in man. In: Troen P, Nankin HR (eds) The testis in normal and infertile men. Raven, New York, pp 213–225

Luboshitzky R, Rosen E, Trestian S, Spitz IM (1979) Hyperprolactinemia and hypogonadism in men: response to exogenous gonadotropins. Clin Endocrinol 11:217–223

Lunenfeld B, Mor A, Mani M (1967) Treatment of male infertility. I. Human gonadotropins. Fertil Steril 18:581–592

Luton JP, Thieblot P, Valcke JC, Mahoudeau JA, Bricaire H (1977) Reversible gonadotropin deficiency in male Cushing's disease. J Clin Endocrinol Metab 45:488–495

Lytton B, Mroueh A (1966) Treatment of oligospermia with urinary human menopausal gonadotrophin: a preliminary report. Fertil Steril 17:696–700

MacDonald PC, Edman CD, Hemsell DL, Porter JC, Siiteri PK (1978) Effect of obesity on conversion of plasma androstenedione to estrone in postmenopausal women with and without endometrial cancer. Am J Obstet Gynecol 130:448–455

MacDonald PC, Madden JD, Brenner PF, Wilson JD, Siiteri PK (1979) Origin of estrogen in normal men and in women with testicular feminization. J Clin Endocrinol Metab 49:905–916

MacLeod J (1970) The effects of urinary gonadotropins following hypophysectomy and in hypogonadotropic eunuchoidism. In: Rosemberg E, Paulsen CA (eds) The human testis. Plenum, New York, pp 577–586

MacLeod J, Pazianos A, Ray BS (1964) Restoration of human spermatogenesis by menopausal gonadotrophins. Lancet 1:1196

Maddock WO, Nelson WO (1952) The effects of chorionic gonadotropin in adult men: increased estrogen and 17-ketosteroid excretion, gynecomastia, Leydig cell stimulation and seminiferous tubule damage. J Clin Endocrinol Metab 12:985–1014

Mancini RE, Seiguer AC, Lloret AP (1969) Effect of gonadotropins on the recovery of spermatogenesis in hypophysectomized patients. J Clin Endocrinol Metab 29:467–478

Maroulis GB, Parlow AF, Marshall JR (1977) Isolated follicle-stimulating hormone deficiency in man. Fertil Steril 28:818–822

Means AR (1973) Specific interaction of ^{3}H-FSH with rat testis binding sites. In: O'Malley BW, Means AR (eds) Receptors for reproductive hormones. Plenum, New York, pp 431–448

Merriam GR, Beitins IZ, Bode HH (1977) Father-to-son transmission of hypogonadism with anosmia. Am J Dis Child 131:1216–1219

Misurale F, Cagnazzo G, Storace A (1969) Asthenospermia and its treatment with hCG. Fertil Steril 20:650–653

Mroueh A, Lytton B, Kase N (1967) Effects of human chorionic gonadotropin and human menopausal gonadotropin (Pergonal) in males with oligospermia. J Clin Endocrinol Metab 27:53–60

Nankin HR, Troen P (1971) Repetitive luteinizing hormone elevations in serum of normal men. J Clin Endocrinol Metab 33:558–560

Nankin HR, Troen P (1976) Endocrine profiles in idiopathic oligozoospermic men. In: Hafez ESE (ed) Human semen and fertility regulation in men. Mosby, St. Louis, pp 370–374

Nankin HR, Castaneda E, Troen P (1977) Endocrine profiles in oligospermic men. In: Troen P, Nankin HR (eds) The testis in normal and infertile men. Raven, New York, pp 529–538

Nankin HR, Lin T, Murono E, Osterman J, Troen P (1980) Testosterone and 17-OH-progesterone responses in men to 3-hour LH infusions. Acta Endocrinol 95:110–116

Odell WD, Swerdloff RS, Jacobs HS, Hescox MA (1973) FSH induction of sensitivity to LH: one cause of sexual maturation in the male rat. Endocrinology 92:160–165

Paulsen CA (1965) The effect of human menopausal gonadotropin on spermatogenesis in hypogonadotrophic hypogonadism. In: Proceedings of the VIth pan-american congress of endocrinology, Mexico City. Excerpta Medica International Congress Series 112:398–407

Paulsen CA, Espeland DH, Michals EL (1970) Effects of hCG, hMG, hLH, and hGH administration on testicular function. In: Rosemberg E, Paulsen CA (eds) The human testis. Plenum, New York, pp 547–562

Polishuk WZ, Palti Z, Laufer A (1967) Treatment of defective spermatogenesis with human gonadotropins. Fertil Steril 18:127–134

Pont A, Shelton R, Odell WD (1979) Prolactin-secreting tumors in men: Surgical cure. Ann Intern Med 91:211–213

Purvis K, Hansson V (1978) Hormonal regulation of Leydig cell function. Mol Cell Endocrinol 12:123–138

Purvis K, Brenner PF, Landgren BM, Cekan Z, Diczfalusy E (1975) Indices of gonadal function in the human male. I. Plasma levels of unconjugated steroids and gonadotropins under normal and pathological conditions. Clin Endocrinol 4:237–246

Rabin D, Spitz I, Berrovici B, Bell J, Laufer A, Benveniste R, Polishuk W (1972) Isolated deficiency of follicle-stimulating hormone. N Engl J Med 287:1313–1317

Reiter EO, Kulin HE, Loriaux DL (1972) FSH suppression during short-term hCG administration: a gonadally mediated process. J Clin Endocrinol Metab 34:1080–1084

Ritzen EM, Hagenas L, Hansson V, French FS (1975) In vitro synthesis of testicular androgen binding protein (ABP): stimulation by FSH and androgen. In: French FS, Hansson V, Ritzen EM, Nayfeh SN (eds) Hormonal regulation of spermatogenesis. Plenum, New York, pp 353–366

Rosemberg E (1976) Gonadotropin therapy of male infertility. In: Hafez ESE (ed) Human semen and fertility regulation in men. Mosby, St. Louis, pp 464–475

Saez JM, Forest MG (1979) Kinetics of human chorionic gonadotropin-induced steroidogenic response of the human testis. I. Plasma testosterone: implications for human chorionic gonadotropin stimulation test. J Clin Endocrinol Metab 49:278–283

Santen RJ (1975) Is aromatization of testosterone to estradiol required for inhibition of luteinizing hormone secretion in man? J Clin Invest 56:1555–1563

Santen RJ, Paulsen CA (1973) Hypogonadotropic eunuchoidism. II. Gonadal responsiveness to exogenous gonadotropins. J Clin Endocrinol Metab 36:55–63

Schill WB (1979) Recent progress in pharmacological therapy of male subfertility: a review. Andrologia 11:77–107

Schoysman R (1964) Essais préliminaires de traitement des oligospermies moyennes par la gonadotrophine humaine extraite de l'urine de femmes ménopausées (HMG). Bull Soc R Belge Gynecol Obstet 34:399–407

Schroffner WG (1978) Restoration of male fertility five years after total hypophysectomy. Hawaii Med J 37:331–334

Schwarzstein L (1974) hMG in the treatment of oligospermic patients. In: Mancini RE, Martini L (eds) Male fertility and sterility. Academic Press, London, pp 567–571

Sherins RJ (1974) Clinical aspects of treatment of male infertility with gonadotropins: testicular response of some men given hCG with and without Pergonal. In: Mancini RE, Martini L (eds) Male fertility and sterility. Academic Press, London, pp 545–565

Sherins RJ, Brightwell D, Sternthal PM (1977a) Longitudinal analysis of semen of fertile and infertile men. In: Troen P, Nankin HR (eds) The testis in normal and infertile men. Raven, New York, pp 473–488

Sherins RJ, Winters SJ, Wachslicht H (1977b) Studies of the role of hCG and low-dose FSH in initiating spermatogenesis in hypogonadotropic men. In: Proceedings of the 59th Annual Meeting of the Endocrine Society (Abstr), p 312

Sina D, Haubert HD, Karschnia R (1974) Humanmenopausen – Gonadotropin bei der Behandlung infertiler Männer. Dtsch Med Wochenschr 99:2639–2643

Smith KD, Steinberger E (1977) What is oligospermia? In: Troen P, Nankin HR (eds) The testis in normal and infertile men. Raven, New York, pp 489–503

Southren AL, Olive J, Gordon GG, Vittek J, Brener J, Rafii F (1974) The conversion of androgens to estrogens in hyperthyroidism. J Clin Endocrinol Metab 38:207–214

Spitz IM, Steiner J, Segal S, Schumert Z, Rosen E, Slonim A, Rabinowitz D (1978) Induction of spermatogenesis in hypogonadotropic hypogonadism. Postgrad Med J 54:694–697

Steinberger E (1971) Hormonal control of mammalian spermatogenesis. Physiol Rev 51:1–22

Steinberger A, Walther J, Heindel JJ, Sanborn BM, Tsai YH, Steinberger E (1979) Hormone interactions in the Sertoli cells. In Vitro 15:23–31

Stewart-Bentley M, Odell WD, Horton R (1974) The feedback control of luteinizing hormone secretion in normal adult men. J Clin Endocrinol Metab 38:545–653

Tcholakian RK, Steinberger A (1978) Progesterone metabolism by cultured Sertoli cells. Endocrinology 103:1335–1343

Troen P, Yanaihara T, Nankin H, Tominaga T, Lever H (1970) Assessment of gonadotropin therapy in infertile males. The human testis. Adv Exp Biol Med 10:591–602

Wildt L, Marshall G, Knobil E (1980) Experimental induction of puberty in the infantile female rhesus monkey. Science 207:1373–1375

Winters SJ, Mecklenburg RS, Sherins RJ (1978) Hypothalamic function in men with hypogonadotrophic hypogonadism. Clin Endocrinol 8:417–426

Winters SJ, Janick JJ, Loriaux DL, Sherins RJ (1979) Studies on the role of sex steroids in the feedback control of gonadotropin concentrations in men. II. Use of the estrogen antagonist clomiphene citrate. J Clin Endocrinol Metab 48:222–227

Wong TW, Straus F, Warner NE (1974) Testicular biopsy in the study of male infertility. III. Pretesticular causes of infertility. Arch Pathol 98:1–8

7 Androgen Therapy in Hypogonadism and Infertility

E. Nieschlag and C. W. Freischem

Whereas the endocrine testicular function is intact in most cases of male infertility, almost all forms of endocrine testicular insufficiency are associated with infertility. While testosterone treatment will effectively alleviate symptoms caused by lack of endogenous androgen production in cases of hypogonadism, infertility in these patients cannot be cured by testosterone. If fertility is desired, patients with hypothalamic or pituitary insufficiency may temporarily be treated with LHRH or hCG + hMG, respectively. However, even in these patients, following treatment with releasing hormones or gonadotropins, long-term testosterone substitution will be required.

Since patients with infertility caused by endocrine insufficiency require testosterone substitution, the principles of testosterone treatment and its clinical applications are discussed here. A consideration of testosterone rebound therapy for treatment of male subfertility is also included.

7.1 Mechanism of Testosterone Action

Testosterone is quantitatively and qualitatively the most important androgen secreted by the testis. It is responsible for the development of male characteristics during fetal life and puberty and for the maintenance of virility in adulthood. Testosterone has a multiplicity of functions in the various organs and organ systems, and a lack of testosterone is accompanied by corresponding symptoms (Table 1). Testosterone reaches the target organs via the blood stream and, to a certain extent, the concentration of the steroid reaching the target cells regulates the intensity of testosterone action. Testosterone appears to enter the cell without an active transport mechanism. In the cells of the various target organs, testosterone develops its functions through different mechanisms of action as follows (Liao 1976):

1. After entry into the cell, testosterone is bound to an androgen receptor and acts in the nucleus to initiate DNA and RNA synthesis. This mechanism is found in the brain, pituitary, muscles, and kidney.
2. Before testosterone can have an effect within the cell, it must be transformed into dihydrotestosterone by means of the specific enzyme 5α-reductase. In order to reach the nucleus and become effective, dihydrotestosterone must be bound to a specific receptor. This transformation is a prerequisite of testosterone action in the

Table 1. Clinical manifestation of testosterone deficiency

	Before puberty	*After puberty*
Skeleton	Eunuchoidal stature	Osteoporosis
Larynx	Lack of deepening of the voice	–
Hair pattern	Horizontal pubic hair line, or lack of pubic and axillary hair, lack of beard, straight frontal hair line	Decrease in beard and pubic hair
Skin	Lack of sebum production, paleness	Atrophy, fine wrinkles, paleness
Erythropoiesis	Moderate anemia	Moderate anemia
Muscles	Underdeveloped	Atrophy
Penis	Infantile	–
Prostate	Underdeveloped	Atrophy
Spermatogenesis	Not initiated	Regression
Libido and potency	Not developed	Loss

germinal epithelium, epididymis, ductus deferens, seminal vesicles, prostate, penis, hair follicles, and sebaceous glands of the skin. The importance of the presence of dihydrotestosterone receptors is illustrated by patients with testicular feminization, whose target organs lack such receptors.

3. Testosterone is aromatized, i.e., transformed into estrogens, and only then develops its effectiveness. This mechanism of action plays a role in the hypothalamic-pituitary system, in which testosterone can also be directly effective (Kato 1977). In humans it was demonstrated that aromatization in blood is not a prerequisite for this mechanism of testosterone action (Marynick et al. 1979), so that the conversion can take place within the cell itself.

Understanding these mechanisms of action is important in choosing an androgen for therapeutic purposes. It becomes clear that to be fully effective an androgen must possess all three capacities of testosterone; the ability to bind directly to receptors, to be reduced to dihydrotestosterone, and to be aromatized.

7.2 Pharmacology of Androgens

7.2.1 Free Testosterone

Free unesterified testosterone, as physiologically secreted by the testis, would appear to be the first choice when considering substitution therapy of endocrine testicular failure. The applicability and effectiveness of the unaltered testosterone molecule have been investigated. When given orally in the free form, testosterone is absorbed well from the gut, but is so effectively metabolized in the liver that it never reaches the target organs (first-pass effect) and, thus, remains ineffective. Only when the dosage is 200 mg, or about 30-fold the amount produced daily by a normal male (approximately 7 mg), is the metabolizing capacity of the liver exceeded. At this point, an increase in peripheral testosterone blood levels becomes measurable and clinical effects can be observed (Dagett et al. 1978; Johnsen et al. 1974; Nieschlag et al. 1975, 1977). The testosterone-metabolizing capacity of the liver, however, is age- and sex-dependent. An oral dose of 60 mg free testosterone does not affect peripheral testosterone levels in normal adult men, but produces a significant rise in prepubertal boys and women (Nieschlag et al. 1977). This demonstrates that testosterone induces liver enzymes responsible for its own metabolism (Johnsen et al. 1976).

In order to substitute effectively with the oral ingestion of testosterone, 0.4–0.6 g testosterone must be administered daily (Johnsen 1978; Johnsen et al. 1974). Besides the fact that such high steroid concentrations are uneconomical, the possibility of toxic side effects of such huge testosterone doses cannot be excluded, especially when given over a long period of time for substitution therapy. However, in a small group of patients treated for as long as 7 years with oral testosterone, such effects have not been observed (Johnsen 1978). For these reasons, oral administration of free testosterone has not become a generally recommended method for therapeutic purposes.

In order for testosterone to become effective in target organs in smaller doses, the liver must be bypassed. This can be achieved by administering testosterone suppositories (Hamburger 1958). A single application of 40 mg testosterone in suppository form resulted in the elevation of plasma testosterone levels for up to 4 h (Fig. 1) and effective plasma levels can be achieved by repeated applications (Nieschlag et

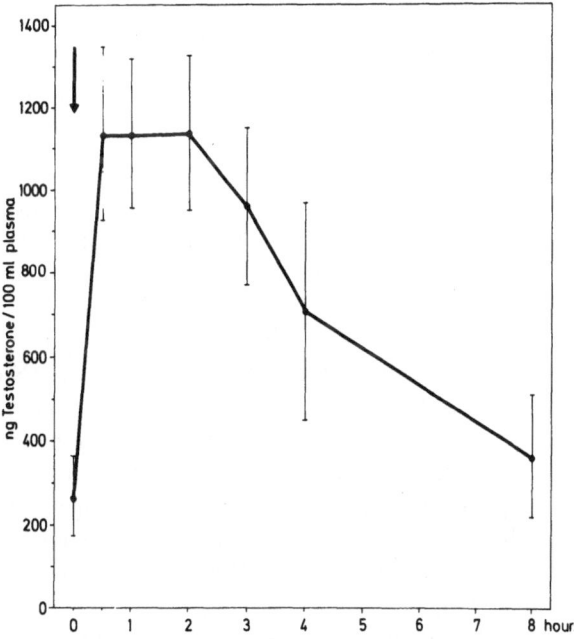

Fig. 1. Plasma testosterone levels in eight men following rectal suppository application of 40 mg testosterone

al. 1976). However, absorption from suppositories two or three times daily is considered inconvenient by most patients. Recently, it has been shown that testosterone is absorbed from the nasal mucosa (Danner and Frick 1980). Whether this route can be used for clinical purposes will be revealed by further trials. The use of subcutaneous implants of pellets containing compressed testosterone crystals has never gained wide usage (Heller and Maddock 1947) and the subcutaneous application of silastic capsules filled with testosterone has not gone beyond experimental use (Frick et al. 1976).

7.2.2 Parenteral Testosterone Esters

The most widely applied parenteral form of testosterone therapy is the intramuscular injection. As pure unesterified testosterone, it has a half-life of only about 10 min and would have to be injected at very short intervals to be therapeutically effective.

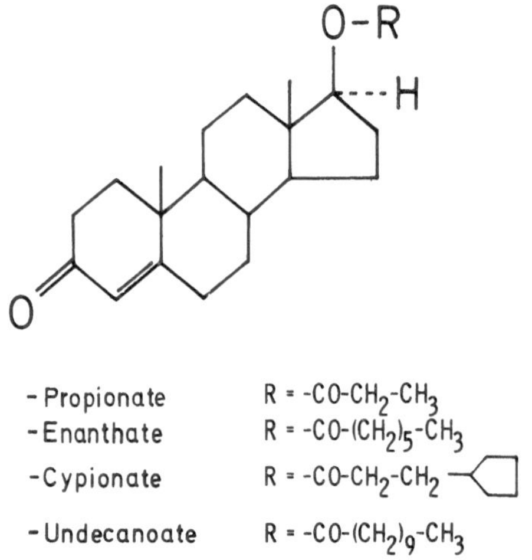

– Propionate	$R = -CO-CH_2-CH_3$
– Enanthate	$R = -CO-(CH_2)_5-CH_3$
– Cypionate	$R = -CO-CH_2-CH_2-\langle\rangle$
– Undecanoate	$R = -CO-(CH_2)_9-CH_3$

Fig. 2. Testosterone esters used in therapy

An increase in effective duration of injected testosterone can be achieved by esterifying the molecule at the 17-hydroxy position (Fig. 2). Several esters have been synthesized of which testosterone propionate, enanthate and cypionate have become most widely used.

Following 25 or 50 mg i.m. *testosterone propionate*, elevated serum testosterone concentrations can be measured for 1 or 2 days (Nieschlag et al. 1976). A longer side-chain increases the length of effectiveness. Thus, following 200 or 250 mg i.m. *testosterone enanthate*, elevated serum testosterone levels can be observed for 12–14 days in normal men and effective serum testosterone levels can be measured for the same period in hypogonadal men (Nieschlag et al. 1976; Schulte-Beerbühl and Nieschlag 1980) (Figs. 3, 4). Therefore, for long-term substitution of an endocrine testicular insufficiency, 200–250 mg testosterone enanthate must be injected intramuscularly every 2, or at least 3 weeks.

In some countries, another ester, *testosterone cypionate,* is available for therapy. It had been believed that testosterone cypionate might have a longer-lasting effect than testosterone enanthate, since its side-chain contains more C atoms. A direct

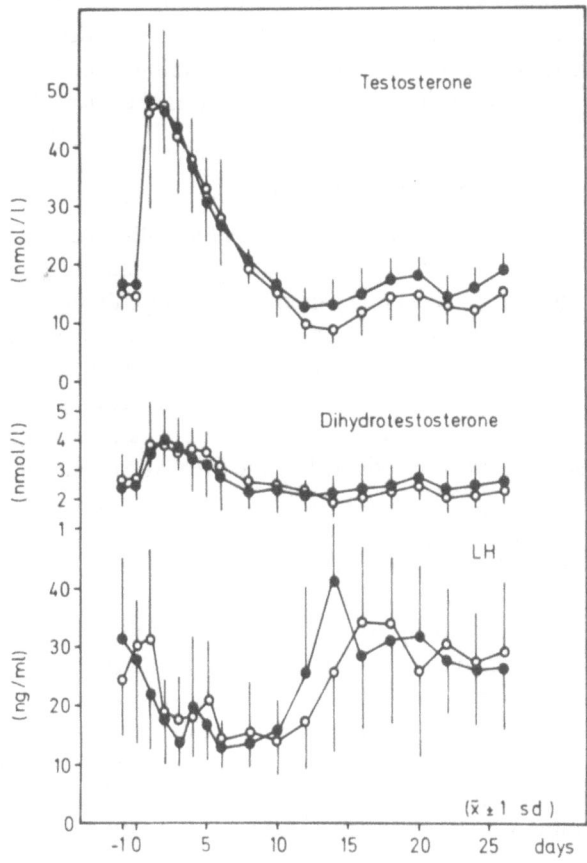

Fig. 3. Effect of 140 mg i.m. testosterone either as enanthate (●) or cypionate (○) ester on serum testosterone, dihydrotestosterone, and LH levels in six normal men (Schulte-Beerbühl and Nieschlag 1980)

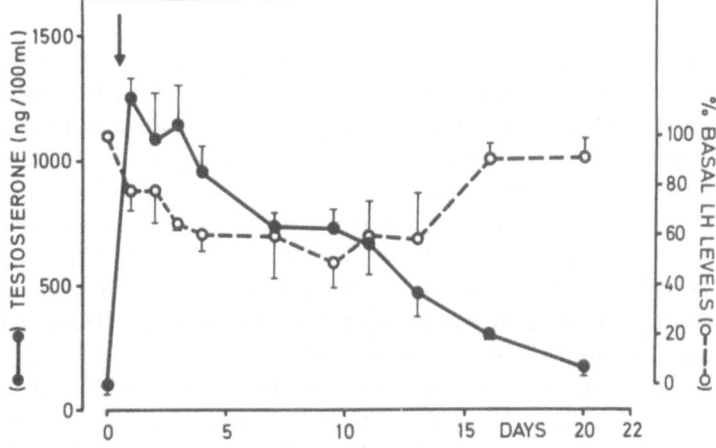

Fig. 4. Serum testosterone levels and suppression of serum LH levels in seven patients with primary hypogonadism following 250 mg i.m. testosterone enanthate (Nieschlag et al. 1976)

comparison of both esters, however, showed that the two preparations are identical with respect to bioavailability and length of effectiveness (Fig. 3) (Schulte-Beerbühl and Nieschlag 1980). Testosterone cypionate and testosterone enanthate can, therefore, be considered equivalent in terms of clinical effectiveness.

7.2.3 Testosterone Undecanoate

While the side-chain in position 17 used for esterification increases the duration and effectiveness of injected testosterone, the introduction of an aliphatic side-chain can result in an effect that can be exploited for therapeutic purposes. When testosterone is esterified with undecanoic acid (11 C atoms) and given orally, the substance is incorporated into chylomicrons in the intestines, absorbed into lymphatic fluid, and reaches the circulation via the ductus thoracicus, as shown in rats (Coert et al. 1975) and in humans (Horst et al. 1976). Thus, the target organs are reached before testosterone is inactivated by the liver. Maximum concentrations in blood are reached 4 h after oral ingestion, falling to basal levels after 8 h (Nieschlag et al. 1975). Absorption is improved if these esters are taken in arachis oil (Nieschlag et al. 1975) and with a meal (Frey et al. 1979).

At present, testosterone undecanoate is only available in several countries in capsules of 40 mg. Sixty-three percent of the preparation is testosterone and the rest is undecanoic acid. Long-term substitution can be achieved by 80–120 mg daily. Because of the relatively short period of effectiveness the dose should be divided into two to three doses per day to achieve satisfactory clinical results (Franchi et al. 1978). However, attempts to use testosterone undecanoate for suppression of spermatogenesis, either to elicit the rebound phenomenon in men with disturbed fertility (Kloer et al. 1980) or for fertility control in normal men (Nieschlag et al. 1978) have failed.

7.2.4 Synthetic Androgens

7.2.4.1 Methyltestosterone

Several attempts have been made to modify the testosterone molecule by chemical means in order to render it orally effective, i.e., to delay metabolism in the liver. In this regard, the longest known testosterone derivative is 17α-methyltestosterone, which is a fully effective oral androgen preparation. Ever since this substance was introduced for clinical use, repeated reports about toxic side effects such as an increase in serum liver enzymes (Carbone et al. 1959), cholestasis of the liver (de Lorimer et al. 1965; Werner et al. 1950), and peliosis of the liver (Westaby et al. 1977) have appeared. It is of interest that humans appear to be more susceptible to the hepatotoxic effects of methyltestosterone than rats (Heywood et al. 1977a) or dogs (Heywood et al. 1977b). The side effects are due to the alkyl group in the 17 position and have also been reported for other steroids with this configuration (Krüskemper and Noell 1967). Because of these side effects, methyltestosterone is being used with increasing reluctance, especially as long-term replacement therapy (Nieschlag 1981). Whether methyltestosterone may also induce hepatoma remains unclear (Farell et al. 1975).

7.2.4.2 Fluoxymesterone

The androgenic activity of fluoxymesterone has been enhanced over that of testosterone by the introduction of fluorine and an additional hydroxy group into the steroid skeleton of testosterone. This substance also contains a 17α-methyl group and accordingly there is a risk of hepatotoxicity with long-term use. Since the substance does not cross-react with the antisera used for radioimmunological testosterone determinations, fluoxymesterone is used for short-term testicular suppression in clinical experiments and tests.

7.2.4.3 Mesterolone

Mesterolone can be considered a derivative of the 5α-reduced testosterone metabolite dihydrotestosterone. In contrast to both previously mentioned synthetic androgen preparations, no hepatotoxicity has been observed with this substance. However, mesterolone, being a derivative of dihydrotestosterone, is only a partially active androgen. In target organs, such as muscle, requiring the direct effect of testosterone and in those requiring aromatiziation to estrogens, such as the hypothalamo-pituitary system, mesterolone is not or only weakly active. Accordingly the pituitary secretion of LH and FSH is hardly affected by the administration of mesterolone (Gordon et al. 1975). Thus, a complete substitution of an endocrine testicular insufficiency cannot be achieved using mesterolone.

7.2.5 Testis Sicca and Testis Extracts

In several countries there are a number of marketed preparations containing testis sicca or testis extracts of animal origin. The manufacturers claim that these preparations are effective in the treatment of endocrine testicular insufficiency, of potency disturbances, and in restoring general activity.

The therapeutic effectiveness of these preparations beyond a placebo effect is highly questionable and no clinical studies on their effectiveness are available. The amount of testosterone present in these preparations does not exceed a few picograms and, hence, cannot be the effective principle. Since the testes synthesize, but do not store testosterone, the concentration of this androgen in the testis is relatively low. Approximately 3 kg of bull testes contain the equivalent of the daily testosterone production of a normal adult man. The testosterone present in the bull testis, when taken orally, could not become effective as it would be completely and rapidly inactivated in the liver. Any other effective agent has so far not been demonstrated in these preparations to date. They are inadequate for replacement therapy of endocrine testicular insufficiency and they should not be included in a therapy based on rational principles.

7.3 Clinical Application

7.3.1 Substitution of Endocrine Testicular Insufficiency

All types of primary testicular failure where the endogenous testosterone production cannot be stimulated sufficiently will require substitution with testosterone. Here the major indications are Klinefelter's syndrome, congenital or acquired defects of both testes, impaired endocrine function due to cryptorchidism, or infections. Some of these diseases may not require testosterone application in the early stages, but the patient must be carefully monitored by both clinical assessment and determination of testosterone in serum in order to guarantee the initiation of testosterone therapy before irreversible effects of androgen deficiency such as osteoporosis are manifested. In cases with secondary hypogonadism due to pituitary or hypothalamic failure fertility may be achieved by hCG + hMG or LHRH treatment. On a long-term basis, however, these patients will also require testosterone substitution.

Long-term substitution therapy is achieved by 200–250 mg testosterone enanthate or cypionate injected intramuscularly every 2–3 weeks. Both esters are clinically equivalent and effects are rapidly noticed by the patients and recognized by the clinician. An occasional estimation of serum testosterone concentrations shortly before the next injection is recommended for control of therapy. This should be done especially in cases where injections are administered every 3 weeks or at shorter intervals but where the response appears to be inadequate. Physical and mental activity, the somatic signs of virility (beard growth, male hair pattern, muscular strength), libido, erections, and potency serve as parameters for the clinical control of therapeutic effectiveness. In particular, sexual activity has proven to be a reliable parameter for the short-term assessment of therapeutic efficacy (Davidson et al. 1979): An example is shown in Fig. 5. The red blood cell count and hemoglobin concentration, as well as the mineralization of the skeleton as determined by X-ray or, more sensitively, by densitometry are useful parameters for monitoring the effectiveness of testosterone treatment on a long-term basis.

7.3.2 Idiopathic Delayed Puberty

Testosterone can also be used in the treatment of idiopathic delayed puberty without influencing the final expected height and without detrimental effects on the germinal epithelium (de Lange et al. 1979; Kaplan et al. 1973). In order to avoid premature epiphyseal closure, testosterone has to be administered carefully. In our experience, monthly injections of 250 mg testosterone enanthate for 3 months is an appropriate regimen for the first course of treatment. If puberty cannot be initiated, another course of three injections may follow 3–6 months later (Fig. 6). The maturation of the hypothalamic-pituitary-testicular axis can be monitored by LHRH tests, which should reveal increasing LH (de Lange et al. 1979).

Other types of delayed puberty may also require testosterone substitution therapy, but in addition treatment of the cause should be undertaken whenever possible, e.g., the removal of a pituitary adenoma or craniopharyngioma.

7.3.3 Excessively Tall Boys

Premature epiphyseal closure can be achieved with high doses of testosterone enanthate or cypionate administered at short intervals. This effect has been exploited to prevent excessive height in boys (Zachman et al. 1976). The treatment should be initiated before the age of 14 years and should last for 1 year. During this treatment the testes cease to grow, but testicular growth resumes quickly after cessation of therapy.

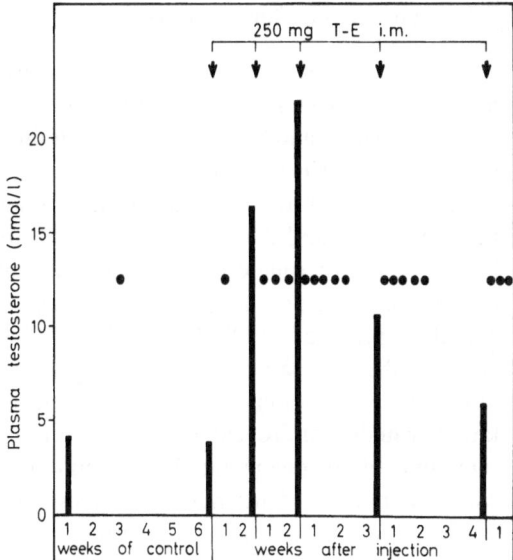

Fig. 5. Effect of spacing of testosterone enanthate injections on frequency of intercourse (●) and on plasma testosterone levels obtained immediately prior to the next injection

Adverse side effects on testicular function after cessation of therapy have not been noted. Since this therapy has been in use for only a few years, it is too early to know whether such high-dose testosterone therapy administered at the time of maturation has long-term side-effects, such as on the prostate or the blood vessels.

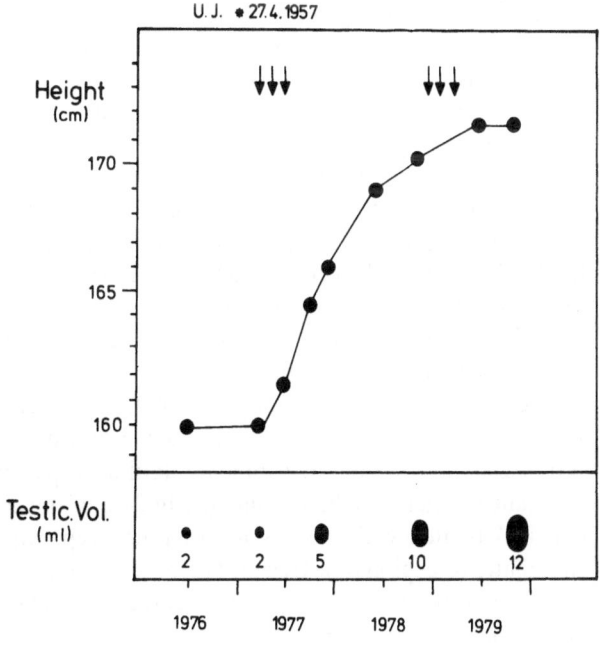

Fig. 6. Treatment of delayed puberty and growth retardation with testosterone enanthate. Each arrow indicates one injection of 250 mg testosterone enanthate given at monthly intervals

7.3.4 Androgens in Advanced Age

The so-called male climacteric cannot be considered as a well-defined pathophysiological entity (Kies 1974). In addition, no correlation between the symptoms of the male climacteric and endocrinological findings, including androgen measurements, has been established. Nevertheless, testosterone has been used for the treatment of symptoms related to advanced age such as sexual disturbances, sweating, nervousness, insomnia, and depression since it became available for therapeutic purposes. Injectable testosterone esters and, more recently, synthetic androgens have mainly been used. There are, however, only occasional reports, mostly positive, of efficacy with these preparations. Well-controlled studies show that androgens have a positive effect on the symptoms of advancing age, yet their effects are not better than those of placebo preparations. Further and conclusive studies appear to be required to establish whether androgens have a role in therapy of patients complaining of the symptoms of advancing age. For the time being, testosterone should only be used when an androgen deficiency has been established by testosterone measurements in serum. Although androgens are not believed to induce prostatic carcinoma, they do enhance the growth of this malignancy and the prostate gland should be regularly investigated in patients receiving testosterone (Nieschlag et al. 1979).

7.3.5 Testosterone Rebound Therapy as Treatment of Male Infertility

For the past 30 years testosterone rebound therapy has sporadically been used to treat infertile men with apparently normal endocrine testicular function. The basic principle of testosterone rebound therapy is to decrease the secretion of gonadotropins with high doses of testosterone, which leads to a suppression of spermatogenesis and to azoospermia. After cessation of testosterone administration, a recovery of sperm counts to higher than pretreatment levels (thus, a "rebound") is expected. The reason for rebound is still obscure. It should be borne in mind that no such effect is observed in normal men participating in testosterone trials for male fertility control (Patanelli 1978 for review).

Heller et al. (1950a, b) first observed that high-dose testosterone administration for up to 3 months improved spermatogenesis as judged by testicular biopsies. Heckel (1951) and Heckel and McDonald (1952) exploited this phenomenon for the treatment of infertile men and observed a rebound of sperm counts in the patients treated. From the wives of 73 patients injected over 4 months with either 50 mg testosterone propionate three times per week or with weekly injections of 200 mg testosterone cypionate, a pregnancy rate of 27% was reported (McDonald and Heckel 1956). Lamensdorf et al. (1975) treated 143 infertile men with weekly injections of 100 or 200 mg testosterone cypionate until azoospermia was reached and reported pregnancies after cessation of therapy in 27% of the couples. In a larger series (840 patients) treated with various testosterone preparations (testosterone propionate, enanthate, or cypionate), Getzoff (1955) found improved sperm counts after cessation of therapy in only 10% of the treated men. The pregnancy rate was only 7% (Table 2).

Other authors attempted to elicit the rebound phenomenon by administering orally effective testosterone preparations. Methyltestosterone did not achieve prom-

Table 2. Representative studies using testosterone (T) rebound therapy for the treatment of male infertility

Reference	T preparation	No. of patients	Pregnancy rate (%)
Getzoff (1955)	Various T preparations	840	7
McDonald and Heckel (1956)	T propionate or T cypionate	73	27
Rowley and Heller (1972)	T enanthate + 17 α-ethyl-19-nor-T	157	43
Lamensdorf et al. (1975)	T cypionate	145	27
Charny and Gordon (1978)	T enanthate or cypionate + 17 α-ethyl-19-nor-T	255	25
	Total	1 470	17

ising results (Spence and Medvei 1959), but should not be used because of toxic effects (see sect. 7.2.4.1). High doses of testosterone undecanoate (3×80 mg daily for 10 weeks) did not lead to uniform suppression of spermatogenesis, however, slightly improved seminal parameters were observed after cessation of therapy (Kloer et al. 1980). Confirmation of this observation in a larger number of patients is required.

The highest pregnancy rate achieved under rebound therapy was reported by Rowley and Heller (1972). These authors administered a combination of 20 mg/day oral norethandrolone (17α-ethyl-19-nor-testosterone) plus 200 mg i.m. testosterone enanthate in weeks 1, 3, and 6 of treatment: a pregnancy rate of 43% was achieved (Table 2). Charny and Gordon (1978), combining testosterone injections with oral norethandrolone, reported a pregnancy rate of 25% in 255 patients. Further studies using this combination cannot be performed, since norethandrolone (Nilevar, G. D. Searle and Co.) has been withdrawn from the market.

A final assessment of rebound therapy is difficult because all studies reported to date were performed as uncontrolled clinical trials, i.e., without a double-blind design or even a placebo group. Moreover, clear guidelines have not emerged for the selection of patients who may benefit from this treatment and the most effective therapeutic regimen has not been identified. Thus, this method for the treatment of male infertility remains equivocal.

7.4 References

Carbone JV, Grodsky GM, Hjelte V (1959) Effect of hepatic dysfunction on circulating levels of sulphobromopthalein and its metabolites. J Clin Invest 38:1989–1996

Charny CW, Gordon JA (1978) Testosterone rebound therapy: a neglected modality. Fertil Steril 29:64–68

Coert A, Geelen J, de Visser J, van der Vies J (1975) The pharmacology and metabolism of testosterone undecanoate (TU), a new orally active androgen. Acta Endocrinol 79:789–800

Daggett PR, Wheeler MJ, Nabarro JDN (1978) Oral testosterone: a reappraisal. Horm Res 9:121–129

Danner Ch, Frick J (1980) Androgen substitution with testosterone-containing nasal drops. Int J Androl 3:429–435

Davidson JM, Camargo CA, Smith ER (1979) Effects of androgens on sexual behaviour in hypogonadal men. J Clin Endocrinol Metab 48:955–958

de Lange WE, Snoep MC, Doorenbos H (1979) The effect of short-term testosterone treatment in boys with delayed puberty. Acta Endocrinol 91:177–183

de Lorimer AA, Gordan GS, Löwe RC, Carbone JV (1965) Methyltestosterone: related steroids and liver function. Arch Intern Med 116:289–294

Farrell GC, Uren RF, Perkins KW, Joshua DE, Baird PJ, Kronenburg H (1975) Androgen-induced hepatoma. Lancet 1:430–432

Franchi F, Luisi M, Kicovic PM (1978) Long-term study of oral testosterone undecanote in hypogonadal males. Int J Androl 3:1–9

Frey H, Aakvaag A, Saanum D, Falch J (1979) Bioavailability of oral testosterone in males. Eur J Clin Pharmacol 16:345–349

Frick J, Bartsch G, Marberger H (1976) Steroidal compounds (injectable and implants) affecting spermatogenesis in men. J Reprod Fertil [Suppl] 24:35–47

Getzoff PL (1955) Clinical evaluation of testicular biopsy and the rebound phenomenon. Fertil Steril 6:465–474

Gordon RD, Thomas MJ, Poynting JM, Stocks AE (1975) Effect of mesterolone on plasma LH, FSH and testosterone. Andrologia 7:287–296

Hamburger C (1958) Testosterone treatment and 17-ketosteroid excretion. Acta Endocrinol 28:529–536

Heckel NJ (1951) Spermatogenic rebound in the human following the administration of testosterone propionate. AMA Arch Surg 53:4–8

Heckel NJ, McDonald JH (1952) The rebound phenomenon of the spermatogenic activity of the human testis following the administration of testosterone propionate. Fertil Steril 3:49–61

Heller CG, Maddock WO (1947) The clinical uses of testosterone in the male. Vitam Horm 5:393–432

Heller CG, Nelson WO, Hill IC, Henderson E, Maddock O, Jungck EC (1950a) The effect of testosterone administration upon the human testis. J Clin Endocrinol 10:816

Heller CG, Nelson WO, Hill IB, Henderson E, Maddock WO, Jungck EC, Paulsen CA, Mortimore GE (1950b) Improvement in spermatogenesis following depression of the human testis with testosterone. Fertil Steril 1:415–422

Heywood R, Hunter B, Green OP, Kennedy SJ (1977a) The toxicity of methyltestosterone in the rat. Toxicol Lett 1:27–31

Heywood R, Chesterman H, Ball SA, Wadsworth PF (1977b) Toxicity of methyltestosterone in the beagle dog. Toxicol Lett 7:357–365

Horst HJ, Höltje WJ, Dennis M, Coert A, Geelen J, Voigt KD (1976) Lymphatic absorption and metabolism of orally administered testosterone undecanoate in man. Klin Wochenschr 54:875–879

Johnsen SG (1978) Long-term androgen therapy with oral testosterone. In: Patanelli DJ (ed) Hormonal control of male fertility. DHEW publication No (NIH) 78-1097, Bethesda, p 123–143

Johnsen SG, Bennet EP, Jensen VG (1974) Therapeutic effectiveness of oral testosterone. Lancet 2:1473–1475

Johnsen SG, Kampmann JP, Bennet EP, Jörgensen F (1976) Enzyme induction by oral testosterone. Clin Pharmacol Ther 20:233–237

Kaplan JG, Moshant T, Bernstein R, Parks JS, Bongiovanni AM (1973) Constitutional delay of growth and development: Effects of treatment with androgens. J Pediatr 82:38–43

Kato J (1977) Steroid hormone receptors in brain, hypothalamus, and hypophysis. In: Pasqualini JR (ed) Receptors and mechanism of action of steroid hormones, vol 8. Dekker, New York Basel, pp 603–672

Kies N (1974) Die klimakterische Symptomatologie aus klinisch-psychologischer Sicht. Med Welt 25:228–235

Kloer H, Hoogen H, Nieschlag E (1980) Trial of high-dose testosterone undecanote in treatment of male infertility. Int J Androl 3:121–129

Krüskemper HL, Noell G (1967) Steroidstruktur und Lebertoxizität. Acta Endocrinol 54:73–80

Lamensdorf H, Compere D, Begley G (1975) Testosterone rebound therapy in the treatment of male infertility. Fertil Steril 26:469–472

Liao S (1976) Receptors in the mechanism of action of androgens. In: Pasqualini JR (ed) Receptors and mechanism of action of steroid hormones, vol 8. Dekker, New York Basel, pp 159–214

Marynick SP, Loriaux DL, Sherins RJ, Pita JC, Lipsett MB (1979) Evidence that testosterone can suppress pituitary gonadotrophin secretion independently of peripheral aromatization. J Clin Endocrinol Metab 49:396–398

McDonald JH, Heckel NJ (1956) Further observations on the rebound phenomenon in the treatment of certain types of spermatogenic dysfunction. J Urol 75:990–992

Nieschlag E (1981) Ist die Anwendung von Methyltestosteron obsolet? Dtsch Med Wochenschr 106:1123–1125

Nieschlag E, Mauss J, Coert A, Kicovic P (1975) Plasma androgen levels in men after oral administration of testosterone or testosterone undecanoate. Acta Endocrinol 79:366–374

Nieschlag E, Cüppers HJ, Wiegelmann W, Wickings EJ (1976) Bioavailability and LH-suppressing effect of different testosterone preparations in normal and hypogonadal men. Horm Res 7:138–145

Nieschlag E, Cüppers HJ, Wickings EJ (1977) Influence of sex, testicular development and liver function on the bioavailability of oral testosterone. Eur J Clin Invest 7:145–147

Nieschlag E, Hoogen H, Bölk M, Schuster H, Wickings EJ (1978) Clinical trial with testosterone undecanoate for male fertility control. Contraception 18:607–614

Nieschlag E, Benkert O, Comhaire F, Doerr P, Schmidt H, Serio M (1979) The male climacteric (workshop report). In: van Keep PA, Serr DM, Greenblatt RB (eds) Female and male climacteric. MTP Press, Lancaster, pp 133–139

Patanelli DJ (ed) (1978) Proceedings of hormonal control of male fertility. DHEW publication No (NIH) 78-1097, Bethesda

Rowley MJ, Heller CG (1972) The testosterone rebound phenomenon in the treatment of male infertility. Fertil Steril 23:498–504

Schulte-Beerbühl M, Nieschlag E (1980) Comparison of testosterone, DHT, LH and FSH in serum after injection of testosterone enanthate or testosterone cypionate. Fertil Steril 33:201–203

Spence AW, Medvei VC (1959) Testosterone in defective spermatogenesis. Lancet 1:124–127

Werner FC, Hamger FM, Kritzler RA (1950) Jaundice during methyltestosterone therapy. Am J Med 8:325–331

Westaby DP, Paradinas FK, Ogle SK, Randell JB, Hurray-Lyon IM (1977) Liver damage from long-term methyltestosterone. Lancet 2:261–263

Zachmann MA, Murset G, Gnehm HE, Prader A (1976) Testosterone treatment of excessively tall boys. J Pediatr 88:116–123

8 Mesterolone: a New Androgen for the Treatment of Male Infertility

B. Norman Barwin

Hormonal treatment of male infertility has mainly involved the use of androgens and gonadotropins for disturbances in spermatogenesis. Mesterolone (17β-hydroxy-1α-methyl-5α-androstan-3-one) is a new androgen for the treatment of male infertility. Up to the present, only the C17-alkylated testosterone- and androstene-diol-derivatives have been used for oral androgen treatment. These steroids, given in higher doses and for longer periods, all have an inhibitory effect on gonadotropin secretion by the hypophysis and on testicular function. Mesterolone does not possess the central blocking effect of testosterone even at high doses.

8.1 Properties of Mesterolone

Mesterolone differs in its chemical structure from 17-methyl-testosterone in two respects; the position of the methyl group and the absence of a double bond between C4 and C5 (Fig. 1). Important from a clinical point of view is the fact that mesterolone, in contrast to other oral active androgens, does not have adverse liver effects and does not suppress pituitary function. The absence of inhibition of gonadotropin secretion by mesterolone could be explained by the fact that the A-ring in the steroid molecule is saturated. This kind of steroid cannot be aromatized to estrogens,

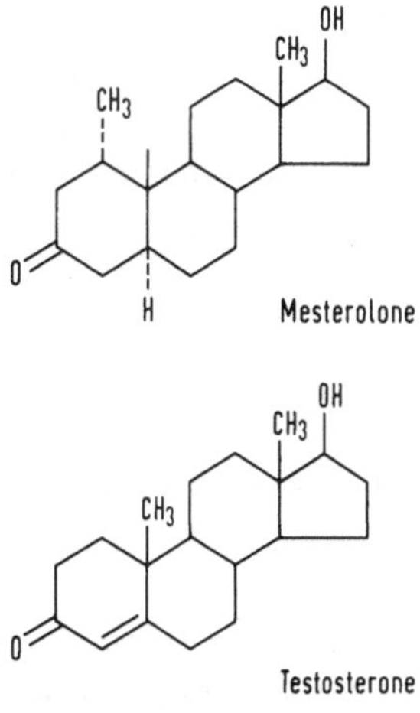

Fig. 1

which have the greatest inhibiting effect on the gonadotropin function of the hypophysis. Typically, androgens are metabolized to a measurable degree by aromatization of the A-ring, and almost certainly the estrogenic metabolites so formed are largely responsible for the negative feedback exerted by androgens on the pituitary. Mesterolone has no estrogenic action in biological systems and aromatized metabolites have never been detected in men (Petry et al. 1968).

This is the rationale for using mesterolone in the treatment of defective spermatogenesis, despite the fact that other androgens have repeatedly been shown to suppress spermatogenesis. How can we explain this rather unusual separation of properties? By far the most potent class of sex hormones in the suppression of gonadotropin secretion is that of androgens. The distinctive feature of estrogens as compared with other classes of hormonal steroids is that the A-ring is aromatic, as in benzene and its compounds. A comparative androgenic effect of other androgens is shown in Table 1.

Table 1. Comparative androgenic effect as determined by the growth of accessory sex organs in castrated male rats (Barwin et al. 1978)

Testosterone propionate	1.0
Mesterolone	0.3 – 0.4
Methyltestosterone	0.2

The possibility that the testis might be a target for its own endocrine secretion was considered years ago, and androgens were readily shown to stimulate spermatogenesis in a wide range of animal experiments (Urry and Cockett 1976). Consequently, attempts were made to do so in subfertile men. Spence and Medvei (1959) reported that 30 cases of defective spermatogenesis treated with various androgen preparations had considerable success in terms of pregnancies, but oddly enough with little change in the quality of the semen. Skepticism about the value of androgens in stimulating spermatogenesis persisted (Schellen 1970). Great interest, therefore, was aroused by the synthesis of mesterolone 1-methyl-5α-dihydrotestosterone (Petry et al. 1968). Mesterolone proved to be a rather weak androgen, but it has the surprising and unique property that, at a dosage sufficient to produce androgenic stimulation of peripheral target tissues, it has little or no effect on gonadotropin secretion (Barwin et al. 1973).

8.2 Literature Review

Hendry et al. (1973) gives fairly convincing evidence that treatment with mesterolone is beneficial. Table 2 shows the response to treatment of 69 patients who received 100 mg mesterolone daily for 1 year. Each figure shows the percentage of patients whose sperm count had risen to more than 40 million/ml. They are divided into four groups on the basis of their sperm count before treatment. Patients with azoospermia showed no response. In terms of ability to raise sperm count above 40

Table 2. Mesterolone 100 mg daily for 1 year: Results obtained in 69 patients with initial counts of less than 40 million/ml, expressed as percentage showing improvement to more than 40 million/ml (Hendry et al. 1973)

	No. of patients	Initial sperm count (millions/ml)			
		Aspermic	1–10	11–20	21–40
		7	24	27	11
3 months	69	0	17%	22%	27%
6 months	63	0	5%	35%	38%
9 months	37	–	29%	47%	50%
12 months	16	–	16%	50%	2/2
Pregnancies		–	7	4	2

Table 3. Mesterolone 100 mg daily for 1 year: Results obtained in 24 patients with initial counts of less than 10 million/ml, expressed as percentage showing improvement to more than 20 million/ml (Hendry et al. 1973)

	Sperm count more than 20 million/ml
3 months	29%
6 months	33%
9 months	57%
12 months	50%

Table 4. Mesterolone treatment: Review of results

Author	Total no. of patients	Sperm counts		Pregnancies
		Less than 10 million/ml	10–20 million/ml	
Schellen (1970)	80	67	13	9
Hendry et al. (1973)	69	31	38	13
Barwin et al. (1973)	12	2	10	3

million/ml, it made little difference whether the patients' initial sperm counts were in the 11–20 million range or in the 21–40 million range, about a quarter having responded to that extent in 3 months, a third within 6 months, and half within 9 months. Although the figures for those whose initial sperm counts were below 10 million were not as good (Table 3), the percentage of those patients whose sperm counts were raised to about 20 million was about the same. Thirteen pregnancies occurred among the wives of these 69 patients, giving a success rate of 15%.

In 12 infertile men that we reviewed (Table 4), testicular biopsy revealed all 12 patients to have normal spermatogenesis on histology (two had complete azoospermia and ten oligoasthenozoospermia). Three of the patients with oligoasthenzoospermia showed a remarkable improvement in semen analysis from pretreatment levels producing counts greater than 20 million with over 50% motility, and in another four patients the count was still in the oligozoospermic range, but there was a marked improvement in motility after 6 months of therapy. Three patients showed no improvement from their pretreatment level. From the group of 12, three pregnancies occurred after 6 months of treatment. This compares with the work of Hendry et al. (1973).

In another study (Schellen 1970), 125 patients were treated with mesterolone and the results showed that in a group of patients with sperm counts less than 5 million/ml there was no change, whereas in 24% of patients with sperm counts of 5–10 million there was a slight improvement in motility. In the last group of patients, with sperm counts of 10–20 million/ml, 16 pregnancies (20%) were subsequently achieved. Schellen concluded that the administration of mesterolone is of little use for the treatment of infertility if the sperm count is very low or zero, and the main indications for mesterolone are: (1) oligozoospermia; (2) high or elevated excretion of gonadotropin hormones; and (3) reduced seminal plasma fructose concentration.

8.3 Toleration and Function of the Liver

Mesterolone was well-tolerated in all cases and we have found no side effects. Bilirubin, transaminases in the serum, and BSP in all cases remained within normal limits. Only one case showed an increase in alkaline phosphatase. Liver biopsy samples of two patients showed no pathological changes before or after treatment with mesterolone, including the patient with increased alkaline phosphatase and LAP in the serum. Even with a dose of 150 mg given to five patients for 4 weeks, an impairment of hepatic function was not observed.

It has been shown that there are steroid receptors in all tubule cells and that labelled steroids can enter the tubule, although the presence of the label within the tubule does not enable us to say in what form it is present (Lacy 1967). However, steroids certainly enter the tubules with different facility, corticosteroids, for example, having little ability to do so (Setchell 1967). But it is not possible to say whether differential ability to penetrate the seminiferous tubules plays any part in the influence of mesterolone on spermatogenesis (Bye 1975).

The most probable explanation relates to the function of Sertoli's cells (Lacy et al. 1969). It has now been clearly established that Sertoli's cells possess all the enzymes necessary for the conversion of various precursors to testosterone, and to synthesize testosterone from cholesterol (Lacy et al. 1973). The fact that cells have the potential to carry out a certain metabolic process does not necessarily mean that, in life, the process is carried out or, if so, to a significant extent. There can be little doubt that these processes do occur, since changes in the intracellular organelles and the concentrations of certain enzymes and sterols, indicative of changing steroid metabolism in Sertoli's cells of many seasonal submammals, follow the pattern of seasonal variation in spermatogenesis (Lofts 1968). Moreover, these changes can be produced in vitro by the direct action of FSH on dissected tubules, whereas LH, which controls the activity of Leydig's cells, has no such effect on the tubules (Dorrington et al. 1973; Lacy 1973). This is in accordance with the generally accepted roles of FSH and LH; that is, that FSH influences gamete production and LH is the hormone required for stimulating secondary sexual functions. So, if there is a separate source of androgens within the seminiferous tubules, it must surely be part of the normal physiological control of spermatogenesis. For the one process unique to the gonads, the meiotic division, androgens are indispensable (Clermont and Harvey 1967).

If the androgens produced by Sertoli's cells are no more than a nonspecific contribution to a pool, the separate control of production outside and inside the tubules by the different gonadotropins would be a very odd mechanism indeed. There was in vivo evidence from the above-mentioned experiments that this difference in gonadotropin control was significant since, in the hypophysectomized rats from which these tubules were dissected, diminished production of androgens by Leydig's cells was shown by a reduction in weight of the seminal vesicles: at the same time, androgen production within the tubules was stimulated by administration of FSH. Conversely, when LH was used, androgen production by Leydig's cells was increased while that within the tubules was generally reduced (Lacy et al. 1973).

The ability of androgens to stimulate spermatogenesis by rebound of the pituitary-testicular axis (Charney and Gordon 1978) lead to the conclusion that the old theory of pituitary-testicular function was wrong, and any new model had to accommodate the idea that the testis was a target tissue for its own endocrine secretion. The evidence that there are two anatomically, and probably functionally separate sources of androgens within the testis (each of which is responsive to a single gonadotropin) returns us to the original model. In this model, LH stimulates the production of androgens from Leydig's cells in the interstitial tissue and FSH, the production of androgens from Sertoli's cells within the seminiferous tubules. The necessary androgenic stimulus to spermatogenesis is provided by the intratubular source rather than by the production of Leydig's cells, which are responsible for development and maintenance of extratesticular androgen functions.

Testosterone and its derivatives are capable of causing damage to the gonads even in therapeutic doses by suppression of gonadotropin secretion. At 24 days after starting the treatment with 25 mg i.m. testosterone daily, damage to the germ cells and reduction of Leydig's cells was already observed (Petry et al. 1968). There was no detectable gonadotropin excretion in the urine and the number of spermatozoa was greatly reduced. The histologic picture of the testes showed that the tubules were greatly reduced in size. There were sclerosis and hyalinization of the basal membrane, tunica propria, and necrosis of germinal epithelium. Leydig's cells could not longer be detected (Petry et al. 1968).

Hendry et al. (1973) showed that mesterolone has no effect on urinary LH and FSH excretion with a dose of up to 60 mg/day. Petry (1968) examined total gonadotropin excretion with a dose of up to 150 mg daily from 3 days to 2.5 months and found no reduction.

It then appears that gonadotropins are not essential for spermatogenesis, in which they play no direct role, and that their place can be taken by androgens. If this is so, some other explanation must be sought for the extremely high potency of mesterolone in stimulating the secondary sexual organs. Two possible explanations seem likely. One is that mesterolone has a superior ability to penetrate the seminiferous tubules, which, of course, an androgen must do in order to stimulate the germinal epithelium. The Sertoli's cells, which for want of a better name, used to be called "supporting cells", do not contribute to the formation of gametes, but clearly have a metabolic function. Electron-microscopy has shown that tight junctions exist between Sertoli's cells so that no germinal cells are in direct contact with the walls of the seminiferous tubules.

8.4 Conclusions

Because most cases of infertility are idiopathic, there is no reason to assume that a large percentage will benefit from androgen therapy. There are two sources of androgen production, and it is the source outside the tubules – the one that is not apparently concerned with spermatogenesis – that produces the systemic manifestations of androgenicity. Those manifestations, when normal, do not in themselves prove that androgen deficiency within the seminiferous tubules is not present. Consider the so-called fertile eunuch, who has normal spermatogenesis, but very little secondary sexual development. Presumably, in such cases the production of androgens by Sertoli's cells within the tubules is normal, while production in Leydig's cells is not.

In patients treated with mesterolone, there were no signs of impairment of hepatic function though this is often caused by C17-alkylated testosterone and antrostenediol derivatives. It can be stated from this investigation, that mesterolone is a steroid with good antrogenic effect. In therapeutic and higher doses it does not have a damaging effect on the liver or any detectable inhibiting effect on pituitary gonadotropin secretion and male gonads.

Lacy et al. (1973) found mesterolone, in the form of an injectable ester, to be successful in fully restoring apparently normal spermatogenesis after long-term suppression of gonadotropin production in the rat. They have not been able to obtain comparable results with other androgens (Lacy et al. 1969).

In maintenance experiments immediately after hypophysectomy or after gonadotropin suppression, the seminiferous tubules retain the capacity to synthesize an androgen (not testosterone) needed for spermatogenesis. Mesterolone is unique among synthetic androgens in being a derivative not of testosterone but of the reduced form, 5α-dihydrotestosterone. Where the natural hormone is of limited effectiveness because of its rapid rate of breakdown, mesterolone, which is methylated in the 1 position, is more stable. Therefore, it may be that, despite mesterolone's advantage in not suppressing gonadotropin production, its ability to obviate certain metabolic steps in the stimulation of spermatogenesis may be of equal, or even greater importance. Lacy's work in the rat remains to be confirmed in the human, but if the same, apparently complete maintenance of spermatogenesis in the absence of gonadotropins can be shown, there will no longer be the need to postulate any direct role of gonadotropins in spermatogenesis. The way would then be open to use oral mesterolone in even larger doses than is recommended at present, since some suppression of gonadotropins would then be unimportant. The toxicity of steroids in large doses exerts restraint on their use, but mesterolone is not alkylated in the 17 position and it may be that doses even higher than those presently used will not induce liver toxicity.

Mesterolone is a new androgen which may prove useful in the treatment of male infertility. It is indicated when there is low sperm count and poor motility. It is also useful in cases of high or elevated gonadotropins. Mesterolone has been found to be well tolerated and offers some hope for the future management of some infertile patients.

8.5 References

Amelar RD, Dubin L (1977) The Management of idiopathic male infertility. J Reprod Med 18:191–197

Barwin BN, Clarke SD, Biggart JD (1973) Mesterolone in the treatment of male infertility. Practitioner 211:669–675

Barwin BN, McKay D, Jolly E, Hudson RW (1978) Pharmacological therapy in male infertility. Prog Reprod Biol 3:131–142

Bye P (1975) Recent advances in the treatment of male sub-fertility. Postgrad Med J 51:215–218

Charny CW, Gordon JA (1978) Testosterone rebound therapy: A neglected modality. Fertil Steril 29:64–79

Check JH, Rakoff AE (1977) Improved fertility in oligospermic males treated with clomiphene citrate. Fertil Steril 28:746–751

Clermont Y, Harvey SC (1967) Endocrinology of the testis. Ciba Found Colloq Endocrinol 16:173–186

Dorrington JH, Vernon RE, Fritz IB (1973) Effect of FSH on the 3',5'-AMP content of seminiferous tubules. In: Proceedings of the IVth international congress of endocrinology, Washington, D.C., 1972 (Abstract 537). Excerpta Medica, Amsterdam

Hendry WF, Sommerville IF, Hall RR, Pugh CB (1973) Investigation and treatment of the subfertile male. Br J Urol 45:670

Lacy D (1967) The seminiferous tubule in mammals. Endeavour 26:101–107

Lacy D (1973) Androgen dependency of spermatogenesis and the physiological significance of steroid metabolism in vitro by the seminiferous tubules. The Endocrine function of the human testis, vol I. Academic Press, New York London

Lacy D, Rotblat J (1958) Effects of ionising radiation on the testis of the rat with some observations on its normal morphology. In: Proceedings of the IVth international congress on electron microscopy, Berlin, vol II. Springer, Berlin Göttingen Heidelberg, pp 484–486

Lacy D, Vinson GP, Collins P, Bell J, Fyson P, Pudney J, Pettitt J (1969) Progress in endocrinology. In: Proceedings of the IIIrd international congress of endocrinology, Mexico, 1968. Excerpta Medica, Amsterdam

Lacy D, Bass JJ, Bell JBG, Collins PM, Fyson P, Pettitt AJ, Pudney J (1973) Steroid metabolism by the seminiferous tubules of mammals and its biological and medical significance. In: Proceedings of the IVth international congress of endocrinology, Washington D.C., 1972 (Abstract 46). Excerpta Medica, Amsterdam

Lofts B (1968) Patterns of testicular activity. In: Barrington EVM, Barker-Jorgensen C (eds) Perspectives in endocrinology. Academic Press, New York London

Petry R, Rausch-Stroomann JG, Heinz HA, Senge T, Mauss J (1968) Androgen treatment without inhibiting effect on hypophysis and male gonads. Acta Endocrinol 59:497–503

Schellen TCM (1970) Results with mesterolone in the treatment of disturbances of spermatogenesis. Andrologia 2:1–9

Setchell BP (1967) The blood testicular fluid in sheep. J Physiol (Lond) 189:63–67

Spence AW, Medrei VC (1959) Testosterone in defective spermatogenesis. Lancet 1:124–127

Urry RL, Cockett TK (1976) Treating the subfertile male patient: improvement in semen characteristics after low-dose androgen therapy. J Urol 116:54–58

9 Kinin-Releasing Pancreatic Proteinase Kallikrein

W. B. Schill

Pancreatic kallikrein, a kinin-releasing proteinase, has recently been demonstrated to be a possible new therapeutic agent in some forms of male infertility (Schill 1979 a). Andrological therapy in general is largely empiric and, therefore, often unsuccessful. However, through the introduction of this tissue hormone-releasing proteinase the spectrum of andrological therapy is broadened, especially in cases of idiopathic normogonadotropic oligozoospermia and asthenozoospermia. This report will summarize the available experimental and clinical data about the efficacy of kallikrein and the kallikrein-kinin system in andrology and will discuss the practical aspects of kallikrein treatment.

9.1 Kallikrein-Kinin System

9.1.1 Biochemistry and Physiology

The kallikrein-kinin system is a complex biological system with four major components (Erdös 1970): kininogen; kininogenases (kallikreins); kinins; and kininases (Fig. 1). The specific effectors of the kallikrein-kinin system are the kinins, which are polypeptides of great biological potential, acting as tissue hormones at the cellular level. The best known kinins are the nonapeptide bradykinin (Bk), the decapeptide kallidin (Lys-Bk), and methionylkallidin (Fig. 2). Methionylkallidin and kallidin are converted by aminopeptidases into bradykinin. Kinins normally have very short life spans due to a rapid degradation by exo- and endopeptidases, the kininases, present in blood plasma, body fluids, and tissue extracts. Two kininases are present in human serum (kininase I and II) and degrade kinins to inactive peptides by cleavage of the C-terminal arginine residue or hydrolysis of the prolyl-phenylalanine bond between positions 7 and 8. Kinins are released from kininogen, occurring ubiquitously in a low and high molecular weight form in serum and in all body fluids. Kinin liberation by limited proteolysis is possible by kininogenases (kallikreins) present in blood plasma (plasma kallikrein) and in tissues (glandular or organ kallikrein). High concentrations of a tissue kallikrein are found especially in the secretory glands (pancreas, submandibular glands) and the kidneys (Dietl et al. 1978; Lemon et al. 1979).

Pancreatic kallikrein (EC 3.4.21.8) is a glycoprotein with a molecular weight of approximately 29,000 and belongs to the serin proteinases. It is isolated from auto-

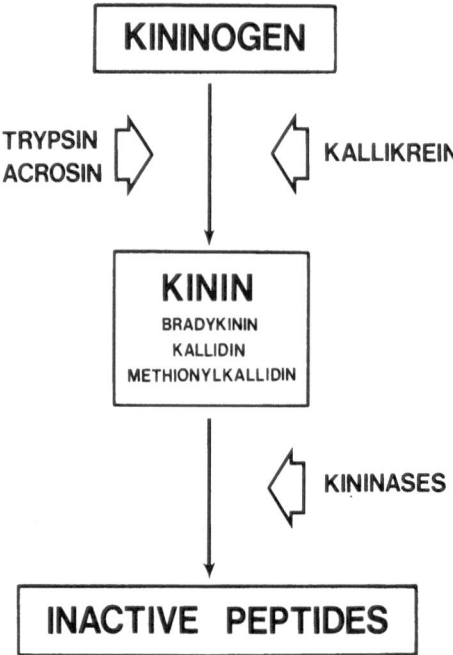

Fig. 1. Pathways of the kallikrein-kinin system

lyzed hog pancreas and shows multiple enzymatic forms at least in part due to a varying carbohydrate content (5%–12%). Commercially available kallikrein preparations contain two molecular forms (kallikrein A and B) which differ only in the composition of the carbohydrate portion, but not in the amino acid composition (232 amino acid residues) and in the enzymatic properties (Fritz 1975). There is a close structural homology between hog pancreatic kallikrein and trypsin (Tschesche et al. 1979). Whereas plasma kallikrein is considered to be an important factor of the blood clotting system, organ kallikreins have high substrate specificity which seems to be limited to the production of kinins from kininogen only. Kallikreins themselves are liberated from inactive precursors called prekallikreins. In the case of pancreatic kallikrein, the enzyme is liberated by trypsin. Other kininogenases with broad substrate specificity are trypsin, plasmin, and acrosin.

Apart from major components of the kallikrein-kinin system, other substrates are directly or indirectly involved in kinin generation or degradation: prekallikrein activator; inhibitors of kallikreins, such as α_2-macroglobulin; C$\bar{\text{I}}$-inactivator; α_1-antitrypsin; and inhibitors of the kininases.

The physiological significance of the kallikrein-kinin system is still not yet completely understood. There is a close inter-relationship between this system and

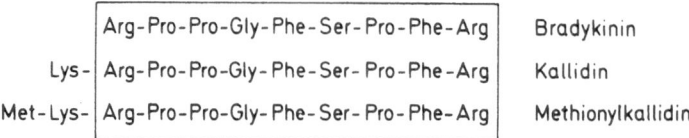

Fig. 2. Primary structure of kinins

coagulation, fibrinolysis and the complement system, the prostaglandin system, and the angiotensin-renin system (Fujii et al. 1979 a, b). Kinins are involved in enhancing vascular permeability and lowering blood pressure; they also have pain-producing properties, stimulate smooth muscle contractions, and improve glucose transport through cell membranes (Erdös 1970; Meng and Haberland 1973; Wicklmayr et al. 1978). They contribute to the muscular reactions of the carcinoid syndrome, hereditary angioedema, and inflammation, where they are effective mediators. The kinin system is also involved in cell proliferation of various tissues (Haberland and Rohen 1973; Haberland et al. 1975 a, b, 1977).

9.1.2 Reproductive Functions

The kallikrein-kinin system may be involved in reproductive function as follows: (1) involvement in the transport of spermatozoa through the female genital tract by smooth muscle contractions of the uterus; (2) stimulation of sperm motility; (3) involvement in spermatogenesis by improving total sperm output.

The kallikrein-kinin system is involved in reproductive functions mainly by its participation in the regulation and stimulation of sperm motility and spermatogenesis. This is supported by the fact that all components of the kinin system are present in male and female genital secretions: low amounts of kininogen as the specific substrate for kallikrein, kininases as the kinin-inactivating enzymes and kinin-liberating proteinases (Palm et al. 1976). As long as these three components are present in the body fluids, generation and inactivation of kinins take place continuously. If this is not so, sperm motility may be impaired and lead to reduced fertility.

Identification of the relevant kininogenase in human seminal plasma and cervical mucus is still necessary. The presence of a potent kininogenase in the coagulating gland of the guinea pig has recently been established (Moriwaki et al. 1975). The following proteinases of human genital secretions may be involved in kinin generation: the sperm specific proteinase acrosin; a tissue kallikrein from the prostate; kallikrein from blood plasma; leukocytic proteinases.

Acrosin released from dead spermatozoa occurs in seminal plasma as an inactive enzyme-inhibitor complex. Thus, acrosin only plays a role as a potent kinin-liberating enzyme in the female genital tract when it is released from desintegrating or dead spermatozoa during intrauterine sperm migration. In the presence of kininogen, kinins will be released, stimulating the motility of the surviving vital spermatozoa (Schill et al. 1979a). The occurrence of a potent kininogenase in human seminal plasma, thus far unidentified, has been demonstrated (Schill and Preissler 1977). This proteinase may be identical with trace amounts of a tissue kallikrein originating from prostatic secretions.

Kininogenase inhibitors may be present in seminal plasma and cervical mucus. Aside from low concentrations of α_1-antitrypsin and α_1-antichymotrypsin, no other plasma proteinase inhibitors are found in seminal plasma (Schill 1976). However, high levels of low molecular weight, acid-stable proteinase inhibitors which inhibit acrosin (acrostatin = HUSI II) and leukocytic proteinases (leucostatin = HUSI I) are present in human seminal plasma (Fritz et al. 1975). For this reason, acrosin released into the seminal plasma from spermatozoa cannot act on kininogen. The same is true for leukocytic proteinases, which are inhibited rapidly and completely by leucostatin. Human cervical mucus contains more kininogenase inhibitors, such as α_1-antitrypsin, α_1-antichymotrypsin, inter-α-trypsin inhibitor, antithrombin III, and $\overline{C_1}$-esterase inhibitor. However, the concentrations of these inhibitors during midcycle are so low that inhibition of kininogenases in ovulatory cervical mucus should occur only very slowly (Schumacher 1973). Measurable amounts of a low molecular weight, acid-stable cervical mucus inhibitor are directed against leukocytic proteinases, but do not interfere with kallikrein.

From these data it can be concluded that alterations of the homeostasis of the kallikrein-kinin system in the male and female reproductive tract have to be considered as pathophysiological. It may, therefore, be mandatory in the future to quantiatively determine components of the kallikrein-kinin system in human genital secretions providing additional diagnostic information.

9.2 Experimental Investigations

9.2.1 In Vitro Studies

The significance of the kallikrein-kinin system in the stimulation and maintenance of sperm motility was established by in vitro studies using fresh and aged semen specimens with populations of spermatozoa showing reduced motility. Pancreatic kallikrein and kinins, respectively, show the following effects on spermatozoa:

1. Increase of the mean sperm velocity, demonstrated by Laser-Doppler-spectroscopy (Fig. 3) (Steiner et al. 1977; Thompson et al. 1980);
2. increase of the percentage of motile spermatozoa (Schill et al. 1974; Sato 1980; Schütte et al. 1981);
3. significant shift of the number of spermatozoa with poor motility to those with very good forward progression (Schill and Haberland 1975);
4. slight improvement of sperm viability (Leidl et al. 1975);
5. stimulation of sperm motility in fresh and 24-h old spermatozoa, as well as in frozen semen specimens (Schill and Haberland 1975; Schill and Pritsch 1976);
6. stimulation of sperm metabolism (increased consumption of fructose and oxygen, increased production of lactic acid and CO_2, small increase of the intracellular cAMP level) (Leidl et al. 1975; Schill 1978a);
7. significant improvement of cervical mucus penetration (Wallner et al. 1975; Schill et al. 1976b; Schill and Preissler 1977; Steiner et al. 1981);
8. inhibition of sperm motility by kinin-inactivating enzymes (kininases) (Schill and Haberland 1975);
9. enhancement of sperm metabolism and motility in bull spermatozoa (Leidl et al. 1975; Bratanov et al. 1978).

Maximal stimulation of sperm motility was obtained with 5 kallikrein units (KU) per ml ejaculate corresponding to 3.5 µg kallikrein. However, there was a wide range of individual variation (0.1–100 KU/ml).

Kinins are the mediators of the kallikrein effect, though an additional indirect effect of kinins via the activation of prostaglandin synthesis should not be excluded (Palm et al. 1976). Figure 4 schematically illustrates the hypothetical mode of action

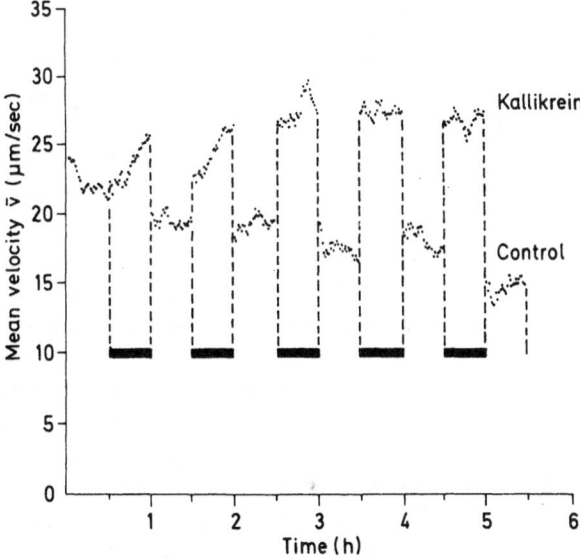

Fig. 3. Mean velocity ($\bar{v}$) of human spermatozoa determined by Laser-Doppler spectroscopy in the presence of 2 IU kallikrein per ml ejaculate. Each point represents one experiment performed within 45 s. Intervals between control and sample, 30 min (Steiner et al. 1977)

of how kallikrein and kinins, respectively, stimulate sperm metabolism at the cellular level. One possibility is the occurrence of kinin receptors at the surface of the plasma membrane of the sperm cell. Another more likely pathway is that kinins accelerate glucose and fructose transport across the sperm cell membrane and, thus, stimulate sperm metabolism.

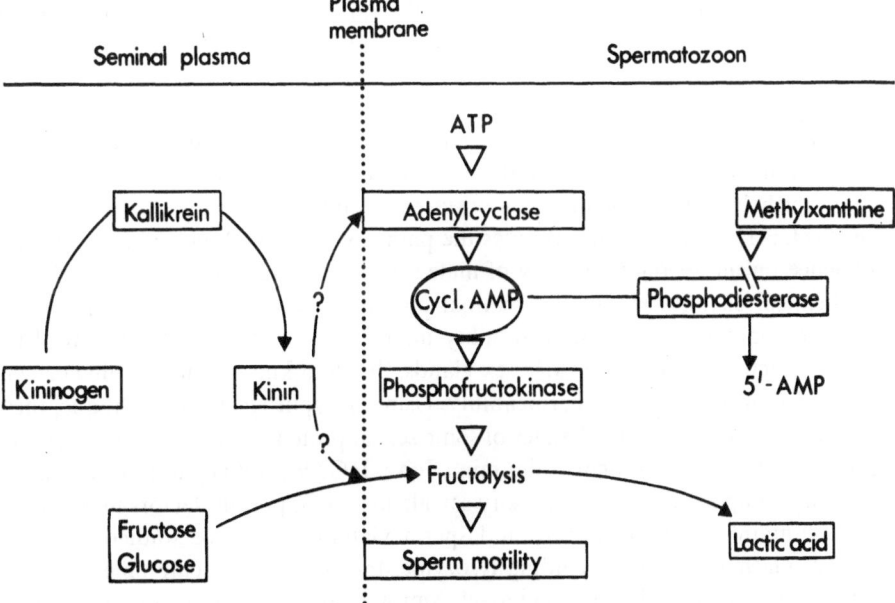

Fig. 4. Hypothetical mode of action of kallikrein and kinins on sperm metabolism

9.2.2 Animal Studies

Involvement of the kallikrein-kinin system in cell proliferation of various tissues (Rixon et al. 1971; Haberland et al. 1977 for summary) triggered clinical studies in subfertile men indicating an effect of kallikrein on the spermatogenic process and sperm motility. These investigations also stimulated several animal studies (primarily in the rat) to investigate the mode of action of pancreatic kallikrein with special reference to spermatogenic function.

The following experimental data were found in the rat: activation of Sertoli's cell function (Rohen and Buschhüter 1975) and increased numbers of supporting cells (Kleeberg et al. 1975); increase of relative number of spermatocytes and first appearance of A-spermatogonia 1–2 days earlier in premature rats (Rohen and Stuttmann 1977); increase of ^{3}H-thymidine incorporation in the DNA of the testicular tissue of adult rats (Matthiessen and Rohen 1975); enhancement of glucose-intake due to an increase of membrane permeability (Dennhardt and Haberich 1973; Meng and Haberland 1973); increase of testicular blood flow (Blümel et al. 1975); selective concentrations of kallikrein in the epithelium of the ductus epididymis (Blasini et al. 1980); high concentrations of kininase II (angiotensin-converting enzyme) demonstrable in testis and epididymis (Cushman and Cheung 1971; Hohlbrugger et al. 1980); intestinal resorption of orally administered kallikrein is 3%–5% (Moriwaki et al. 1973). Additional uptake of kallikrein by the ductus thoracicus was recently described (Fink et al. 1980).

In conclusion, although some of the available data are still preliminary, there is increasing experimental evidence demonstrating involvement of the kallikrein-kinin system in reproductive functions.

9.2.3 Biochemical and Endocrinological Studies in Men

In addition to the experimental studies in the rat, Dietze et al. (1977) showed that the kallikrein-kinin system participates in the physiological regulation of muscular substrate metabolism during muscular work and hypoxia. According to these studies, using the human forearm as a model to study muscular metabolism, kinins seem to increase muscular glucose uptake in an insulin-like manner by means of an acceleration of the glucose transport across the cell membranes.

Nevertheless, the mode of action of systemic kallikrein therapy in subfertile men (see Sect. 3.1) is still obscure. Besides the pathways already discussed (see Sect. 2.), influence on the secretory activity of male sex glands might be feasible, leading to biochemical changes within the seminal plasma. Tauber et al. (1977) speculated whether improvement of sperm motility might be possible via stimulation of the secretory activity of the accessory sex glands, due to a kinin-induced enhancement of blood flow and capillary permeability. Using the split-ejaculate technique, these authors showed significant changes of some serum proteins found in seminal plasma during kallikrein treatment (albumin, IgA, IgG, α_1-antichymotrypsin). Since secretory components of the accessory sex glands are important factors in triggering and maintaining sperm motility and sperm viability, we have studied the same seminal plasma proteins, including lysozyme, transferrin, the acute-phase proteins CRP (C-reacting protein) and acid α_1-glycoprotein and two seminal plasma proteinases (seminin, BAEE-splitting enzyme) (Schill et al. 1980). A significant increase only in α_1-antichymotrypsin during oral kallikrein therapy could be demonstrated. It is concluded that kallikrein treatment affects, at least to a certain degree, the secretory activity of the male sex glands and the blood-seminal plasma barrier, respectively. However, it is still speculative whether changes of the secretory components of the accessory sex glands are one of the mechanisms stimulating sperm motility.

Another mode of action of systemic kallikrein therapy might be its interference with the pituitary-gonadal system, as suspected by Hartenbach (1954) and Igarashi et al. (1962) using crude bioassay methods. Radioimmunological investigations performed by Török et al. (1978) showed no changes of LH, FSH, and testosterone levels in patients treated orally with a daily dose of 300 IU kallikrein for 7 weeks. In contrast, recent radioimmunological investigations by Schill and Rjosk (1979) in subfertile men (600 KU/day kallikrein for 3 months) showed a significant increase of serum LH, prolactin, and testosterone levels, whereas FSH levels were not affected. In contrast, LH and prolactin, determined in the seminal plasma of the same patients, showed no change. Growth hormone and serum cortisol levels also remained constant (Schill and Braun 1981). These findings indicate an influence of systemic kallikrein administration on the hormonal balance of the pituitary-gonadal axis, possibly leading to an increased intratesticular testosterone level necessary to maintain and accelerate spermatogenesis. In addition, locally increased testosterone levels might favor epididymal sperm maturation with an improvement of sperm viability and sperm motility. However, besides the observed increase of the strictly target-cell-oriented sex hormones, the local action of kinins as biologically active tissue hormones involved in cell proliferation of various tissues has to be considered as primarily responsible for the observed spermatogenic effects.

9.3 Clinical Investigations and Application

9.3.1 Systemic Kallikrein Treatment

Clinical studies performed during recent years in several independent andrological centers around the world have shown that kallikrein therapy can be used in cases of idiopathic asthenozoospermia (Schill 1975 a; Lunglmayr 1976; Schütte and Schirren 1977; Homonnai et al. 1978; Kamidono et al. 1981), idiopathic normogonadotropic oligozoospermia (Hofmann et al. 1975; Schill 1975 b; Török 1979; Schill et al. 1980), oligozoospermia due to primary testicular failure with slightly elevated FSH levels (Schill 1978 b; Schirren 1978; Sato et al. 1979), oligoasthenoteratozoospermia of unknown origin (Stüttgen 1973; Schill 1975 b; Schirren et al. 1975), polyzoospermia (Stüttgen 1975), and teratozoospermia (Hofmann et al. 1975; Schill 1975 b).

Kallikrein therapy is empirically based and there are no parameters available to predict for a single patient whether it will be successful. Best results are obtained in idiopathic forms of oligozoospermia and asthenozoospermia, whereas in spermatogenic arrest or severe testicular failure no effects are seen. In some men with polyzoospermia normalization of sperm numbers is found; in men with mild teratozoospermia the number of morphologically abnormal spermatozoa is sometimes reduced.

9.3.1.1 Open Clinical Trials

Several open clinical trials have shown that kallikrein treatment leads to a quantitative and qualitative improvement of sperm motility, an increase in the number of spermatozoa and a slight improvement of the percentage of morphologically normal spermatozoa in about 30%–50% of infertile men with idiopathic fertility disturbances. In asthenozoospermia, an improvement of sperm motility will be the primary effect. In oligozoospermia and oligoasthenozoospermia, the number and motility of spermatozoa will be improved. Interestingly, in asthenozoospermia, in contrast to an improvement of sperm motility, a decrease of sperm number is sometimes found. Mean sperm count, however, will still be within the normal range and there will be sperm recovery within 3 months after cessation of therapy.

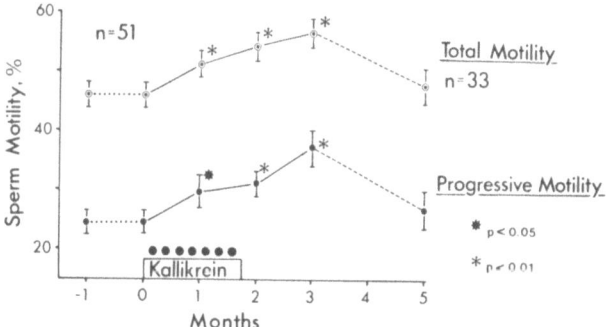

Fig. 5. Kallikrein therapy in 51 subfertile men with idiopathic asthenozoospermia. Daily oral administration of 600 IU pancreatic kallikrein over a period of 7 weeks. Mean ±SEM values of total and progressive sperm motility are plotted (Kienitz and Schill 1977)

Figure 5 shows an example of the results obtained with oral administration of kallikrein in 51 men with idiopathic asthenozoospermia treated over a period of 7 weeks (Kienitz and Schill 1977). Quantitative and qualitative sperm motility increased 1 month after initiation of therapy, reaching a maximum 1 month after withdrawal of kallikrein medication, and followed by a decline to pretreatment values. In individual cases, however, improved motility was observed for several weeks and months. The reason for this long-term effect is not known. It may come from a direct effect of kallikrein on epididymal function. Of the asthenozoospermic men, 65% responded with a distinct improvement of progressive sperm motility, whereas 14% showed no change and 21% even showed impaired motility. Conception rate within 1 year after the start of kallikrein treatment was 31%. Most of the conceptions occurred within the first 5 months after initiation of therapy, with a maximum around the second and the third months. The abortion rate was 9%. Similar results with improvement of semen parameters (sperm motility, sperm number) were found in subfertile men suffering from idiopathic oligozoospermia (Fig. 6).

9.3.1.2 Double-Blind Studies

The clinical trials were confirmed by the results of a double-blind study in 90 subfertile male subjects with idiopathic oligozoospermia (Fig. 7) showing a significant

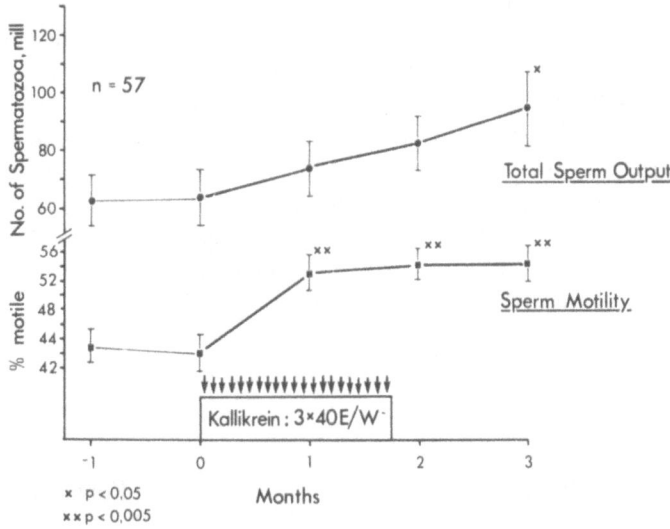

Fig. 6. Kallikrein therapy in 57 subfertile men with idiopathic oligozoospermia. One injection of 40 IU i.m. pancreatic kallikrein was given three times weekly over a period of 7 weeks. Mean ±SEM values of total sperm output and progressive sperm motility are plotted (Schill 1978b)

increase in the number of spermatozoa (average increase 31 million per ejaculate) with a maximum at 2–3 months after onset of the trial (Schill 1979b). In addition, quantitative and qualitative sperm motility was improved, reaching a maximum at the end of the treatment period (Fig. 8). Conception rates within a period of 1 year were 16% for placebo and 38% for kallikrein (p < 0.05). Abortion rates were similar in both groups (20% placebo, 14% kallikrein). No abnormalities were reported in the

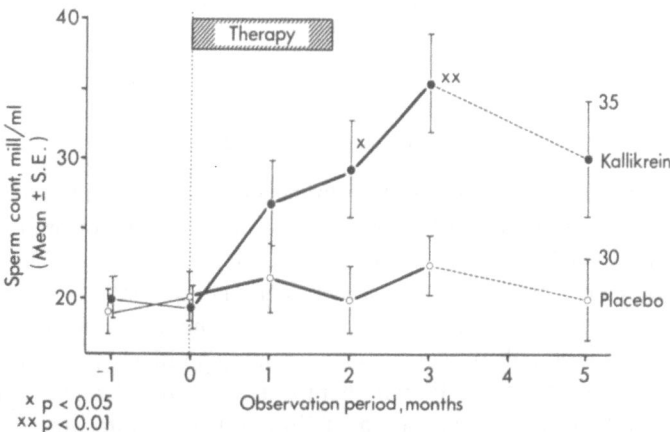

Fig. 7. Mean ±SEM sperm count in million per ml obtained during a double-blind study in 90 men with idiopathic oligozoospermia (placebo, 42 men; kallikrein, 48 men) during a treatment period of 7 weeks. The number of semen analyses performed 5 months after onset of the treatment are 35 in the kallikrein group and 30 in the placebo group (Schill 1979b)

babies after delivery. When the time of conception was investigated and correlated with the onset of therapy, conceptions accumulated within the first 6 months after initiation of kallikrein therapy, whereas, in the placebo group, conceptions occurred randomly during the observation period of 1 year. The significant increase in the conception rate in the kallikrein group was supported during a double-blind crossover study by Propping et al. (1978). Furthermore, the increase of the sperm number was very recently confirmed in a double-blind crossover study by Bedford and Elstein (1981). In contrast, Nürnberger and Grassow (1977) were unable to show any effect of systemic kallikrein administration, however, the patient group was too small to draw conclusions.

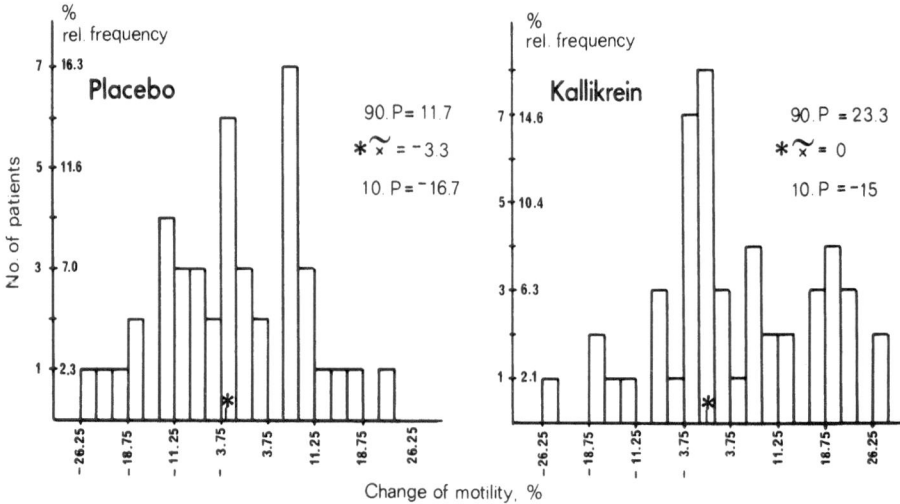

Fig. 8. Mean values and level differences between pre- and post-treatment levels of the total sperm motility in the placebo and kallikrein group (see Fig. 7). There are significant differences in the size of the distribution curves between both groups (Schill 1979 b)

9.3.1.3 Routes of Administration and Side Effects

Pancreatic kallikrein can be administered either parenterally (Fig. 9) in the form of intramuscular injections (40 IU three times weekly) or orally in the form of coated tablets (600 IU daily). Oral administration seems to give better results compared to parenteral treatment. A treatment period of 3 months is more effective than shorter treatment periods (Fig. 10). Long-term administration for 6–12 months is a possibility, especially in those cases responding positively to 3-months treatment.

Side effects of kallikrein therapy are rare; they include vertigo, diarrhea, allergic eruptions, and exacerbation of chronic male genital tract infections with the development of acute prostatitis or epididymitis due to kinin liberation. Therefore, male genital tract inflammation is an absolute contraindication to kallikrein therapy. A positive effect of kallikrein on libido and sexual behavior has not been established.

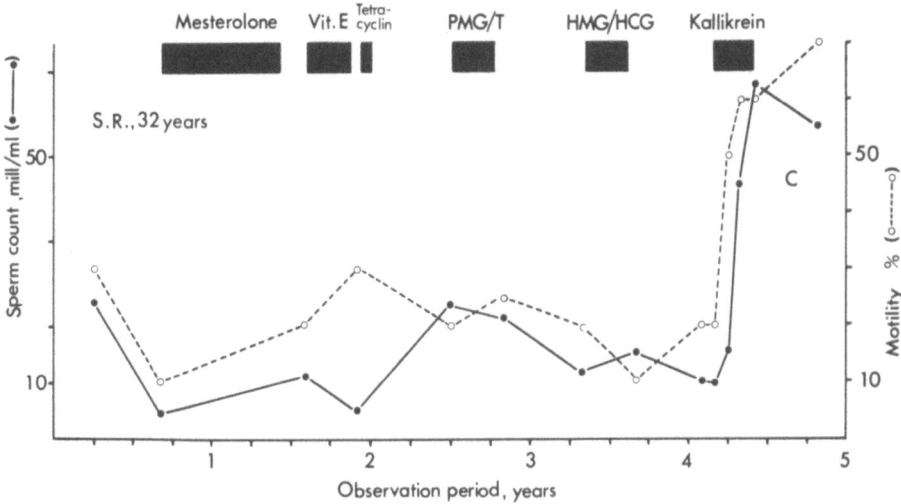

Fig. 9. Parenteral administration of 40 IU i.m. pancreatic kallikrein three times weekly over a period of 3 months in a 32-year-old man with idiopathic normogonadotropic oligozoospermia. The patient had suffered from primary sterility for 3 years and was followed-up for 5 years. Within this follow-up period, the following different treatment schedules were performed without any significant improvement of semen parameters: mesterolone; vitamin E; tetracycline; a combination of pregnant mare's gonadotropin and testosterone; and a combined human gonadotropin therapy. In contrast, kallikrein application led to a dramatic improvement of sperm count and sperm motility. A conception (c) occurred 3 months after withdrawal of the medication

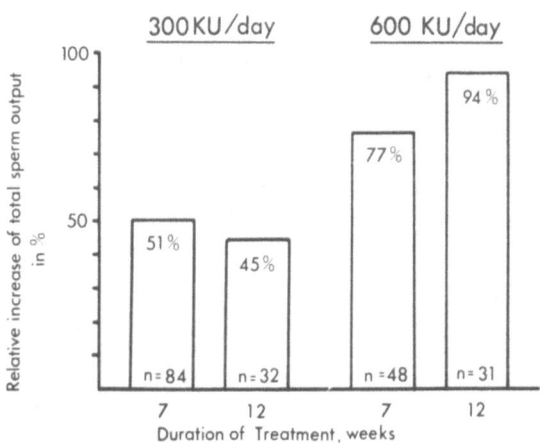

Fig. 10. Efficacy of the different regimens of oral kallikrein therapy in men with idiopathic oligozoospermia. Total sperm output as determined 3 months after initiation of therapy was used for comparison (Schill et al. 1980)

9.3.2 In Vitro Improvement of Human Semen

Since impaired sperm motility is a major factor causing infertility, improvement of motility is an important therapeutic goal in the treatment of male subfertility. In patients with reduced sperm motility (asthenozoospermia, oligoasthenozoospermia) who are unresponsive to medical treatment, topical administration of kallikrein to semen in combination with instrumental insemination may be a promising ap-

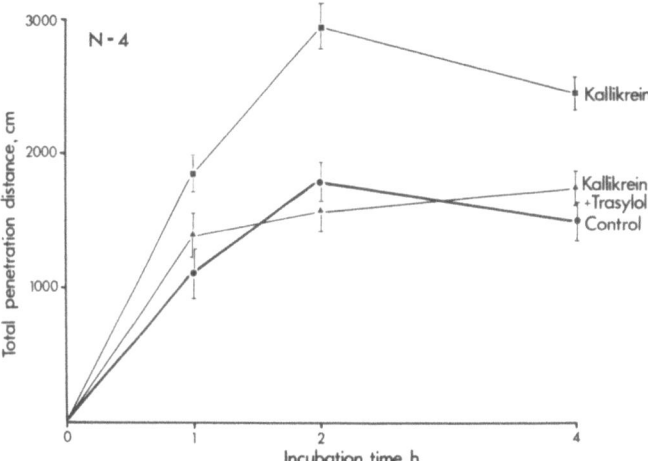

Fig. 11. Kallikrein-induced enhancement of cervical mucus sperm penetration through human midcycle determined by the Kremer capillary tube test. The mean values of four typical experiments using oligozoospermic ejaculates are shown (Schill and Preissler 1977)

proach to increasing the probability of conception. This possibility is supported by a significant improvement of cervical mucus penetration by kallikrein-stimulated spermatozoa (Fig. 11).

However, before considering insemination with kallikrein, it is mandatory to perform an in vitro stimulation test in a test tube, to check whether kallikrein is capable of improving sperm motility in an individual semen sample (Schill and Preissler 1977). If not, other possibilities have to be investigated, for example, the addition of caffeine or inseminations with the sperm-rich fraction of the split ejaculate.

First clinical results with the addition of kallikrein to the semen of subfertile men suffering from a male factor (reduced sperm motility) showed that, after paracervical insemination by vacuum cap twice at the time of ovulation (9–11 cycles), the Sims-Huhner test was still positive 36 h after insemination in contrast to control

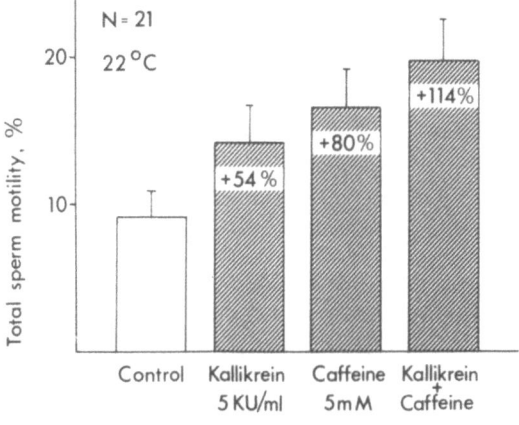

Fig. 12. Effect of pancreatic kallikrein and caffeine on the post-thaw motility of cryopreserved human spermatozoa. Mean ± SEM values of 21 semen specimens after 4-h incubation of frozen, then thawed semen samples at room temperature (22 °C) (Schill et al. 1979 b)

periods without kallikrein addition. In 52 childless couples, homologous insemination during a period of 1 year yielded a conception rate of 38.5% (Littich and Schill 1979). No side effects were observed. The abortion rate was 15%. Of the 17 children born, six were boys and 11 were girls. All delivered babies were healthy and showed no abnormalities. A crossover, blind study is currently being performed to critically evaluate these data. First data indicate the beneficial effect of topical addition of kallikrein for the improvement of semen quality in cases of isolated athenozoospermia (Schill and Littich 1981).

Kallikrein may also be used to improve sperm viability and motility of frozen semen samples (Schill and Pritsch 1976). For this purpose, it is recommended that kallikrein is added in a final concentration of 5 KU to the frozen semen samples immediately after thawing (Fig. 12). If it is added before freezing, there may be loss of enzymatic activity due to the freezing procedure. In this case it is necessary to add 10 KU to the semen samples before cryopreservation (Kaden and Grossgebauer 1980).

Investigations with frozen semen show a significant improvement of total and progressive motility after the addition of kallikrein. This is confirmed by a small increase of the post-thaw fructose consumption in these semen specimens (Schill et al. 1979b; Maier and Lunglmayr, to be published).

9.4 Conclusions

According to various in vitro experiments, animal studies, and clinical trials, evidence indicates that the kallikrein-kinin system is involved in reproductive, as well as other functions. In reproduction, the effects are primarily on the stimulation and regulation of sperm motility and migration. In addition, kinins seem to have stimulatory effects on the spermatogenic functions of the testis. Hence, administration of the pancreatic proteinase kallikrein to subfertile men may be a promising approach to improvement of fertility, either by systemic administration or addition of kallikrein to human semen in combination with instrumental insemination. However, for this kind of therapy, it is absolutely necessary to develop better criteria for patient selection in order to have more specific treatment. Particularly, it is mandatory to study the quantitative distribution of all components of the kallikrein-kinin system in human genital secretions. Hopefully, this would help to select those men who, due to a lack of one of these components, show an alteration of homeostasis of the kinin system that possibly leads to significant impairment of sperm motility and spermatogenesis.

As stated, systemic kallikrein treatment is presently absolutely empirically based. Oral administration is preferred to parenteral injections, the dosage being 600 IU/day kallikrein taken shortly before a meal. According to our clinical experience (2400 infertile men/year), kallikrein is at the moment the medication of first choice in idiopathic normogonadotropic oligozoospermia and asthenozoospermia. If it is not effective within a medication period of 3–6 months, however, other pharmacological therapy should be considered.

Very recently, it was demonstrated that systemic kallikrein medication particularly improved semen parameters in men with idiopathic varicocele proven by a reno-testicular reflux (Hofmann and Ebert 1981; Schill 1981). This indicates an improvement of the testicular and the epididymal functions, possibly because kallikrein is a vasoactive substance that leads to a vasodilatation of the testicular arteries. This is of particular interest, since an arterial component in the pathophysiology of varicocele has been demonstrated by histopathological methods and technetium scintigraphy. On the basis of these facts, Hofmann and Ebert (1981) suggest a kallikrein test in men with varicocele to differentiate varicocele orchiopathy against other causes of testicular disturbances. In addition, from a practical point of view, long-term therapy with kallikrein in varicocele may be considered in those men who refuse surgical therapy (Schill 1981).

Another aspect might be of importance: it would be of interest to study systemic kallikrein administration in infertile women during ovulation. Theoretically, it is conceivable that through systemic kallikrein administration an improvement of sperm migration within the female genital tract is possible. To answer all these questions depends to a large degree on further fundamental research in reproductive biochemistry, since there is still much to learn about the mode of action and the pharmacokinetics of this natural compound.

Acknowledgements. Supported in part by Deutsche Forschungsgemeinschaft (Schi 86/5, 86/6, 86/7-2) Bonn-Bad Godesberg, West Germany.

9.5 References

Bedford NA, Elstein M (1981) The effect of kallikrein on male infertility: a double-blind study. In: Insler V, Bettendorf G (eds) Diagnosis and treatment of infertility. Elsevier North Holland, New York Amsterdam Oxford, pp 339–344

Blasini R, Schmeller ML, Pfeiffer C, Wriedt-Lübbe J, Huber P, Blümel G (1980) Experimental investigations concerning the specific concentration of kininogenases in testis and epididymis (in German). Andrologia 12:199–205

Blümel G, Erhardt W, Rupp N, Huber P (1975) Microangiographic investigations following kallikrein application. In: Haberland GL, Rohen JW, Schirren C, Huber P (eds) Kininogenases. Kallikrein 2. Schattauer, Stuttgart New York, pp 107–108

Bratanov K, Somlev B, Doycheva M, Tornyor A, Efremova V (1978) Effect of kallikrein on bull sperm motility in vitro. Int J Fertil 23:73–75

Cushman DW, Cheung HS (1971) Concentrations of angiotensin-converting enzyme in tissues of the rat. Biochim Biophys Acta 250:261–265

Dennhardt R, Haberich FJ (1973) Effect of kallikrein on the absorption of water, electrolytes, and hexoses in the intestine of rats. In: Haberland GL, Rohen JW (eds) Kininogenases. Kallikrein 1. Schattauer, Stuttgart New York, pp 81–88

Dietl T, Kruck J, Fritz H (1978) Localization of kallikrein in porcine pancreas and submandibular gland as revealed by the indirect immunofluorescence technique. Hoppe-Seylers Z Physiol Chem 359:499–505

Dietze G, Wicklmayr M, Mayer L (1977) Evidence for a participation of the kallikrein-kinin system in the regulation of muscle metabolism during hypoxia. Hoppe-Seylers Z Physiol Chem 358:633

Erdös EG (ed) (1970) Bradykinin, kallidin and kallikrein. (Handbook of experimental pharmacology, vol XXV). Springer, Berlin Heidelberg New York

Fink E, Geiger R, Witte J, Biedermann S, Seifert J, Fritz H (1980) Biochemical, pharmacological and functional aspects of glandular kallikreins. In: Gross F, Vogel G (eds) Enzymatic release of vasoactive peptides. Raven, New York, pp 101–115

Fritz H (1975) The kallikrein-kinin system in reproduction: Biochemical aspects. In: Haberland GL, Rohen JW, Schirren C, Huber P (eds) Kininogenases. Kallikrein 2. Schattauer, Stuttgart New York, pp 9–16

Fritz H, Schiessler H, Schill W-B, Tschesche H, Heimburger N, Wallner O (1975) Low molecular weight proteinase (acrosin) inhibitors from human and boar seminal plasma and spermatozoa and human cervical mucus-isolation, properties and biological aspects. In: Reich E, Rifkin DB, Shaw E (eds) Proteases and biological control. Cold Spring Harbor Laboratory, Cold Spring Harbor, pp 737–766

Fujii S, Moriya H, Suzuki T (1979a) Kinins II: Biochemistry, pathophysiology and clinical aspects. Plenum, New York

Fujii S, Moriya H, Suzuki T (1979b) Kinins II: Systemic proteases and cellular function. Plenum, New York

Haberland GL, Rohen JW (1973) Kininogenases. Kallikrein 1. Schattauer, Stuttgart New York

Haberland GL, Rohen JW, Schirren C, Huber P (eds) (1975a) Kininogenases. Kallikrein 2. Schattauer, Stuttgart New York

Haberland GL, Rohen JW, Blümel G, Huber P (1975b) Kininogenases. Kallikrein 3. Schattauer, Stuttgart New York

Haberland GL, Rohen JW, Suzuki T (1977) Kininogenases. Kallikrein 4. Schattauer, Stuttgart New York

Hartenbach W (1954) Über den heutigen Stand der experimentellen und klinischen Untersuchungen der Wirkung der Anwendungsmöglichkeiten von Padutin. Muench Med Wochenschr 96:429–431

Hofmann N, Ebert L (1981) Kallikrein as a diagnostic test in cases of varicocele. In: Haberland GL, Rohen JW (eds) Kininogenases. Kallikrein 5. Schattauer, Stuttgart New York, pp 93–98

Hofmann N, Schönberger A, Gall H (1975) Investigations on kallikrein treatment of male infertility disturbances (in German). Z Hautkr 50:1003–1012

Hohlbrugger G, Schweisfurth H, Knonsalla M, Dahlheim H (1980) Experimental approach to the physiological role of gonadal angiotensin I-converting enzyme. Pfluegers Arch 384:R28

Homonnai ZT, Shilon M, Paz G (1978) Evaluation of semen quality following kallikrein treatment. Gynecol Obstet Invest 9:132–138

Igarashi M, Sato S, Kubo H, Sato T (1962) Über die Wirkung von Kallikrein auf die Funktion des Hypophysen-Gonaden-Systems. Endocrinol Jpn 9:81–89

Kaden R, Grossgebauer K (1980) Enhancement of motility in fresh and preserved semen by kallikrein and caffeine. Arch Androl 5:36

Kamidono S, Hazama M, Matsumoto O, Takada KJ, Tomioka O, Ishigami J (1981) Kallikrein and male subfertility. Usefulness of high-unit kallikrein tablets. Andrologia 13:108–120

Kienitz T, Schill WB (1977) Oral kallikrein therapy in asthenozoospermia (in German). Fortschr Med 95:2102–2106

Kleeberg S, Prinzen R, Leidl W (1975) Effect of kallikrein on the gonads of premature male rats. In: Haberland GL, Rohen JW, Schirren C, Huber P (eds) Kininogenases. Kallikrein 2. Schattauer, Stuttgart New York, pp 99–105

Leidl W, Prinzen R, Schill WB, Fritz H (1975) The effect of kallikrein in motility and metabolism of spermatozoa in vitro. In: Haberland GL, Rohen JW, Schirren C, Huber P (eds) Kininogenases. Kallikrein 2. Schattauer, Stuttgart New York, pp 33–40

Lemon M, Fiedler F, Förg-Brey B, Hirschauer C, Leysath G, Fritz H (1979) The isolation and properties of pig submandibular kallikrein. Biochem J 177:159–168

Littich M, Schill WB (1979) Homologous insemination with the addition of pancreatic kallikrein. In: Fujii S, Moriya H, Suzuki T (eds) Kinins II. Systemic proteases and cellular function. Plenum, New York, pp 685–690

Lunglmayr G (1976) Sperm motility during kallikrein treatment (in German). Wien Klin Wochenschr 88:709–711

Maier U, Lunglmayr G (to be published) Influence of highly purified kallikrein on sperm motility after semen preservation (in German). Urologe

Mathiessen PF, Rohen JW (1975) ^{3}H-Thymidine-incorporation in the testis of the albino rat after migration of the pancreatic duct. In: Haberland GL, Rohen JW, Schirren C, Huber P (eds) Kininogenases. Kallikrein 2. Schattauer, Stuttgart New York, pp 75–83

Meng K, Haberland GL (1973) Influence of kallikrein on glucose transport in the isolated rat intestine. In: Haberland GL, Rohen JM (eds) Kininogenases. Kallikrein 1. Schattauer, Stuttgart New York, pp 75–80

Moriwaki C, Moriya H, Yamaguchi K, Kizuki K, Fujimori H (1973) Intestinal absorption of pancreatic kallikrein and some aspects of its physiological role. In: Haberland GL, Rohen JW (eds) Kininogenases. Kallikrein 1. Schattauer, Stuttgart New York, pp 57–66

Moriwaki C, Kiszuki K, Moriya H (1975) Kininogenase from the coagulating gland. In: Haberland GL, Rohen JW, Schirren C, Huber P (eds) Kininogenases. Kallikrein 2. Schattauer, Stuttgart New York, pp 23–31

Nürnberger F, Grassow J (1977) Kallikrein therapy in oligozoospermia and asthenozoospermia during a double-blind trial (in German). Hautarzt [Suppl II] 28:308–312

Palm S, Schill WB, Wallner O, Prinzen R, Fritz H (1976) Occurrence of components of the kallikrein-kinin system in human genital secretions and their possible function in stimulation of sperm motility and migration. In: Sicuteri F, Back N, Haberland GL (eds) Kinins: Pharmacodynamics and biological roles. Plenum, New York, pp 271–279

Propping D, Tauber PF, Plewa G, Katzorke T (1978) Kallikrein treatment of the subfertile male: results of a double-blind cross-over study. Vth European Congress Fertility Sterility, Oct. 1978, Venice Italy (Abstr), p 93

Rixon RH, Whitfield JF, Bayliss J (1971) The stimulation of mitotic activity in the thymus and bone narrow of rats by kallikrein. Horm Metab Res 3:279–284

Rohen JW, Buschhüter H (1975) Karyometric measurements on the Sertoli cell nuclei in kallikrein-treated albino rats. In: Haberland GL, Rohen JW, Schirren C, Huber P (eds) Kininogenases. Kallikrein 2. Schattauer, Stuttgart New York, pp 85–97

Rohen JW, Stuttmann R (1977) The early postnatal development of the germinative epithelium of the testis in the albino rat under the influence of kallikrein. In: Haberland GL, Rohen JW, Suzuki T (eds) Kininogenases. Kallikrein 4. Schattauer, Stuttgart New York, pp 217–223

Sato H (1980) Studies on the components of kallikrein-kinin system and treatment of male infertility. Keio J Med 29:19–38

Sato H, Mochimaru F, Kobayashi T, Jizuka R, Kaneko S, Moriwaki C (1979) Kallikrein treatment of male infertility. In: Fujii S, Moriya H, Suzuki T (eds) Kinins II: Biochemistry, pathophysiology and clinical aspects. Plenum, New York, pp 529–536

Schill WB (1975 a) Improvement of sperm motility in patients with asthenozoospermia by kallikrein treatment. Int J Fertil 20:61–63

Schill WB (1975 b) Influence of kallikrein on sperm count and sperm motility in patients with infertility problems: Preliminary results during parenteral and oral application with special reference to asthenozoospermia and oligozoospermia. In: Haberland GL, Rohen JW, Schirren C, Huber P (eds) Kininogenases. Kallikrein 2. Schattauer, Stuttgart New York, pp 129–146

Schill WB (1976) Quantitative determination of high molecular weight serum proteinase inhibitors in human semen. Andrologia 8:359–364

Schill WB (1978 a) Effect of kallikrein on the motility of fresh and frozen human semen. In: Emperaire JC, Audebert A (eds) Proceeding of the First International Symposium Artificial Insemination Homologous and Male Subfertility. Institut Aquitain de Recherches sur la Reproduction Humaine, Bordeaux, pp 222–235

Schill WB (1978 b) Clinical experience with kallikrein in the treatment of oligozoospermia and asthenozoospermia (in German). Fortschr Androl 6:52–72

Schill WB (1979 a) Recent progress in pharmacological therapy of male subfertility: a review. Andrologia 11:77–107

Schill WB (1979 b) Treatment of idiopathic oligozoospermia by kallikrein: results of a double-blind study. Arch Androl 2:163–170

Schill WB (1981) Kallikrein administration in subfertile men with varicocele. IIIrd World Congress of Human Reproduction, Berlin Germany March 22–26 (Abstr), p 437

Schill WB, Braun S (1981) Serum levels of growth hormone and cortisol in subfertile men during kallikrein treatment. In: Haberland GL, Rohen JW (eds) Kininogenases. Kallikrein 5. Schattauer, Stuttgart New York, pp 99–102
Schill WB, Haberland GL (1975) Effects of different components of the kallikrein-kinin system on sperm motility in vitro (in German). Klin Wochenschr 53:73–79
Schill WB, Littich M (1981) Split-ejaculate insemination with and without the addition of kallikrein. Andrologia 13:121–126
Schill WB, Preissler G (1977) Improvement of cervical mucus spermatozoal penetration by kinins: A possible therapeutic approach in the treatment of male subfertility. In: Insler V, Bettendorf G (eds) The uterine cervix in reproduction. Thieme, Stuttgart, pp 134–146
Schill WB, Pritsch W (1976) Kinin-induced enhancement of sperm motility in cryo-preserved human spermatozoa. In: Tischner M, Pilch J (eds) Proceedings of the VIIth International Congress Animal Reproduction Artificial Insemination, Krakow July 12–16, Wroclawska Drukarnia Naukowa, Krakow, vol IV, pp 1071–1074
Schill WB, Rjosk H-K (1979) Serum levels of LH, FSH, prolactin and testosterone in oligo- and asthenozoospermic men during kallikrein treatment. Acta Endocrinol [Suppl] 225:96
Schill WB, Braun-Falco O, Haberland GL (1974) The possible role of kinins in sperm motility. Int J Fertil 19:163–167
Schill WB, Wallner O, Palm S, Fritz H (1976) Kinin stimulation of spermatozoa motility and migration in cervical mucus. In: Hafez ESE (ed) Human semen and fertility regulation in man. Mosby, St. Louis, pp 442–451
Schill WB, Preissler G, Dittmann B, Müller WP (1979a) Effect of pancreatic kallikrein, sperm acrosin and high molecular weight (HMW) kininogen on cervical mucus penetration ability of seminal plasma-free human spermatozoa. In: Fujii S, Moriya H, Suzuki T (eds) Kinins II: Systemic protease and cellular function. Plenum, New York, pp 305–310
Schill WB, Pritsch W, Preissler G (1979b) Effect of caffeine and kallikrein on cryo-preserved human spermatozoa. Int J Fertil 24:27–32
Schill WB, Rjosk H-K, Križić A (1980) Andrological, biochemical and endocrinological investigations in subfertile men during kallikrein-kinin treatment (in German). Hautarzt 31:191–197
Schirren C (1978) Kallikrein in andrology (in German). Fortschr Androl, Volume 6, Grosse, Berlin
Schirren C, Schill WB, Hofmann N (1975) The influence of kallikrein on semen parameters of subfertile patients. In: Haberland GL, Rohen JW, Schirren C, Huber P (eds) Kininogenases. Kallikrein 2. Schattauer, Stuttgart New York, pp 111–127
Schütte B, Schirren C (1977) Therapeutic administration of kallikrein in patients with sperm motility disturbances (in German). Z Hautkr 52:930–934
Schütte B, Eckmann B, Wirsig H, Schirren C (1981) The influence of kallikrein on sperm motility: in vitro and in vivo investigations. In: Haberland GL, Rohen JW (eds) Kininogenases. Kallikrein 5. Schattauer, Stuttgart New York, pp 33–39
Schumacher GFB (1973) Soluble proteins of human cervical mucus. In: Elstein M, Moghissi KS, Borth R (eds) Cervical mucus in reproduction. Scriptor, Copenhagen, pp 93–113
Steiner R, Hofmann N, Kaufmann R, Hartmann R (1977) The influence of kallikrein on the velocity of human spermatozoa measured by Laser-Doppler-spectroscopy. In: Haberland GL, Rohen JW, Suzuki T (eds) Kininogenases. Kallikrein 4. Schattauer, Stuttgart New York, pp 229–235
Steiner R, Hofmann N, Hartmann R, Kaufmann R (1981) Kallikrein-enhanced human sperm motility in different media and cervical mucus measured with Laser-Doppler-spectroscopy. In: Haberland GL, Rohen JW (eds) Kininogenases. Kallikrein 5. Schattauer, Stuttgart New York, pp 17–26
Stüttgen G (1973) Clinical substantiation of the effect of kallikrein. In: Haberland GL, Rohen JW (eds) Kininogenases. Kallikrein 1. Schattauer, Stuttgart New York, pp 189–193
Stüttgen G (1975) Kallikrein effects: a short comment. In: Haberland GL, Rohen JW, Schirren C, Huber P (eds) Kininogenases. Kallikrein 2. Schattauer, Stuttgart New York, pp 171–172
Tauber PF, Propping D, Niesel A, Kurz E, Zaneveld LJD (1977) Effect of kallikrein treatment on the composition of human split ejaculates. In: Haberland GL, Rohen JW, Suzuki T (eds) Kininogenases. Kallikrein 4. Schattauer, Stuttgart New York, pp 237–245

Thompson W, Traub AJ, Earnshaw JC (1980) Effect of kallikrein on sperm motility. Arch Androl [Suppl] 5: A 117

Török L (1979) Behandlung der Subfertilität des Mannes mit Kallikrein. Muench Med Wochenschr 121: 1047–1049

Török L, Morvay J, Sas M (1978) Untersuchungen über Serum-FSH, -LH und -Testosteron bei der Behandlung subfertiler Männer mit Kallikrein. Fortschr Androl 6: 84–87

Tschesche H, Mair G, Godec G, Fiedler F, Ehret W, Hirschauer C, Lemon M, Fritz H (1979) The primary structure of porcine glandular kallikrein. In: Fujii S, Moriya H, Suzuki T (eds) Kinins I: Biochemistry, pathophysiology and clinical aspects. Plenum, New York, pp 245–260

Wallner O, Schill WB, Grösser A, Fritz H (1975) Participation of the kallikrein-kinin system in sperm penetration through cervical mucus: in vitro studies. In: Haberland GL, Rohen JW, Schirren C, Huber P (eds) Kininogenases. Kallikrein 2. Schattauer, Stuttgart New York, pp 63–70

Wicklmayr M, Dietze G, Günther B, Mayer L, Böttger J, Geiger R, Schultis K (1978) Improvement of pathological glucose tolerance by bradykinin in diabetic and in surgical patients (in German). Klin Wochenschr 56: 1077–1083

10 Treatment of Male Infertility with Nucleotides

G. F. Menchini-Fabris and M. Mariani

Some nucleotides, such as adenosine triphosphate (ATP), adenosine diphosphate (ADP), and adenosine monophosphate (AMP), have the capacity to stimulate sperm motility and are especially useful in causing flagellar rotation. These nucleotides provide energy for metabolic processes of the germ cell (respiration, movement) (Nelson 1975). Other nucleotides [guanosine monophosphate (GMP), guanosine diphosphate (GDP), guanosine triphosphate (GTP), uridine monophosphate (UMP), uridine diphosphate (UDP), uridine triphosphate (UTP)] are important during the first phase of sperm formation at the level of the germinal cell (for epididymal maturation and capacitation of the spermatozoon), providing the energy necessary for protein synthesis (Hoskins and Casillas 1975).

These effects have aroused the interest of various authors who have studied these compounds to determine their usefulness in the therapy of human oligozoospermia with bradykinesis, since a reduction of sperm number and/or motility causes a decrease of male fertilizing capacity (Bianchi et al. 1978).

10.1 Structure and Metabolism

Complete acid hydrolysis of a nucleic acid yields a mixture of basic substances called purines and pyrimidines, a sugar (ribose or deoxyribose), and phosphoric acid.

After partial hydrolysis of nucleic acids, nucleotides and nucleosides can be obtained (Fig. 1). Each nucleoside consists of a base acid and a sugar component. The nucleotides yield, on hydrolysis, the same components as well as phosphoric acid. Nucleotides are, therefore, phosphoric esters of the nucleosides. These are considered strong acids (adenylic, guanylic, thymidylic, cytidylic, and uridylic acids) in which the phosphate is always esterified to the sugar moiety. The phosphorylation of the sugar can be at C $3'$ or C $5'$ (Fig. 2).

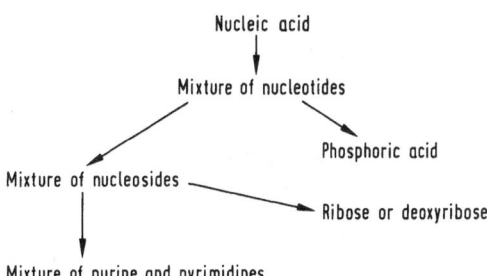

Fig. 1. Nucleic acid metabolism

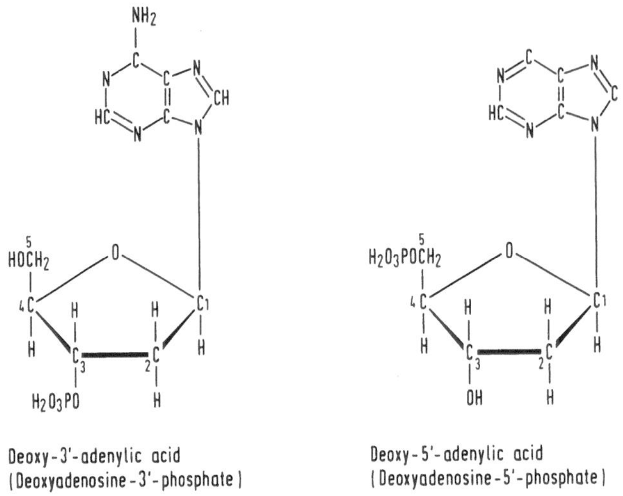

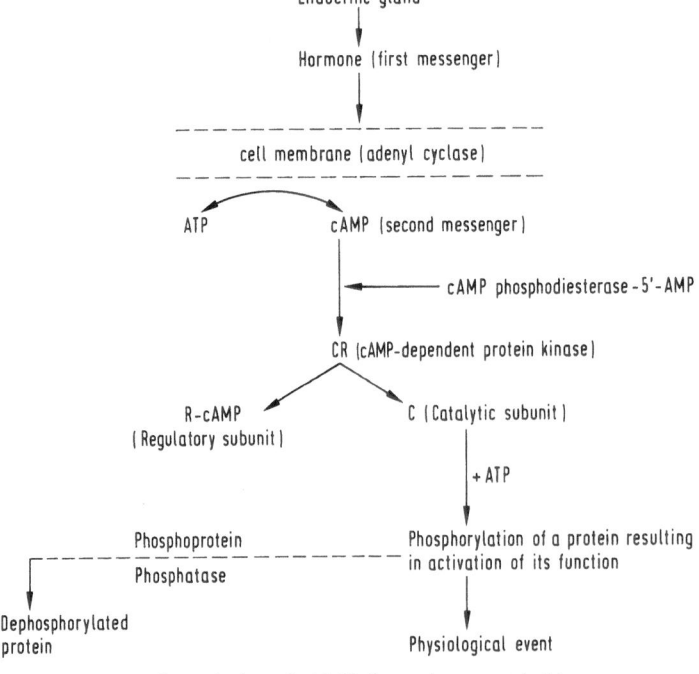

Deoxy-3'-adenylic acid
(Deoxyadenosine-3'-phosphate)

Deoxy-5'-adenylic acid
(Deoxyadenosine-5'-phosphate)

Fig. 2. Adenylic acid phosphorylation at the C3' or C5' positions

Nucleotide synthesis involves the coupling of orotic acid with 5-phosphoribosil-1-pyrophosphate, a reaction catalyzed by orotidine-5'-phosphate pyrophosphory-lase. These compounds are utilized in every metabolic process of the body, such as muscular contraction, nervous stimulus transmission, and ciliary movements.

A partial list of important nucleotides is shown in Table 1, while in Fig. 3 the probable hormonal regulation of synthesis through cyclic AMP (cAMP) and cAMP-

Endocrine gland

Hormone (first messenger)

cell membrane (adenyl cyclase)

ATP   cAMP (second messenger)

cAMP phosphodiesterase-5'-AMP

CR (cAMP-dependent protein kinase)

R-cAMP   C (Catalytic subunit)
(Regulatory subunit)

+ ATP

Phosphoprotein   Phosphorylation of a protein resulting in activation of its function

Phosphatase

Dephosphorylated protein   Physiological event

Fig. 3. Hormonal regulation of cAMP-dependent protein kinase

Table 1. List of some important nucleotides: The triphosphate compounds are important because they are more energetic

Adenosine monophosphate (adenylic acid)	AMP
Adenosine diphosphate	ADP
Adenosine triphosphate	ATP
Guanosine monophosphate (guanylic acid)	GMP
Guanosine diphosphate	GDP
Guanosine triphosphate	GTP
Cytidine monophosphate (cytidylic acid)	CMP
Cytidine diphosphate	CDP
Cytidine triphosphate	CTP
Uridine monophosphate (uridylic acid)	UMP
Uridine diphosphate	UDP
Uridine triphosphate	UTP
Thymidine monophosphate (thymidylic acid)	TMP
Thymidine diphosphate	TDP
Thymidine triphosphate	TTP

dependent protein kinase (Monesi 1974; Menchini-Fabris et al. 1975; Baccetti et al. 1976).

10.2 Clinical Studies

Our assessment of the role of nucleotides in the treatment of male infertility was based on observations of other authors (Hicks et al. 1972; White 1973), who have shown the importance of cyclic nucleotides in spermatozoan metabolism as related to its environment in the male reproductive tract and in follicular fluid. For our studies, we tried to evaluate the potential effects of Diamantil (Istituto Chemioterapico Italiano, Milano), a neonatal calf extract derived from heart-lymph node tissue preparations. The chemical composition of Diamantil is shown in Table 2. This drug was used due to its richness in amino acids and deoxyribosil nucleotides.

The study was carried out during January to April 1980, using 227 men (20–60 years old, mean 30 years) as subjects. The efficacy of Diamantil in the treatment of male infertility was assessed. We examined normal men and subjects affected by various andrological pathologies. The subjects were selected on the basis of age,

Table 2. Chemical composition of diamantil. The total amount of deoxyribosilnucleotides/ml is 20 µg

Amino acids	(µmol/ml)	Amino acids	(µmol/ml)
Lysine	(2.8)	Glycine	(6.17)
Arginine	(1.2)	Alanine	(5.65)
Aspartic acid	(1.0)	Valine	(3.66)
Threonine	(2.6)	Isoleucine	(1.92)
Serine	(2.15)	Leucine	(5.07)
Glutamic acid	(8.72)	Phenylalanine	(1.20)
Proline	(3.17)		

pathology, general and genital objective examinations, medical history, and the results of seminal fluid examination, karyotype and basal blood plasma levels of FSH, LH, prolactin (PRL), and testosterone (T). The criteria for patient selection were as follows: 20–60 years old, no azoospermia, all previous treatments discontinued for at least 6 months.

The 227 men were divided into the following groups: ten normal subjects having the characteristics shown in Table 3 (six were given drug, four received a placebo; 79 patients with oligozoospermia and/or bradykinesis due to genital inflammation, such as prostatitis or epididymitis (57 received drug and 22 a placebo);

Table 3. Characteristics of normal subjects

Signs and symptoms of disease	None
Proven fertility	One or more children
Semen volume	2.0 – 4.5 ml
pH	7.0 – 8.5
Density	Normal
Viscosity	Normal
Color	Yellowish
Odor	Chestnut
Sperm count	$\geq 40 \times 10^6$ /ml
Basal normokinetic motility	$\geq 60\%$
Normokinetic motility after 2 h	$\geq 55\%$

39 patients with oligozoospermia and/or bradykinesis due to left varicocele (19 received drug, 20 a placebo); 20 patients with oligozoospermia and/or bradykinesis due to cryptorchidism (ten received drug, ten a placebo); 35 patients with oligozoospermia and/or bradykinesis due to hypospermatogenesis (25 received drug, 10 placebo); 28 patients with oligozoospermia and/or bradykinesis due to immunologic pathology (14 received drug, 14 a placebo); 16 patients with idiopathic oligozoospermia and/or bradykinesis (eight received drug, eight a placebo).

10.2.1 Procedure

We defined oligozoospermia as a sperm count of less than 40 million spermatozoa/ml and bradykinesis as less than 60% normokinetic spermatozoa with linear and progressive movements, as determined 30 min after ejaculation.

For immunologic studies we used cell-mediated immunity assays based on Clausen's test for leukocyte migration inhibition on agarose (Polidori et al. 1980). We used a standardized form for the collection of data (Mariani et al. 1977).

For each patient, the average value of two seminal fluid examinations was used. Sperm number/ml was evaluated by counting in a Thomas-Zeiss chamber after immobilization in a 1% acetic acid solution: the motility was given in percent of normokinetic spermatozoa as compared to the percent of spermatozoa with abnormal motility (circular and nonprogressive movements). The count was made 30 min after ejaculation and then again after 2 h. For optical evaluation, a binocular micro-

Table 4. Average of seminal fluid parameters before and after treatment with placebo and diamantil in all the patients (227 men)

Seminal fluid parameters	ml		pH		Millions of spermatozoa/ml		Percent basal normo-kinetic spermatozoa		Percent normokinetic spermatozoa after 2 h	
Placebo										
Normal subjects	3.3	3.2	7.8	7.9	52.6	51.2	61.3	62.0	55.5	55.3
Genital inflammation	3.4	3.2	7.7	7.8	26.0	18.7[a]	23.9	20.4[a]	17.8	13.6[a]
Left varicocele	3.2	3.2	7.8	7.8	16.0	14.3[a]	24.0	20.0[a]	21.5	18.7[a]
Cryptorchidism	3.5	3.5	7.8	7.8	13.0	11.7	18.4	15.2	11.9	11.2
Hypospermatogenesis	3.1	3.0	7.9	7.8	5.8	4.9	14.1	12.9	10.8	9.9
Immunologic	2.8	2.9	7.7	7.8	34.3	30.1	17.2	18.0	12.1	14.2
Idiopathic	2.9	3.0	7.8	7.8	33.7	35.0[a]	18.1	18.0[a]	13.2	13.0[a]
Diamantil										
Normal subjects	3.1	3.4	7.7	7.8	53.9	67.3	61.6	62.9	56.5	56.1
Genital inflammation	3.5	3.5	7.8	7.8	25.7	28.5	24.4	33.1[a]	19.9	27.1[a]
Left varicocele	3.3	3.2	7.8	7.8	15.4	22.8[a]	23.7	27.0	19.1	23.1
Cryptorchidism	3.6	3.6	7.8	7.9	11.7	10.9	17.1	14.6	12.5	10.5
Hypospermatogenesis	3.2	3.4	7.7	7.8	4.6	6.7	13.4	11.8	10.3	8.5
Immunologic	3.0	3.1	7.8	7.8	16.3	21.9	16.0	15.0	11.4	11.1
Idiopathic	2.6	2.7	7.7	7.8	33.9	54.8[a]	16.8	30.4[a]	11.1	24.4[a]

[a] $P < 0.05$

scope (40×10) was used and the pH determination was made with a digital device. Serum hormone levels of FSH, LH, PRL, and T were determined by standard radioimmunoassays. All these examinations were made such that interferences due to one or more diseases in the same patient were avoided, since such interferences could have altered the results of the treatment.

An IBM 370/168 computer and an Olivetti TC 485 terminal with a SPSS program were used for statistical analyses of the data.

10.2.2 Treatment

The drug dose was one i.m. injection vial of 2 ml/day every morning for 20 days, followed by a rest period of 10 days. This scheme was repeated over a 3-month period. The placebo (distilled water) was administered in the same manner. It was not possible to assess other ways of administration, as only the intramuscular preparation of the drug is available. Also, different dosages and drug regimens were not tested because of varying pathologies and insufficient numbers of subjects.

10.3 Results

There were no adverse effects related to the treatment with Diamantil, as assessed by physical examination or biochemical and hematological tests.

Table 4 shows the evaluation of results obtained in all 227 patients treated with placebo and Diamantil. No significant changes in seminal plasma volume and pH were noted. However, the number of spermatozoa/ml and percent of normokinetic spermatozoa at 30 min and 2 h from the time of ejaculation demonstrated the following statistically significant variations:

1. In the ten normal subjects (Table 5), placebo treatment of four patients revealed decreased numbers of spermatozoa in two, an increase in one, and no change in

Table 5. Normal subjects

		Placebo treatment (n = 4)			Diamantil treatment (n = 6)		
		>	=	<	>	=	<
N o r m o k i n e t i c	Millions of spermatozoa/ml	50% [a]	25%	25% [a]	83% [a]	17%	0%
	Basal motility	50% [a]	25%	25% [a]	33% [a]	67%	0%
	Motility after 2 h	50% [a]	25%	25% [a]	33% [a]	67%	0%

[a] $P > 0.05$

Table 6. Effect of placebo treatment. (The numbers in the table refer to the percentage.) > improved; = not improved; < deteriorated

	Pathology						
	Inflammation	Left varicocele	Cryptorchidism	Hypospermato-genesis	Immunologic	Idiopathic	Total
No. of patients	22	20	10	10	14	8	84
Millions of spermatozoa/ml	9 / 9 / 82[a]	10 / 5 / 85[a]	10 / 10 / 80[a]	10 / 10 / 80[a]	14 / 7 / 79[a]	25[a] / 12 / 63[a]	12 / 8 / 80[a]
Basal motility	4 / 4 / 92[a]	5 / 5 / 90[a]	10 / 10 / 80[a]	20 / 10 / 70[a]	7 / 7 / 86[a]	25 / 12 / 63[a]	10 / 7 / 83[a]
Motility after 2 h	4 / 4 / 92[a]	5 / 5 / 90[a]	10 / 10 / 80[a]	20 / 10 / 70[a]	7 / 7 / 86[a]	25 / 12 / 63[a]	10 / 7 / 83[a]
% of	> / = / <	> / = / <	> / = / <	> / = / <	> / = / <	> / = / <	

[a] $P > 0.05$

Table 7. Effect of Diamantil treatment. The numbers in the table refer to the percentages. > improved; = not improved; < deteriorated

	Pathology																				
	Inflammation			Left varicocele			Cryptorchidism			Hypospermatogenesis			Immunologic			Idiopathic			Total 133		
No. of patients	57			19			10			25			14			8					
Millions of spermatozoa/ml	47[a]	6	47	78[a]	10	12	40	20	40	48[a]	32	20	79[a]	0	21	88[a]	12	0	56[a]	12	32
Basal motility	64[a]	3	33	47[a]	16	37	30	10	60[a]	40	16	44	36	14	50[a]	88[a]	0	12	53[a]	9	38
Motility after 2 h	61[a]	8	31	58[a]	5	37	30	20	50[a]	36	20	44	36	14	50[a]	88[a]	0	12	53[a]	10	37
% of	>	=	<	>	=	<	>	=	<	>	=	<	>	=	<	>	=	<			

[a] $P < 0.05$

one. In all four placebo-treated subjects, sperm motility remained unchanged. In the six Diamantil-treated patients, five showed a numeric increase of spermatozoa, while the sixth showed no significant variation. In two of the Diamantil-treated patients, both basal motility and that observed after 2 h, increased while the remaining four showed no significant variations.

2. *In the group of 217 patients with various pathology,* we observed that, in 84 subjects treated with placebo (Table 6), the number of spermatozoa showed no statistically significant increase, but motility was significantly diminished. In 133 patients treated with Diamantil (Table 7), the number of spermatozoa increased significantly in 56% and motility increased in 53% (Table 8). For both groups of patients, the variations of pH and ejaculate volume were not significant. Pregnancies that may have occurred during the course of treatment were not evaluated in the normal subjects since the wives of these men were taken contraceptive measures.

Table 8. Mean seminal fluid parameters before and after Diamantil treatment (improved pathologic patients) (n = 70)

Pathology	ml		pH		Millions of spermatozoa/ml		Percent of basal normokinetic spermatozoa		Percent of normokinetic spermatozoa after 2 h	
	Before	After	Before	After	Before	After	Before	After	Before	After
Genital inflammation	4.5	4.0	8.5	8.0	19	37[a]	22	42[a]	18	36[a]
Left varicocele	4.0	3.9	7.7	7.8	17	24[a]	23	34[a]	20	27
Cryptorchism	3.6	3.8	7.9	8.0	3	7	21	28	20	22
Hypospermatogenesis	3.2	3.5	7.8	7.9	4	11[a]	5	18	4	14
Immunologic	3.0	3.3	7.8	7.8	13	20[a]	13	23	12	22
Idiopathic	3.0	3.0	7.8	8.0	38	62[a]	14	30[a]	9	26[a]

[a] $P < 0.05$

Table 9. Number of pregnancies under placebo and Diamantil treatment. In the normal group no pregnancy occurred because of the use of contraceptive pills by the women

Pathology	Placebo 5/84 (6%)	Diamantil 24/133 (18%)
	Contraceptive pill	
Genital inflammation	3	16
Left varicocele	1	4
Cryptorchidism	0	1
Hypospermatogenesis	0	0
Immunologic	0	0
Idiopathic	1	3

In infertile couples where the female was healthy and capable of normal pregnancy, administration of placebo (Table 9) to 84 infertile men resulted in five pregnancies (6%), while treatment with Diamantil in 133 patients increased the number of pregnancies to 24 (18%). The most significant increase occurred in the wives of men with genital inflammations.

10.4 Conclusion

The results suggest that Diamantil may have an effect on sperm count and motility. Diamantil appears to exert its action by providing a substrate for the meiotic process, thus affecting protein synthesis in the differentiation phase of the germinal cell. With respect to its effect on motility, it may provide energy-rich compounds utilized in flagellar movement. Whether the observed increase in pregnancies in the Diamantil-treated group is truly a consequence of the treatment remains to be determined by future studies.

10.5 References

Baccetti B, Afzelius BA (1976) The biology of the sperm cell, vol. X. Karger, Basel

Bianchi B, Mariani M, Menchini-Fabris GF (1978) Modificazioni dei parametri seminologici in 140 pazienti dispermici dopo trattamento con TBM78. In: Pacini (ed) Giornate endocrinologiche Pisane. Pacini, Pisa, pp 599–605

Hicks JJ, Pedron N, Rosado A (1972) Modifications of human spermatozoa glycolysis by AMP, estrogens and follicular fluid. Fertil Steril 23:886–893

Hoskins DD, Casillas ER (1975) Function of cyclic nucleotides in mammalian spermatozoa. In: Greep RO, Astwood EB, Hamilton DW, Geiger SR (eds) Endocrinology. Waverly, Baltimore (Handbook of physiology, section 7, vol V, pp 453–460)

Mariani M, Bianchi B, Basile-Fasolo C, Menchini-Fabris GF (1977) Considerazioni sulla gestione di dati raccolti mediante una cartella andrologica standardizzata. In: Cofese (ed) Istituzioni di sessuologia. Cofese, Palermo, pp 571–576

Menchini-Fabris GF, Giannotti P, Moggi G, Giorgi G, Panetta R, Bianchi B (1975) Andrological procedures used in the diagnosis of infertility in the married couple. Clin Exp Obstet Gynecol 2:61–67

Monesi V (1974) Nucleoprotein synthesis in spermatogenesis. In: Mancini RE, Martini L (eds) Male fertility and sterility. Academic Press, New York, pp 59–87

Nelson L (1975) Spermatozoan motility. In: Greep RO, Astwood EB, Hamilton DW, Geiger SR (eds) Endocrinology. Waverly, Baltimore (Handbook of physiology, section 7, vol V) pp 421–435

Polidori R, Ambrogi F, Izzo PL, Mariani M, Grassi B, Menchini-Fabris GF (1980) Cell-mediated immunity in male fertility. Andrologia 12:141–145

White IG (1973) Biochemical aspects of spermatozoa and their environment in the male reproductive tract. J Reprod Fertil [Suppl] 18:225–235

11 Immunological Infertility in Men: Clinical and Therapeutic Considerations

J. Friberg

The antigenicity of spermatozoa and the seminal fluid has been known since the turn of the century. That immunization of both male and female animals with semen, testicular cells, and spermatozoa could render them temporarily or permanently sterile boosted research in immunoreproduction. As a result of these studies, a complex of antigenic substances has been described in semen. These antigens can be broadly classified into those found in the seminal fluid and those found in or on the spermatozoa (Fig. 1). Proteins, blood-group substances, HL-A antigens, and lactoferrin are examples of potent antigens found in the seminal fluid. In the group of antigens demonstrated with the spermatozoa, hyaluronidase, acrosin, protamine, and LDH-X can be mentioned, the first three originating from the sperm head and the last in the middle piece. In addition, a lipoglycoprotein present on the sperm surface appears to constitute at least one of the antigens that induces sperm agglutination and sperm immobilization. To further complicate the picture, spermatozoa have been shown to be potent antigen absorbers. Lactoferrin, for example, can be

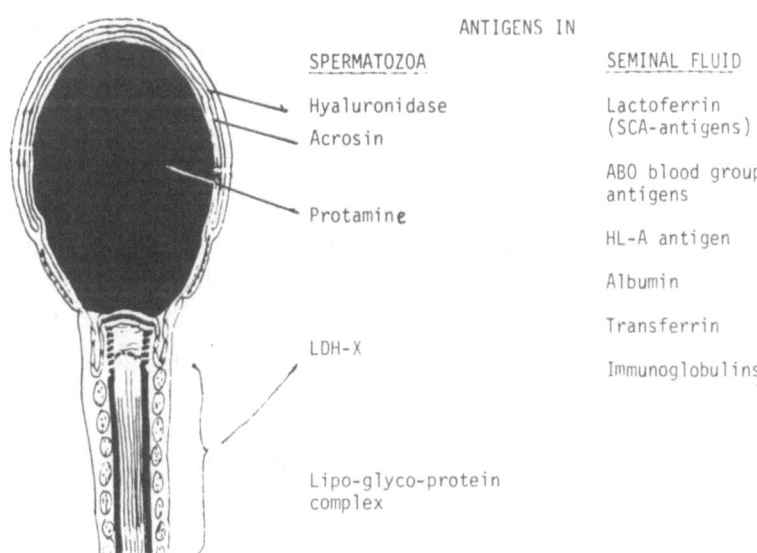

Fig. 1. Localization of some seminal antigens on spermatozoa and in seminal fluid

demonstrated in both the seminal fluid and on the ejaculated spermatozoa whereas it is absent from epididymal spermatozoa. Sperm-coating antigen (SCA antigen) was also the first name given to seminal lactoferrin.

Tolerance to "self" antigens is developed during embryonic and early fetal life. Substances not in contact with the immune system during this period will be considered "foreign" and the host will be able to respond with antibody formation. The seminal antigens are not present in the organism during the fetal period of life and, therefore, these antigens will be handled by the body as foreign. To avoid the induction of antibodies under normal conditions against substances from the reproductive system, the body has developed two sophisticated mechanisms.

First, a barrier has been developed that separates secretions of the male reproductive tract from the general circulation. This barrier, the "blood-testis" barrier, was first demonstrated in the testis where it was shown to prevent the entrance of certain substances from the blood into the seminiferous tubules (Setchell 1980 for review). This barrier appears to exist all along the male reproductive tract, where it not only prevents the passage of substances such as antibodies from the blood into the seminal fluid, but also interferes with the escape of seminal antigens into the general circulation. An appropriate name for this barrier, therefore, appears to be the "blood-male genital tract" barrier or "blood-semen" barrier.

The second mechanism involves an immunosuppressive action of semen. It has recently been demonstrated that both spermatozoa and seminal fluid can inhibit blast transformation of peripheral blood lymphocytes (Stites and Erickson 1975; Marcus et al. 1978). Such a phenomenon could effectively inhibit production of antibodies against seminal substances even if an extravasation of seminal content took place. However, the role of this mechanism under normal circumstances has not been investigated.

11.1 The Different Types of Sperm Antibodies Observed in Men

In spite of the blood-male genital tract barrier and the immunosuppressive properties of semen, antibody formation against spermatozoa can take place under certain circumstances. The first observations of circulating sperm-agglutinating antibodies in men were made by Wilson (1954) and Rümke (1954). Intensive research has thereafter demonstrated the presence of several types of both cell-mediated and

Table 1. Different types of antibodies against human spermatozoa observed in serum and seminal fluid

Humoral	Agglutinating	Against surface antigens
	Immobilizing	
	Cytotoxic	
	Immunofluorescent	Against sub-surface antigens
Cell-mediated	Lymphocyte transformation	
	Lymphocyte migration inhibition	
	Lymphocytotoxic	

humoral antibodies against spermatozoa in both serum and seminal fluid from men (Table 1). Such antibodies have also been demonstrated in women, but they will not be the subject of the present review.

The sperm antibodies demonstrated with agglutinating and immobilizing techniques have been implicated in male infertility. Some evidence indicates that, in male sera, the techniques used for the demonstration of sperm immobilization and sperm cytotoxicity detects the same antibody (Husted and Ingerslev 1975). The significance of cellular immunity to spermatozoa in male infertility has not been established. Also, the subsurface antigen-antibody reactions demonstrated with the immunofluorescent sperm antibody technique appear not directly correlated with infertility (Husted 1975; Husted and Hjort 1975).

Sperm-agglutinating activity in male sera can be demonstrated with Kibrick macroagglutination, as well as the Franklin-Dukes and the tray microagglutination techniques. An excellent reproducibility between the Kibrick and tray microagglutination techniques, as well as correlation between the different titers observed in the two techniques have been reported (Friberg 1974; Hellema and Rümke 1976). An advantage with the tray microagglutination technique over the Kibrick macroagglutination technique is that, not only the titer, but also the type of agglutination can easily be recorded. The Franklin-Dukes microagglutination technique, which has only occasionally been used in the study of sera from men, appears to suffer from poor reproducibility and correlation with other agglutination techniques has also been reported to be low (Mettler and Gradl 1975; Boettcher et al. 1977). The two most commonly observed types of agglutination have been designated head-to-head (H-H) and tail-to-tail (T-T) agglutination. In H-H agglutination, various parts of the sperm heads are involved in the agglutinates and with T-T agglutination different parts of the heads, middle pieces, tails, and end pieces make up the agglutinates. Other names for T-T agglutination have, therefore, been head-to-tail, mixed, or tangled agglutination.

Sperm immobilization and sperm cytotoxicity can be demonstrated using the techniques described by Fjällbrant (1965), Isojima et al. (1968), and Husted and Hjort (1975).

For the practical performance of the tests to demonstrate sperm antibodies the reader is referred to the review of Rose et al. (1976). When the tests are performed, it is important to fulfill certain criteria, such as the use of diluted sera, inclusion of known positive and negative control sera, as well as the use of semen with excellent characteristics from a reference donor. Since a low concentration of circulating antibodies in some men apparently does not interfere with their fertility, it is important not only to demonstrate the presence or absence of sperm antibodies but also to quantitate the concentration of antibodies present (usually expressed as a titer or index).

11.2 Antibody Nature of Sperm-Agglutinating and Sperm-Immobilizing Activities

Fractionation and absorption experiments performed by Rümke and Hellinga (1959) and Fjällbrant (1969), both using the Kibrick macroscopic sperm-agglutinating technique, indicated that both the sperm-agglutinating and sperm-immobilizing activities observed in *serum* from men were caused by true antibodies, mainly of the 7S IgG type. Further fractionation experiments, using the tray microagglutination technique for demonstration of sperm-agglutination, indicated that the H-H sperm-agglutination was usually caused by IgM antibodies (Table 2), whereas the T-T sperm-agglutination was mainly caused by IgG antibodies (Friberg 1974; Husted and Hjort 1975). In a few sera, a small proportion of H-H sperm-agglutinating activity was caused by IgG antibodies and, in a few other sera, part of the T-T sperm-agglutination was demonstrated with the IgA antibodies (Friberg 1974).

Table 2. Antibody classes of tail-to-tail and head-to-head spermagglutinating antibodies in human serum and seminal fluid

	Serum		Seminal fluid	
Tail-to-tail agglutination	IgG (common)	IgA (rare)	IgA/secr. IgA (common)	IgG (uncommon)
Head-to-head agglutination	IgM (common)	IgG (rare)	Absent	

Studies on the T-T sperm-agglutination observed in *seminal fluid* indicated that most of this activity was caused by IgA and/or secretory IgA antibodies. A few seminal fluid samples also contained some sperm-agglutinating activity caused by IgG antibodies (Friberg 1974). T-T sperm-agglutinating antibodies were only demonstrated in the seminal fluid from men who also had high titers of such antibodies in serum. The seminal fluid titers were usually 2–4 2-log titers steps lower than the serum titer (Rümke 1974a; Friberg 1974).

Men with IgM H-H sperm-agglutination in serum demonstrated no antibody-mediated sperm-agglutination in their ejaculates (Friberg and Tilly-Friberg 1977). Also, IgM appears to be absent from the seminal fluid (Rümke 1974b).

11.3 Causes of Sperm Antibody Production

Clinical evaluation and physical examination of men with circulating sperm antibodies only reveal a likely cause for the antibody formation in about 50% of the cases (Table 3). Among these patients, events that can lead to a temporary or permanent obstruction in the ejaculatory ducts, vas deferens, or epididymis play a prominent role. On the testicular side of an obstruction in the efferent sperm transportation pathway, the lumen becomes distended and the accumulation of fluid may cause breaks in the barrier, with extravasation of spermatozoa and eventual sperm antibody production. Granuloma formation does not seem to be correlated with the presence of sperm antibodies (Alexander and Schmidt 1977). In cases of obstruction, extravasation of spermatozoa into the surrounding tissues appears to be an uncommon phenomenon and, in these men, the spermatozoa are usually phagocytized in the lumen of, for example, the vas deferens (Phadke 1964). Incomplete

Table 3. Clinical evaluation of sperm antibody formation in 99 men with circulating head-to-head or tail-to-tail sperm-agglutinating antibodies. The men underwent clinical examination and their past medical history was reviewed to obtain the most likely event that could have caused sperm antibody production

No significant findings	47
Previous inguinal herniorraphy	17
History orchiepididymitis	9
Gonorrhea	6
Prostatitis	5
Urinary tract infection	3
Mumps orchitis	3
Urethritis	2
Varicocele-variococelectomy	2
Hematuria	1
Testicular trauma	1
Status postoperative hydrocele	1
Status postoperative retentio testis	1
Status postoperative vasovasostomy	1
Total	99

degradation of spermatozoa in the lumen with subsequent absorption of antigenic fragments may lead to sperm antibody production.

A prerequisite for the formation of sperm antibodies is the presence of mature spermatozoa in the testis. In obstructive azoospermia, about 60% of the men will develop sperm antibodies whereas in men with azoospermia, in whom various degrees of deranged spermatogenesis and no mature spermatozoa are observed by testicular biopsy, sperm antibodies do not form (Friberg 1980a). In obstructive azoospermia as well as following vasectomy, the serum titers are quite elevated, but the seminal fluid titers are absent or low. In contrast, patients with normal sperm counts and circulating sperm antibodies often have high titers of antibodies both in serum and seminal fluid.

11.4 The Significance of Sperm Antibodies in Men

The first comprehensive study of sperm antibodies in sera from men was published by Rümke and Hellinga (1959). They examined sera from 2015 unselected infertile and 416 fertile men and found sperm-agglutinating antibodies using the Kibrick technique in 4% of the infertile men and in 1% of the fertile men. There was a significant difference between the infertile and the fertile men at the titers 1:16 and 1:32: titers higher than 1:16 were only encountered among the infertile men. These findings were essentially confirmed by Fjällbrant (1968a, 1973) who compared the presence and titers of sperm-agglutinating antibodies in a large group of men, unselected with regard to infertility, with findings in men of recently delivered spouses. In some of the fertile men, titers above 1:32 were found but only two of the men had a titer above 1:128. These studies demonstrate that in infertile men, approximately 4% will have a serum titer of 1:32 or more and 2% will have a serum titer of 1:512 or more. In male partners of selected couples with *unexplained infertility*, the corresponding figures may be as high as 17%–19% and 6%–10%, respectively (Friberg 1974; Schoenfeld et al. 1976; Koskimies 1979).

The significance of high serum titers of sperm-agglutinating antibodies has been well documented in a follow-up study of couples where the husbands were found to be positive for such antibodies 2–16 years earlier (Rümke et al. 1974). With low titets in the husband's serum, 28% of the couples were reported to have children, with titers of 1:32–1:128 this figure dropped to 12%, and with titers above 1:128 only 8% of the couples had children. Of special importance was the observation that no conceptions were reported from couples where the husband had serum titers above 1:512.

Men with low serum titers (1:32 or less) of sperm-agglutinating antibodies rarely have any demonstrable antibody titers in the seminal fluid. With higher serum titers, a seminal fluid titer is more commonly observed and with serum titers of 1:512 or more the presence of a seminal fluid titer is the rule (Rümke 1974a; Friberg 1974). With *serum titers* of sperm-agglutinating antibodies above 1:32, a marked decrease of the sperm migration in the in vitro cervical mucus penetration tests is noted (Fjällbrant 1968b; Morgan et al. 1977) and in the postcoital tests the same phenomenon is observed (Friberg 1980b). Sperm invasion in the post-coital test also appears to be markedly affected when the *seminal fluid titer* is 1:16 or more and, therefore, it has been suggested that determination of the seminal fluid titer of antibodies would be of a better prognostic value than the determination of the serum titer. Preliminary findings (Husted and Hjort 1975) appear to favor such an assumption, but more comprehensive studies with demonstration of both serum and seminal fluid titers of sperm-agglutinating antibodies in infertile and fertile men are necessary.

In the evaluation of men with sperm-agglutinating antibodies in serum, the following guidelines can be followed (Table 4). Men with low titers (1:32 or less) of sperm-agglutinating antibodies in serum probably only have an insignificant reduction of their fertilizing capacity. Men with moderate titers (1:64–1:512) of sperm-agglutinating antibodies appear to have a marked reduction of their fertility but, although long-standing infertility is the rule, conceptions may occasionally be encountered in couples where the husband fits into this category. With high serum titers (more than 1:512) conceptions take place so rarely that the man has to be con-

Table 4. Clinical significance of different titers of sperm-agglutinating antibodies in serum and seminal fluid

Antibody titer in serum		
≦1:32	1:64 – 1:512	>1:512
Probably only minor effects on fertility	Markedly decreased fertility, but not sterility	Probably sterility
Antibody titer in seminal fluid		
≦1:16	≧1:32	
Markedly decreased fertility, but not sterility	Probably sterility	

sidered clinically sterile. Men with sperm-immobilizing antibodies in serum usually also have high titers of circulating sperm-agglutinating antibodies and their fertility is, therefore, classified according to the titer of sperm-agglutinating antibodies observed. The presence of sperm-agglutinating antibodies in the seminal fluid appears to worsen the prognosis. If the seminal fluid titer is 1:16 or less, even if the serum titer is low, the fertility of the patient is considered to be in the same category as with a moderate serum titer. If the seminal fluid titer is 1:32 or more, the prognosis is as bad as if the serum titer is more than 1:512.

These guidelines can only be considered for men with a sperm concentration of more than 20 million/ml. Varying degrees of oligozoospermia indicates a poorer prognosis, since the agglutinating effect of the antibodies drastically reduces the number of spermatozoa that can ascend into the female genital tract.

11.5 Treatment of Men with Sperm Antibodies

The treatment of men with sperm antibodies must at present be considered experimental and no approach can be considered as the "treatment of choice". The results of several types of therapy are discussed in Sects. 5.1–5.5.

11.5.1 Treatment of Men with Genital Infections

During the course of a prostatitis, vasitis, or epididymitis, the swelling and edema in the periluminal tissue quite often cause temporary obstruction of the efferent sperm transportation pathway. During such an obstruction, formation of sperm antibodies appears to be a reality: a past history of a genital infection is not uncommon in men with sperm-agglutinating antibodies. Also the scarring observed after an infection can lead to permanent obstruction. The obstruction may be one-sided, which means that the number of spermatozoa in the ejaculate remains normal. Not all patients with an infection develop sperm antibodies, but the factors responsible and the possible adjuvant effects of an infection are currently unknown. After an infection has healed, the antibodies may disappear spontaneously: The sperm antibody titers have also been reported to fall following intensive antibiotic treatment of chronic prostatitis (Bandhauer 1966; Quesada et al. 1968; Fjällbrant 1973).

The reduction in the titers of sperm-agglutinating antibodies after intensive treatment of chronic prostatitis using antibiotics and low doses of testosterone has recently been described in eight men (Fjällbrant and Nilsson 1977). These patients had high serum titers (1:128–1:1024) of sperm-agglutinating antibodies before treatment: during the course of treatment and the follow-up, a significant titer reduction (i.e., more than two titer steps) was noted (Fig. 2). Five of these men whose titers had fallen to between 1:4 and 1:128 after the treatment also impregnated their wives.

The decrease in antibody titers with subsequent conceptions following the treatment of genital infections should encourage physicians to evaluate patients with circulating sperm antibodies for the possible presence of a nonsymptomatic (prostatic) infection. If signs of an infection are found, i.e., a swollen and tender prostatic gland and/or aggregates of a large number of leukocytes in prostatic secretions, the in-

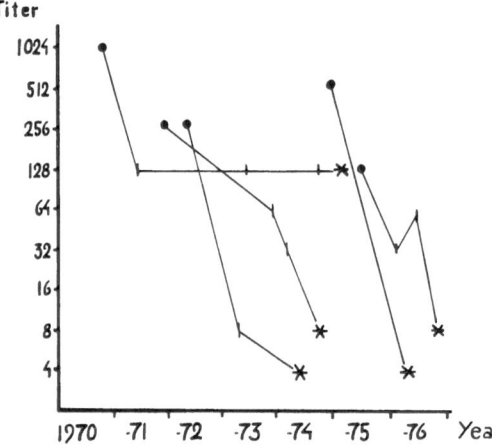

Fig. 2. Sperm-agglutinating antibody titers in the sera of five men at the time when treatment of their chronic prostatitis was started (•) and about the time of their wives' conception (*) (Fjällbrant and Nilsson 1977)

fection should be treated vigorously for an appropriate length of time; several months if necessary. The possibility of a simultaneous infection in the wife should also be considered and she should receive adequate therapy.

11.5.2 Surgical Treatment

Surgical removal of impaired organs from the male genital tract as a treatment for men with sperm antibodies was first attempted by Rümke and Hellinga (1959), who described the removal of a testis from an infertile man. This man had experienced atrophy of one testicle following a surgical accident nine years earlier. The orchiectomy was not followed by any change in the antibody titer. However, other reports have been more optimistic. Circulating sperm antibodies were, for example, reported to disappear from one patient following removal of an epididymal cyst and in another patient after an epididymectomy for a tuberculous epididymitis (Bandhauer 1966). These two patients had not complained of infertility and, therefore, the effect of the disappearing antibodies on their fertility is not known. In another patient who was found to have cytotoxic sperm antibodies in serum following epididymoorchitis, the antibody titer decreased after orchiectomy and 9 months later the antibodies had disappeared. At the same time, the spermiogram improved from pronounced asthenoteratozoospermia to normal (Laurenti et al. 1978).

These few isolated case reports are of interest, but the long-term follow-up as well as the influence of surgical procedure on fertility is not known. Therefore, surgical removal of diseased genital organs from men with circulating sperm antibodies must be considered experimental.

11.5.3 Sperm Washing and Intrauterine Inseminations

Most of the IgG and IgA antibodies present in the seminal fluid enter into the ejaculate with the prostatic secretion (Rümke 1974b). Therefore, mixing of the antibodies and the spermatozoa does not take place until the moment of ejaculation. Although ejaculates from men with sperm-agglutinating antibodies usually demonstrate a pronounced autoagglutination directly after ejaculation, it was hoped that immediate dilution, centrifugation, and removal of the seminal fluid would remove enough antibodies to allow some of the spermatozoa to ascend into the female genital tract. Since the migration of spermatozoa through cervical mucus in men with high titers of sperm-agglutinating antibodies is severely impaired (Kremer and Jager 1976), bypassing the cervical mucus with an intrauterine insemination might increase the possibility of pregnancy.

Sperm washing and insemination was first tried by Halim et al. (1973) who reported three pregnancies in 12 treated couples. The method was later used by Shulman et al. (1977, 1978a) who had success with pregnancy in one of seven treated couples. Only the presence of antibody and not the titers from the men in these couples were reported and consequently a full interpretation of the results cannot be given.

Kremer et al. (1978a, b) performed intrauterine inseminations in 15 couples where the husbands had serum titers of sperm-agglutinating antibodies of 1:32–1:4096, high seminal fluid titers, and a poor sperm penetration of cervical mucus both in vitro and in vivo. Three couples reported conception after this treatment. According to the titer evaluations described earlier, these men would be considered to have markedly reduced fertility. Intrauterine inseminations in cases with high titers of sperm-agglutinating antibodies may, therefore, be worth trying.

11.5.4 Immunosuppressive Treatment

11.5.4.1 Low-Dose Corticosteroids

Antibody formation against spermatozoa in men is an autoimmune phenomenon. Symptoms as well as immunological events associated with autoimmune diseases have long been known to respond to corticosteroid treatment (Parrillo and Fauci 1979). Soon after the demonstration of autoantibodies against spermatozoa in men, corticosteroid therapy was attempted. The doses administered were fairly low and usually of 15–20 mg/day prednisone. With this dose regimen, treatment for up to 30 or 60 days did not affect the serum or seminal fluid titer, nor did the degree of autoagglutination in the ejaculates decrease (Rümke and Hellinga 1959; Bandhauer 1966). Not until treatment periods of 3–12 months had been employed did any titer changes in the sperm antibodies occur with subsequent conceptions. Hendry et al. (1979) treated 29 men with sperm-agglutinating antibodies (15 oligozoospermic and 14 normozoospermic men) using 5 mg prednisone three times daily for an average of 6–7 months and found a decrease in sperm antibodies, but the titers never fell below 1:32. In ten of the oligozoospermic men, the sperm counts normalized and two conceptions occurred. In addition, two more patients conceived when sperm washing and insemination were used after the corticosteroid treatment. In the group of men with normal sperm counts, two pregnancies were obtained and one more patient became pregnant when sperm washing and insemination was added to the treatment. De Almeida and Soufir (1977) gave 2 mg dexamethasone to a man with a serum antibody titer of 1:160 and a seminal fluid titer of 1:32, as well as pronounced autoagglutination in the ejaculate. During 6 months of treatment, the sperm counts remained stable in the normal range and after 5 months of therapy, a con-

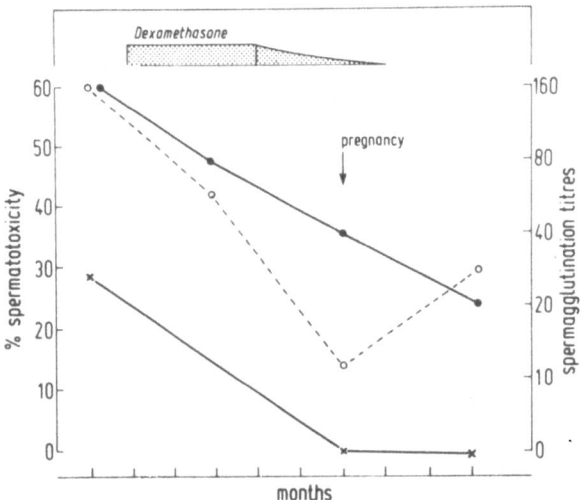

Fig. 3. Decrease of sperm-agglutinating and cytotoxic sperm antibody titers in a man treated with dexamethasone for 6 months. ●—●= Serum spermagglutinins, ○—○= Serum spermacytotoxins, ×—× = Seminal plasma cytotoxins (De Almeida and Soufir 1977)

ception occurred when the serum titer had declined to 1:40 and the seminal fluid titer was no longer demonstrable (Fig. 3).

11.5.4.2 High-Dose Corticosteroids

"High doses" of the newer synthetic corticosteroids seem to affect immune responses in humans much more dramatically than the low-dose therapy. Butler and Rossen (1973) gave 96 mg methyl prednisolone to male volunteers and noted a significant decrease of serum IgG in 86% and of IgA in 43% of the men; for IgM the decrease was much more limited. The decrease of IgG was quite pronounced with a mean drop of 22% compared to untreated controls. The maximum decrease occurred 2 weeks after a 3-day course and 3 weeks after a 5-day course of the drug (Fig. 4). This high-dose corticosteroid treatment was first tried in men with circulating sperm-agglutinating antibodies by Shulman (1976): He treated a patient with a serum antibody titer of 1:512 and a seminal fluid titer of 1:16 with methylprednisolone for 7 days and observed a drop in the serum titer to 1:16 and the disappearance of the seminal fluid titer within 4 weeks after initiation of therapy (Fig. 5). Conception occurred at the time of the wife's next ovulation. Shulman et al. (1978a,b) later reported a success rate of 22% (four pregnancies from 18 treated men) and 33% (five conceptions from 15 men with circulating sperm antibodies).

Kremer et al. (1976, 1978a) reported the treatment of two men with circulating sperm antibodies using high-dose methylprednisolone for 1 week, but saw no significant decrease in the titer and these men remained infertile. In a later report (Kremer et al. 1978b), they used an extended treatment program where the high-dose of methylprednisolone was given repeatedly for 7 days a month for several months if no titer changes were noted. In a series of five patients with serum titers of

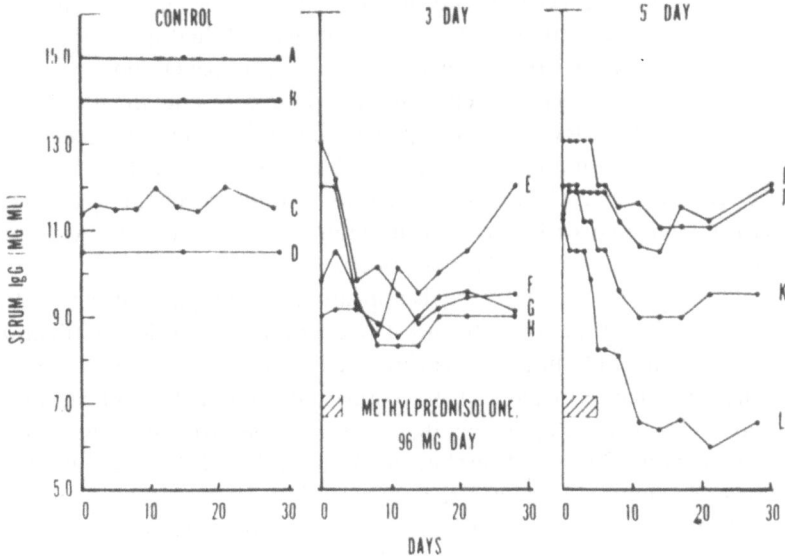

Fig. 4. Decrease of IgG concentrations after treatment with 96 mg methylprednisolone for 3 and 5 days. Serial IgG determinations demonstrate the lag-phase before the IgG concentrations begin to decline rapidly and the delayed onset of recovery in the 5 days treatment group. Code letters represent individual volunteers (Butler and Rossen 1973)

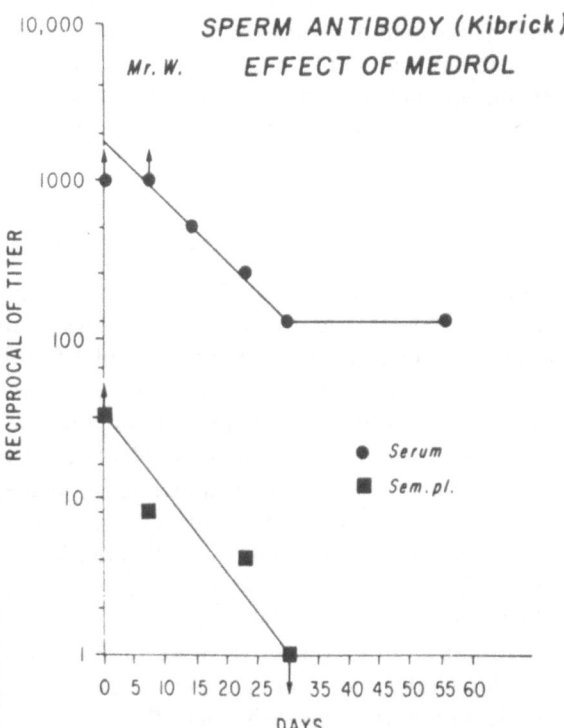

Fig. 5. Decline of serum and seminal fluid sperm-agglutinating antibody titers in relation to time (days) after treatment with 96 mg methylprednisolone for 7 days. (Shulman et al. 1978b)

1:32–1:2048, a conception was obtained in a couple where the man experienced a drop from only 1:1024–1:512, a constant seminal fluid titer but a pronounced improvement in the spermiogram and cervical mucus penetration.

Hendry et al. (1979) felt that high-dose cortisone treatment was more advantageous than the low-dose regimen and noted a more pronounced drop in the antibody titers with high-doses than with the low-dose treatment. Some patients received one course whereas others had two or three treatments synchronized with the wife's menstrual cycle. From their series of 18 treated men they obtained seven pregnancies, i.e., a conception rate of 39%.

Therapy using corticosteroids appears to have a place in the treatment of men with circulating sperm antibodies. The use of high-doses for short periods with repetition at monthly intervals synchronized with the wife's menstrual cycle, in cases where no change of the titer is recorded after the first treatment, appears to be a more advantageous approach. If a 5-day course is given, the optimal drop would be expected after 3 weeks. Therefore, medication should be given during days 21–26 of the cycle and, if a 7-day course is employed, the steroid is given slightly later in the cycle, for example, during days 15–21 after the first day of menstruation. Few complications have been reported and they have been limited to slight euphoria, water retention, and red flushings of the face.

11.5.4.3 Azathioprine

Profound immunological effects have been observed with the immunosuppressive drug azathioprine, and during such treatment the titer of circulating sperm-agglutinating antibodies has also been reported to be affected. However, only a single case report is available in the literature. Krause and Meyhöfer (1973) described the treatment of an infertile man with azathioprine for almost 1 year. His serum titer of 1:512 became negative and, shortly thereafter a conception was reported (Krause 1974).

11.5.5 The Testosterone Rebound Phenomenon and Sperm Antibodies

Once sperm antibody production has been initiated, it is maintained at a high level and the spontaneous disappearance of these antibodies appears to be very uncommon (Rümke et al. 1974). If the stimulus for sperm antibody formation (i.e., the spermatozoa) could be removed, then the titer would probably diminish and perhaps eventually disappear. High doses of testosterone will suppress spermatogenesis and cause azoospermia. Schoysman (1968) treated 17 men with high serum titers (1:64 or more) of sperm-agglutinating antibodies using 250 mg testosterone intramuscularly every 2 weeks, and in all cases the men became azoospermic. A reduction of the antibody titer was observed in all men during the course of 6–12 months of treatment. Following cessation of therapy, the spermatozoa returned in the ejaculates of all men, but in a majority of the men the antibodies returned at the same time as the spermatozoa. However, in seven men, the antibodies remained absent for various lengths of time and five of these men were reported to have become fertile. In a later report (Schoyman 1971), the treatment was described in more detail. The original group consisted of 29 men with serum titers of 1:64–1:512 of sperm-agglutinating antibodies and pronounced autoagglutination in the ejaculates. In 17 men, a titer reduction was noted after at least 6 months of treatment and a titer below 1:32 was noted after 8–13 months of treatment. As previously mentioned, treatment was successful in seven men and five conceptions occurred, four resulted in full-term pregnancies and one in a spontaneous abortion. Re-evaluation of these seven men 1 year after termination of treatment indicated that the agglutination phenomenon had returned in all cases.

After this promising report, Rümke et al. (1973) treated 12 men with high titers of sperm-agglutinating antibodies for 6.5–14.5 months using high-doses of testosterone. No decrease in the serum titers were observed, but in three men a reduction of the seminal fluid titer was noted. Two of these men reported conception 8–9 months after the treatment, but it was not clearly established that these pregnancies were related to the treatment.

In a recent report, 48 men with sperm-agglutinating antibodies were treated with 250 mg depot-testosterone once a week until azoospermia had been maintained for 1–2 months, after which they were treated with a moderate dose of methylprednisolone for 8 weeks (Dondero et al. 1979). In 19 of the men, this treatment did not result in any titer change, and in another seven a decrease in titer was noted, but a prompt return of both antibodies and spermatozoa was seen after stopping the medication. However, in 22 men the titer disappeared and remained absent for at least 1 year following the therapy, despite the return of spermatozoa in the ejaculate. Follow-up 1 year after termination of therapy showed that conception had occurred in 12 couples.

The testosterone rebound phenomenon has usually been used to improve sperm counts in oligozoospermic men, but the therapy has not been unanimously accepted (Walsh and Amelar 1977). In a small proportion of patients, usually those with severe oligozoospermia or abnormal hyalinization of the basement membrane shown by testicular biopsy, permanent and irreversible azoospermia may result (Lamensdorf et al. 1975). Although it may be said that men with very high titers of sperm antibodies are sterile anyhow, the risk of subsequent azoospermia following testosterone rebound treatment, although low, must be considered. Therefore, the success of this therapy has to be weighed against the positive reports seen with other types of treatment for immunological infertility in men.

11.6 Conclusions

Some guidelines for the treatment of men with sperm antibodies can be given in spite of the experimental nature of most of the suggested therapies (Table 5). In the clinical examination of men with sperm antibodies, a genital infection should be sought and, if one is found, adequate antibiotic therapy should be instituted for an appropriate length of time. In case the clinical examination reveals that the patient has an abnormality in the genital tract, e.g., a spermatocele, epididymal cyst, or an atrophic testis, surgical removal may be considered although it has to be remembered that no positive influence on fertility has been documented. If neither of these conditions are present or treatment has not resulted in lowering the antibody titer or pregnancy, sperm washing and intrauterine insemination should be the next step. If

Table 5. Recommendation and guidelines for treatment of men with circulating sperm antibodies

---

1. Presence of genital infection – prostatitis = Treatment!
2. Clinical demonstration of an abnormal organ in the male genital
   tract = Surgery??
3. Sperm washing and intrauterine insemination = Try for 3–6 months
4. Corticosteroids
   a) A low-dose cortisone = 15 mg prednisone daily for 3–6 months
   b) High-dose cortisone = 96 mg oral methylprednisolone to the husband on
      day 15–21 of the wife's menstrual cycle; treat for 3 consecutive months
5. Testosterone rebound = 250 mg i.m. depottestosterone every 2 weeks – azoospermia
   for 2 months – then 16 mg (1 month) and 8 mg (next month)
   methylprednisolone.

Follow up with regular determinations of concentrations of sperm antibodies!

no conception occurs after 3–6 months of this treatment, therapy should continue with high- or low doses of corticosteroids. Testosterone rebound therapy may be tried as the last resort of treatment.

It is hoped that the ongoing studies of immunological infertility in the male will give insight into the causative factors and enable us to come up with preventive measures to avoid the production of sperm antibodies in situations where antibody formation otherwise would be at risk. Also the current evaluations and experimentations with different types of therapy will also hopefully give us an idea of the "treatment of choice", instead of the multiple treatment approach that we must presently suggest.

11.7 References

Alexander NJ, Schmidt SS (1977) Incidence of antisperm antibody levels and granulomas in men. Fertil Steril 28:655–657

Bandhauer K (1966) Immunreaktionen bei Fertilitätsstörungen des Mannes. Urol Int 21:247–282

Boettcher B, Hjort T, Rümke P, Shulman S, Vyazov OE (1977) Auto- and isoantibodies to antigens of the human reproductive system. I. Results of an international comparative study. Clin Exp Immunol 30:173–180

Butler WT, Rossen RD (1973) Effects of cortico-steroids on immunity in man. I. Decreased serum IgG concentration caused by 3 or 5 days of high-doses of methylprednisolone. J Clin Invest 52:2629–2640

De Almeida M, Soufir JC (1977) Corticosteroid therapy for male autoimmune infertility. Lancet II:815–816

Dondero F, Isidori A, Lenzi A, Cerasaro M, Mazzilli F, Giovenco P, Conti C (1979) Treatment and follow-up of patients with infertility due to spermagglutinins. Fertil Steril 31:48–51

Fjällbrant B (1965) Immunoagglutination of sperm in cases of sterility. Acta Obstet Gynecol Scand 44:474–490

Fjällbrant B (1968a) Sperm agglutinins in sterile and fertile men. Acta Obstet Gynecol Scand 47:89–101

Fjällbrant B (1968b) Interrelation between high levels of sperm antibodies, reduced penetration of cervical mucus by spermatozoa, and sterility in men. Acta Obstet Gynecol Scand 47:102–118

Fjällbrant B (1969) Studies on sera from men with sperm antibodies. Acta Obstet Gynecol Scand 48:131–146

Fjällbrant B (1973) Antibodies affecting fertility in males. In: Hesegawa T, Hagashi M, Ebling FJG, Henderson IW (eds) Proceedings of the VIIth World Congress Fertility and Sterility, Tokyo 1971. Excerpta Medica, Amsterdam, pp 99–104

Fjällbrant B, Nilsson S (1977) Decrease of sperm antibody titer in males, and conception after treatment of chronic prostatitis. Int J Fertil 22:255–256

Friberg J (1974) Clinical and immunological studies on sperm-agglutinating antibodies in serum and seminal fluid. Acta Obstet Gynecol Scand [Suppl] 36:1–76

Friberg J (1980a) Serum and seminal fluid immunoglobulins in relation to testicular morphology. J Androl 1:133–137

Friberg J (1980b) Post-coital tests and sperm-agglutinating antibodies in men. Am J Obstet Gynecol 141:76–80

Friberg J, Friberg-Tilly I (1977) Spontaneous sperm-agglutination in ejaculates from men with head-to-head or tail-to-tail sperm-agglutinating antibodies in serum. Fertil Steril 28:657–662

Halim A, Antoniou D, Leedham PW, Blandy JP, Tresidder GC (1973) Investigation and treatment of the infertile male. Proc R Soc Med 66:373–378

Hellema HWJ, Rümke P (1976) Comparison of the tray agglutination technique with the gelatin agglutination technique for the detection of sperm-agglutinating activity in human sera. Fertil Steril 27:284–292

Hendry WF, Stedronska J, Hughes L, Cameron KM, Pugh RCB (1979) Steroid treatment of male subfertility caused by anti-sperm antibodies. Lancet II:498–501

Husted S (1975) Sperm antibodies in men from infertile couples. Analysis of sperm-agglutinins and immuno-fluorescent antibodies in 657 men. Int J Fertil 20:113–121

Husted S, Hjort T (1975) Sperm antibodies in serum and seminal plasma. Int J Fertil 20:97–105

Husted S, Ingerslev HJ (1975) Comparison of methods for the detection of immobilizing and cytotoxic sperm antibodies. Acta Pathol Microbiol Scand Sect C 83:347–353

Isojima S, Li TS, Ashitaka Y (1968) Immunologic analysis of sperm-immobilizing factor found in sera of women with unexplained sterility. Am J Obstet Gynecol 101:677–683

Koskimies AI (1979) Sperm-agglutinating antibodies in infertile couples. Arch Androl 2:241–245

Krause W (1974) Autorennotiz zum Beitrag „Unterdrückung spermagglutinierender Autoantikörper mit Imurek". Hautarzt 25:574

Krause W, Meyhöfer W (1973) Unterdrückung spermagglutinierender Autoantikörper im Serum durch Azathioprin (Imurek). Hautarzt 24:551–552

Kremer J, Jager S (1976) The sperm-cervical mucus contact test: A preliminary report. Fertil Steril 27:335–340

Kremer J, Jager S, Kuiken J (1978a) Treatment of infertility caused by anti-sperm antibodies. Int J Fertil 23:270–276

Kremer J, Jager S, Kuiken J, van Slochteren-Draaisma T (1978b) Recent advances in diagnosis and treatment of infertility due to anti-sperm antibodies. In: Cohen J, Hendry WF (eds) Spermatozoa, antibodies and infertility. Blackwell Scientific Publications, Oxford, pp 117–127

Lamensdorf H, Compere D, Begley G (1975) Testosterone rebound therapy in the treatment of male infertility. Fertil Steril 26:469–472

Laurenti C, Fagioli A, Lenzi A, Dondero F (1978) Anti-sperm antibodies in a case of secondary unilateral testicular atrophy. Br J Urol 50:352

Marcus ZH, Freisheim JH, Houk JL, Herman JH, Hess EV (1978) In vitro studies in reproductive immunology. 1. Suppression of cell-mediated immune response by human spermatozoa and fractions isolated from human seminal plasma. Clin Immunol Immunopathol 9:318–326

Mettler L, Gradl T (1975) Difficulty of obtaining reproducibility in the Franklin and Dukes test for the detection of sperm-agglutinating antibodies in human sera. J Reprod Fertil 44:217–221

Morgan H, Stedronska J, Hendry WF, Chamberlain GVP, Dewhurst CJ (1977) Sperm-cervical mucus crossed-hostility testing and anti-sperm antibodies in the husband. Lancet I:1228–1230

168   J. Friberg

Parrillo JE, Fauci AS (1979) Mechanisms of glucocorticoid action on immune processes. Annu Rev Pharmacol Toxicol 19:179–201

Phadke AM (1964) Fate of spermatozoa in cases of obstructive azoospermia and after ligation of vas deferens in man. Fertil Steril 7:1–12

Quesada EM, Dukes CD, Deen GH, Franklin RR (1968) Genital infection and sperm-agglutinating antibodies in infertile men. J Urol 99:106–108

Rose NR, Hjort T, Rümke P, Harper MJK, Vyazov O (1976) Techniques for detection of iso- and auto-antibodies to human spermatozoa. Clin Exp Immunol 23:175–199

Rümke P (1954) The presence of sperm antibodies in the serum of two patients with oligozoospermia. Vox Sang 4:135–140

Rümke P (1974a) Autoantibodies against spermatozoa in infertile men: Some unsolved problems. In: Centaro A, Carretti N (eds) Immunology in obstetrics and gynecology. Proceedings of the First International Congress, Padua 1973. Excerpta Medica, Amsterdam, pp 26–35

Rümke P (1974b) The origin of immunoglobulins in semen. Clin Exp Immunol 17:287–297

Rümke P, Hellinga G (1959) Autoantibodies against spermatozoa in sterile men. Am J Clin Pathol 32:357–363

Rümke P, van Amstel N, Messer EN, Bezemer PD (1973) Prognosis of men with auto-sperm-agglutinins in the serum and the unsuccessful treatment with testosterone. In: Bratanov K, Edwards RG, Vulchanov VH, Dikov V, Somlev B (eds) Immunology of reproduction. Proceedings of the Second International Symposium, Varna Bulgaria 1971. Bulgarian Academy of Sciences, Sofia, pp 319–324

Rümke P, van Amstel N, Messer EN, Bezemer PD (1974) Prognosis of fertility of men with sperm-agglutinins in the serum. Fertil Steril 25:393–398

Schoenfeld C, Amelar RD, Dubin L (1976) Clinical experience with sperm antibody testing. Fertil Steril 27:1199–1203

Schoysman R (1968) Treatment of male infertility due to auto-agglutination of spermatozoa. In: VIth World Congress Fertility and Sterility, Tel Aviv (Abstr), pp 112–113

Schoysman R (1971) Immunologie du testicle et des spermatozoides. In: Endocrinopathies et immunologie. Masson, Paris, pp 345–365

Setchell BP (1980) The functional significance of the blood-testis barrier. J Androl 1:3–10

Shulman S (1976) Treatment of immune male infertility with methylprednisolone. Lancet II:1243

Shulman S, Davis P, Lade P, Reyniak JV (1977) Immune infertility and new approaches to treatment. In: Boettcher B (ed) Immunological influence on human fertility. Academic Press, Sydney, pp 281–288

Shulman S, Harlin B, Davis P, Reyniak JV (1978a) Immune infertility and new approaches to treatment. Fertil Steril 29:309–313

Shulman S, Mininberg DT, Davis JE (1978b) Significant immunologic factors in male infertility. J Urol 119:231–234

Stites DP, Erickson RP (1975) Suppressive effect of seminal plasma on lymphocyte activation. Nature (Lond) 253:727–729

Walsh PC, Amelar RD (1977) Medical management of male infertility. In: Amelar RD, Dubin L, Walsh PC (eds) Male infertility. Saunders, Philadelphia, pp 179–190

Wilson L (1954) Sperm-agglutinins in human semen and blood. Proc Soc Exp Biol Med 85:652–655

12 Nonsurgical Treatment of Varicocele

M. P. P. de Castro

In the past, the varicocele has been managed in various ways. Until the middle of this century, it was generally accepted that varicosities of the scrotal veins were an innocuous condition which rarely needed treatment. During the last 25 years, however, surgical treatment has been stressed in the management of male infertility.

It was not until 1978 that Lima et al. described a new nonsurgical method for the treatment of varicocele, namely, sclerosis of the spermatic veins immediately after diagnostic selective retrograde venography.

A study of 88 infertile men with varicocele who underwent transcatheter sclerosis of spermatic veins is presented. The results suggest that this technique may provide an alternate method of varicocele treatment.

12.1 Historical Background

In the 16th century, Ambroisé Paré (cited by Ivanissevich 1960) defined varicocele as a "block of vessels filled by melancholic blood" and this was almost all that one could find in the medical literature for the following 300 years. In 1889, Bennet (cited by Greenberg 1977) observed the relationship between the presence of a varicocele and diminished sperm production.

Ivanissevich and Gregorini (1918) defined varicocele as an anatomoclinical syndrome anatomically characterized by varices inside the scrotum, and clinically by venous reflux. They proposed high ligation of the left spermatic vein to effect a cure.

Tulloch (1952) reported the restoration of fertility in a previously azoospermic man after varicocele ligation. The increased incidence of varicocele in men with poor semen quality was subsequently recognized (Russel 1954): e.g., "Where a varicocele is associated with subfertility the varicocele should be cured" (Tulloch 1955). These observations led to the demonstration of the efficacy and safety of high ligation of the spermatic veins (Ivanissevich 1960).

Seminal changes of infertile men with varicocele were described as similar to the "seminal stress pattern" found in men subjected to various noxious agents; namely, a low sperm concentration with low motility and increased numbers of abnormal sperm forms (MacLeod 1965).

The histological description of bilateral testicular injury in the presence of varicocele (Charny 1962; Dubin and Hotchkiss 1969) indicated that the varicocele may not have been the innocuous entity it was once thought to be.

12.1.1 Diagnosis of Varicocele

Diagnosis of the varicocele depends upon detecting blood reflux into the spermatic veins. Unfortunately, there is no universal agreement on the criteria for reflux detection.

A varicocele incidence of 9.2% in infertile men with poor semen quality was found when the varicocele was palpable and there was visible enlargement of the pampiniform plexus (Russell 1954). An incidence of 39% was reported when the patients were examined in the standing position during a Valsalva's maneuver (Dubin and Amelar 1971).

There are differences in varicocele incidence in men from different races. In Brazil, anatomical study of the left spermatic vein in both black and white men led to the conclusion that there is a low incidence of varicocele in black men, because of the adequate number and efficacy of valves found in their spermatic veins (Goulart 1935). The low incidence of varicocele in black men was also pointed out in France (Adjiman 1972).

On the basis of clinical examination, varicoceles can be graded according to the facility of detection. Verstoppen and Steeno (1977) summarize the problem as follows:

"a) all systems for classification involve subjective judgements on the part of the examiner, and the results are likely to vary from one person to another; b) the size of varicocele may differ depending on the previous activity of the patient and whether or not the patient performs a Valsalva maneuver; c) the position of the patient during the examination (sitting, lying or standing) affects the observed results; d) there is no way of comparing the results, obtained using the various systems of classification, with each other; and e) all the systems have divided the varicocele condition into three distinct groups, where in reality there is a gradual transition from the most minor to the most severe situation."

Early radiological studies on varicocele patients were done in Brazil by Cotrim (1940): By in vivo injection of a contrast medium into the scrotal veins, he could conclusively demonstrate that the varicocele is characterized by blood reflux from the renal veins. The existing anastomoses between the left and the right pampiniform plexus were demonstrated by radiological studies during varicocele operation (El-Sadr and Mina 1950).

The development of techniques for selective catheterization of the regional veins demonstrated that retrograde spermatic venography was a useful method in detecting and evaluating the varicocele (Ahlberg et al. 1966). Although a non-invasive method for varicocele diagnosis (scrotal thermography) was described by Kormano et al. (1970), it was by means of retrograde venography that the varicocele could be recognized without palpable distension of the pampiniform veins, i.e., a subclinical grade of varicocele (Comhaire and Kunnen 1976; Castro and Lima 1976).

12.1.2 Treatment of Varicocele

Tulloch (1955), Davidson (1954), and Young (1956) demonstrated that surgical treatment of the varicocele in infertile patients is both effective and basically free of undesirable side-effects. Since the results of medical treatment of male infertility are very poor, varicocele treatment rose to "hit parade" heights and ligation of spermatic veins was performed even in infertile patients without varicocele on the assumption that it could be of value (Palti et al. 1968). The 55% pregnancy rate and the 71% semen quality improvement obtained after surgical ligation of spermatic veins on the 504 infertile men studied by Dubin and Amelar (1975) might have helped to change the scepticism about male infertility therapy.

The first non-surgical attempt to eliminate varicosities of the scrotal veins using injections of alcohol or a 20% dextrose-glycerin solution plus partial scrotum resection was not associated with adhesions (Riedl 1979). During a study of the blood flow direction in patients with varicocele by antegrade venography, in five patients the contrast substance was accidentally injected outside the pampiniform veins and, in three of these, the varicoceles presumably disappeared by perivascular fibrosis reaction (Cotrim 1940).

12.2 Transcatheter Sclerosis of the Spermatic Veins

The feasibility of using the diagnostic technique of selective spermatic venography as a curative procedure was demonstrated by the injection of sclerosing substances (75% hypertonic glucose solution and monoethanolamine oleate) into the catheterized veins (Lima et al. 1978). In this study, three infertile men in whom clinical varicocele was evident had their left spermatic veins catheterized under local anesthesia. After a radiographic demonstration of dilated and tortuous veins in which the flow was retrograde, the veins were sclerosed. Mild local pain was the only complaint and no additional anesthesia was required. Venography immediately after the sclerosing procedure showed a complete occlusion of the veins; the patients were kept resting in bed for only 4 h and then discharged. Follow-up examinations failed to demonstrate recurrence of the varicocele. Although no complications were documented, it was suggested that a potential complication would be the migration of a thrombus from the sclerosed veins to the lungs.

We subsequently studied 20 subfertile patients with varicoceles and treated them by the transcatheter sclerosing technique. Fourteen of these patients, followed-up for approximately 12 months, had a significant increase in the sperm count, motility rate, and percentage of oval sperm forms. The mean sperm count for those 14 patients rose from 8.15 million/ml to 33.12 million/ml. Seven of their wives became pregnant (Castro and Lima 1978).

In view of these results we undertook further studies to determine the efficacy of spermatic vein sclerosis as a mode of treating varicoceles in subfertile men.

From October, 1975, to December, 1979, at the Services of Vascular Radiology (headed by Sérgio Santos Lima) of the Hospital Sírio Libanes and the Hospital Albert Einstein in São Paulo, a total of 163 scleroses of the spermatic veins were performed. At the beginning of the study and in only two cases was the complication of slight pampiniform phlebitis observed. This was clearly related to several repeated injections of 10 ml 75% glucose solution. A modification in the procedure was then introduced by avoiding glucose injection.

12.3 Technique

Spermatic veins are catheterized by the Seldinger technique (Ahlberg et al. 1966). With the patient in the supine position, the catheter (BD Formocath, I.D. 0.047 in.) is introduced into the right femoral vein, under local anesthesia with 2% xylocaine. The catheter is introduced into the inferior vena cava and the renal veins. The spermatic veins are catheterized and 10 ml sodium diatrizoate (50%) is injected manually in the proximal portion of the veins. Films are obtained at the velocity of 1/s for 10 s. The contrast injection permits visualization of the retrograde flow into the spermatic veins, opacifying the pampiniform plexus.

To sclerose the veins, 2 ml monoethanolamine oleate (0.1 g) is injected into the spermatic veins. Usually, the right spermatic vein is catheterized prior to the left one.

After injection of the sclerosing substance, the catheter is kept in the vein for 60 min with an intravenous saline infusion, and the venography is then repeated to assess the vein occlusion. If the vein remains patent, another sclerosing injection is required. As shown by the immediate control venography, complete occlusion of the vein occurred in all cases (Fig. 1–5).

12.4 Observations in 88 Patients

As of December, 1979, a group of 88 men who underwent transcatheter sclerosis of spermatic veins had been followed-up by the author. All of the men consulted for infertility of 17–98 months.

In 33 subjects, varicoceles were palpable, while in 55 cases a subclinical varicocele was detected. Subclinical varicocele was suspected because of persistent oligoteratoasthenozoospermia and/or abnormal scrotal thermography. For the whole

Table 1. Varicocele detection by retrograde venography. Numbers in parentheses indicate those detected by clinical examination

	No. of patients	Retrograde venography		
		Left	Bilateral	Right
Palpable varicocele	33	20 (26)	12 (5)	1 (2)
Subclinical varicocele[a]	55	38	10	7
Total	88 100%	58 66%	22 25%	8 9%

[a] At the beginning of the study the main effort was to catheterize the left spermatic vein. After introduction of thermography into our routine male infertility evaluation, a systematic attempt to catheterize both spermatic veins was carried out

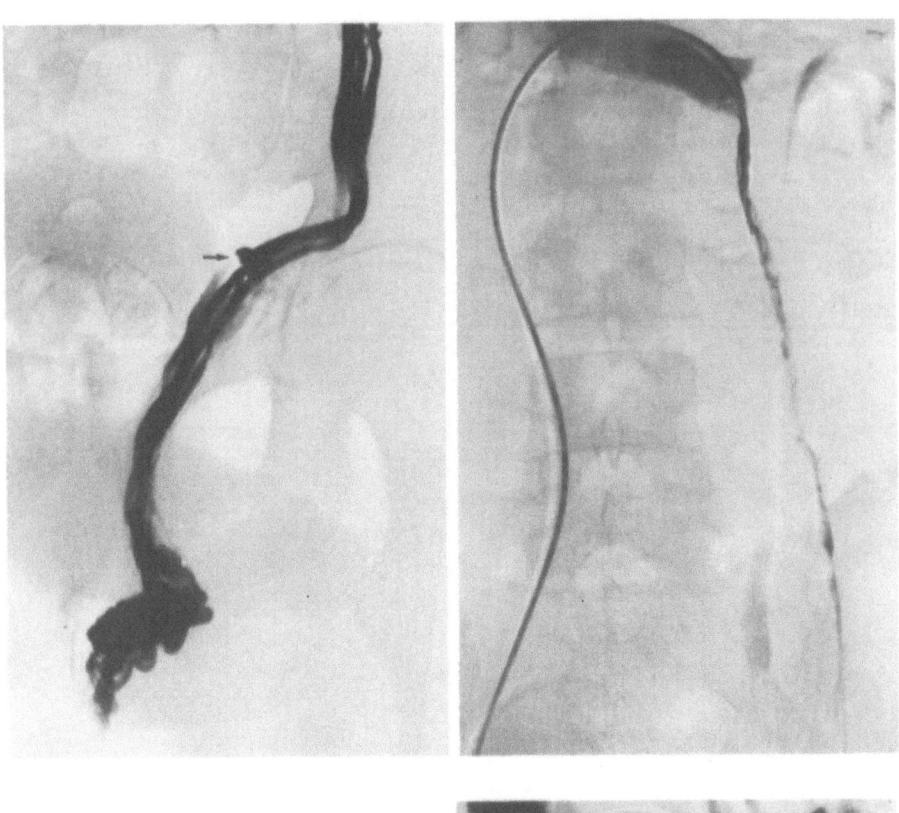

Fig. 1a. Venography in patient with palpable left varicocele. Note three branches of vessels, one of which shows a competent valvule (*arrow*). Other branches fill enlarged and tortuous vessels of pampiniform plexus. **b** Venography showing vessel constriction approximately 30 min after single injection of monoethanolamine oleate into the left spermatic vein. Note irregular distribution of contrast medium due to thrombus formation. **c** Final result of sclerosis. Tip of catheter introduced at the proximal portion of the left spermatic vein. See Fig. 2 for comparison

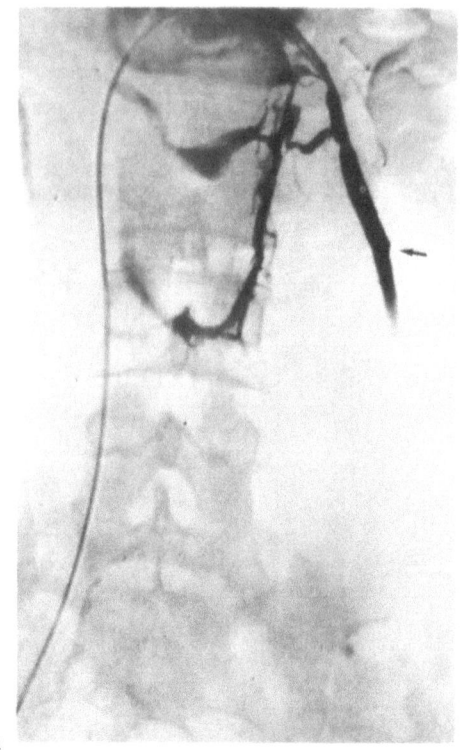

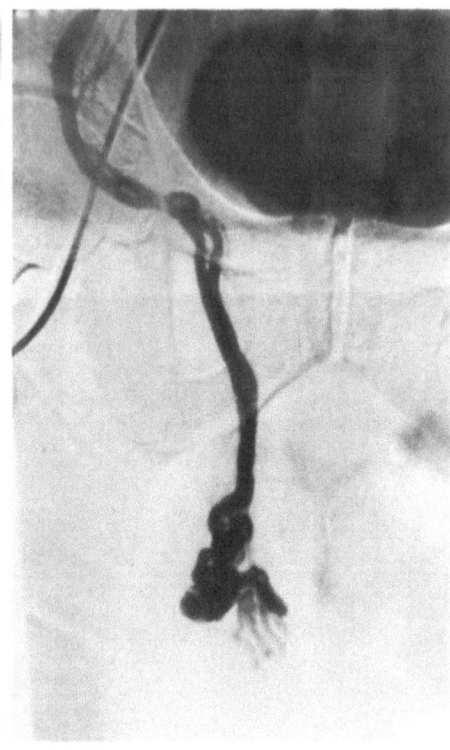

2

3

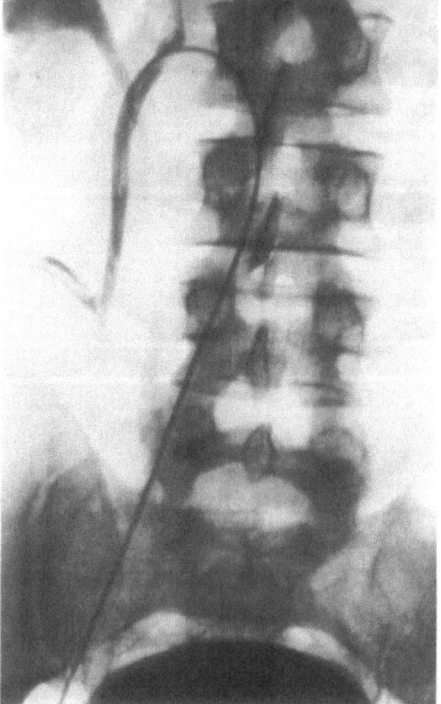

Fig. 2. Venography in man with no varicocele. Contrast medium introduced into left spermatic vein showing valvule situated at approximately 5 cm near renal vein (*arrow*)

Fig. 3. Subclinical right-side varicocele, diagnosed by retrograde venography

Fig. 4. Picture taken 1 h after sclerosing injection for treatment of a right varicocele. Full occlusion of the vein has occurred, thus preventing retrograde blood flow

4

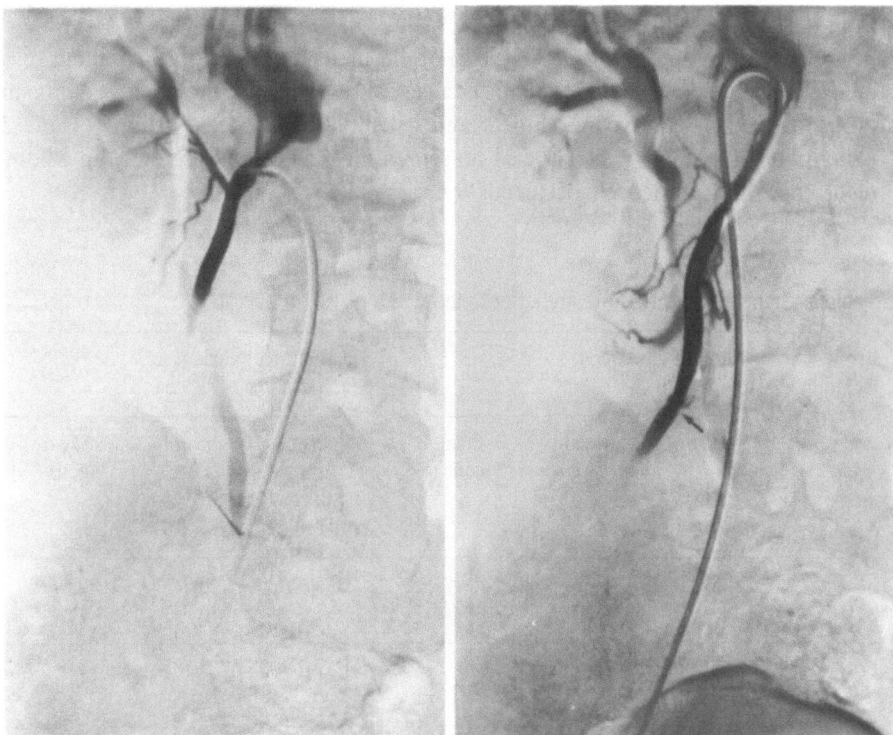

a   b

Fig. 5a. Picture shown to illustrate normal situation in right spermatic vein. Tip of catheter barely introduced into the orifice of vessel. Blood flow is ascendent. **b** In the same man, looped catheter for deeper introduction into right spermatic vein. Arrow pointing in proximal valvule

group, a definite diagnosis was established by retrograde selective spermatic venography (Table 1).

In all but two of the 88 patients, it was possible to sclerose the spermatic varicose veins at the same time. Of these two patients, the one with palpable bilateral varicoceles could only have the right spermatic vein catheterized and underwent surgery for left varicocele ligation. In the other patient, although the blood reflux could be demonstrated in both right and left spermatic veins, due to technical reasons only the left vein could be satisfactorily catheterized and then sclerosed. Six months later the right spermatic vein was uneventfully sclerosed. Patients were followed-up for at least 12 months and no complications, including hydrocele, were observed.

There were seven documented recurrences. In two cases of formerly palpable varicocele, recurrence was clinically detected on the left side. In the five other patients, all with subclinical left-side varicocele, recurrence was shown by scrotal thermography. Recurrences were detected 6–9 months after sclerosing procedure.

For each patient semen analysis was performed at least on two occasions before treatment and on three occasions after the therapeutic procedure. None were azoospermic. The criteria for semen improvement were: a doubling of the mean pretreatment value or an improvement reaching a mean sperm count higher than 20 million/ml; mean motility of 60% or more; and oval cells in excess of 60% (adapted from Fernando et al. 1976).

According to these criteria, 58 (66%) of the men showed an improvement of semen quality, and no significant differences were observed in semen quality improvement when comparing clinical and subclinical varicocele groups (Table 2). Among the 30 patients who showed no semen improvement were those in whom a recurrence of the varicocele occurred.

Table 2. Semen analysis before and after treatment

Pre-treatment	Clinical varicocele 33 patients			Subclinical varicocele 55 patients		
	Sperm count (million/ml)	Motility (%)	Oval cells (%)	Sperm count (million/ml)	Motility (%)	Oval cells (%)
Mean	14.8	47.3	46.4	10.5	43.3	53.7
SD	10.3	18.2	14.9	9.7	16.3	16.4
Post-treatment	Improved = 21 patients			Improved = 37 patients		
Mean	36.0[a]	56.2[a]	61.4[a]	43.4[a]	57.8[a]	65.3[a]
SD	12.4	22.4	11.4	28.3	27.7	10.6
	Not improved = 12 patients			Not improved = 18 patients		
Mean	11.6	21.7	49.1	9.3	23.9	54.0
SD	3.6	15.3	5.8	5.5	17.8	15.3

[a] In comparison with pretreatment values, $P < 0.01$

The wives of 34 men (39%) became pregnant. The time from sclerosis to pregnancy was 2–21 months. Pregnancies resulted only where men showed semen improvement. Thus, this 39% pregnancy rate is probably a result of successful treatment.

12.5 Conclusions

Non-surgical treatment of varicocele is now a practical and feasible therapeutic modality. This was recently confirmed by Zeitler et al. (1980) who performed sclerosis of the spermatic vein in 84 patients. The results in terms of varicocele cure, improved semen quality, and the achievement of pregnancy lead us to conclude that this is a possible process for all patients with a subclinical varicocele who undergo a selective retrograde venography. Furthermore it could be a treatment for selected patients with clinically diagnosed varicocele, e.g., the overweight and those presenting a high surgical risk.

The advantages of this technique are that the process is non-surgical and involves no general anesthesia, hospitalization is reduced to a minimum, and the treatment is supported by a high precision diagnostic method and can be thouroughly checked during the same intervention.

12.6 References

Adjiman M (1972) Le varicocèle et la stérilité masculine. In: Thibault C (ed) Fécondité et stérilité du mâle. Acquisitions récentes. Masson, Paris, pp 293–304

Ahlberg NE, Bartley O, Chidekel N, Fritjofsson A (1966) Phlebography in varicocele scroti. Acta Radiol [Diagn] 4:517–528

Castro MPP, Lima SS (1976) Selective spermatic venography in male infertility. Presented at the 1st International Congress of Andrology – Barcelona, Spain. Int J Androl [Suppl] 1:169

Castro MPP, Lima SS (1978) Results of varicocele transcatheter sclerosing treatment. Presentation at 3rd Annual Meeting American Society of Andrology. Nashville, Tennessee USA, p 20

Charny CW (1962) Effects of varicocele on fertility. Results of varicocelectomy. Fertil Steril 13:47–56

Comhaire F, Kunnen M (1976) Selective retrograde venography of the internal spermatic vein: a conclusive approach to the diagnosis of varicocele. Andrologia 8:11–24

Cotrim ES (1940) Contribution to the radiologic study of the circulation in varicocele (in Portuguese). Med. thesis, University of São Paulo, Brazil

Davidson HA (1954) Treatment of male subfertility. Testicular temperature and varicoceles. Practitioner 173:703–708

Dubin L, Amelar RD (1971) Etiologic factors in 1294 consecutive cases of male infertility. Fertil Steril 22:469–474

Dubin L, Amelar RD (1975) Varicocelectomy as therapy in male infertility: a study of 504 cases. Fertil Steril 26:217–220

Dubin L, Hotchkiss RS (1969) Testis biopsy in subfertile men with varicocele. Fertil Steril 20:50–57

El-Sadr AR, Mina E (1950) Anatomical and surgical aspects in the operative management of varicocele. Urol Cutan Rev 54:257–262

Fernando N, Leonard JM, Paulsen CA (1976) The role of varicocele in male fertility. Andrologia 8:1–9

Goulart TD (1935) How to explain the low incidence of varicocele in black race: Experimental study (in Portuguese). Rev Bras Cir 4:531–538

Greenberg SH (1977) Varicocele and male fertility. Fertil Steril 28:699–706

Ivanissevich O (1960) Left varicocele due to reflux. Experience with 4470 operative cases in 42 years. J Int Coll Surg 34:742–753

Ivanissevich O, Gregorini H (1918) Una nueva operación para curar el varicocele. Sem Med (Buenos Aires) 25:575–579

Kormano M, Kahanpää K, Svinhufvud U, Tähti E (1970) Thermography of varicocele. Fertil Steril 21:558–564

Lima SS, Castro MPP, Costa OF (1978) A new method for the treatment of varicocele. Andrologia 10:101–106

MacLeod J (1965) Seminal cytology in the presence of varicocele. Fertil Steril 16:735–757

Palti Z, Kedar S, Polishuk WZ (1968) Ligature of the left spermatic vein in the treatment of oligozoospermia. Fertil Steril 19:631–636

Riedl P (1979) Selektive Phlebographie und Katheterthrombosierung der Vena testicularis bei primärer Varikocele. Wien Klin Wochenschr 91 (99):3–20

Russell JK (1954) Varicocele in groups of fertile and subfertile males. Br Med J 1:1231–1233
Tulloch WS (1952) A consideration of sterility factors in the light of subsequent pregnancies. II. Subfertility in the male. Trans Edinburgh Obstet Soc 104:29–34
Tulloch WS (1955) Varicocele in subfertility: Results of treatment. Br Med J 2:356–358
Verstoppen GR, Steeno OP (1977) Varicocele and the pathogenesis of the associated subfertility. A review of the various theories. II. Results of surgery. Andrologia 9:293–305
Young D (1956) The influence of varicocele on human spermatogenesis. Br J Urol 28:426–427
Zeitler E, Jecht E, Richter EJ, Seyferth W (1980) Perkutane Behandlung männlicher Infertilität im Rahmen der selektiven Spermatikaphlebographie mit Katheter. Fortschr Roentgenstr 132:294–300

13 Retrograde Ejaculation

J. P. Collins

Retrograde ejaculation is the propulsion of seminal fluid from the posterior urethra into the bladder. Its incidence is unknown, but it is undoubtedly more common than is thought (Sandler 1979). It may be associated with diseases like diabetes mellitus and with the use of certain drugs (Ellenberg and Weber 1966; Hughes 1964). Most cases, however, are iatrogenic or secondary to diseases that occur after the reproductive years (Potts 1975); therefore, retrograde ejaculation is most often an interesting clinical observation, but a relatively uncommon cause of male infertility.

13.1 Anatomy of the Male Urethra and Internal Genitalia

The posterior urethra is a two-layered muscular tube formed as a direct continuation of the smooth muscle layers of the bladder wall. The inner and outer longitudinal smooth muscle layers of the bladder become, respectively, the inner longitudinal and the outer circular layers of the urethra. These muscular layers sweep over the vesicourethral junction and end near the urogenital diaphragm (Hutch and Rambo 1967). Striated muscle extends upward from the urogenital diaphragm and is incorporated into the urethral wall distally (Fig. 1).

The predominantly autonomic innervation of the posterior urethra and internal genitalia is unique (Birmingham and Wilson 1963; Richardson 1962). A dual sympathetic and parasympathetic network of short, interdigitating postganglionic neurons forms the final link of the innervation (Elbadawi and Schenk 1974; Kedia and Markland 1975). Their synapses are placed at ganglion cells near the urethra and internal genitalia. This unusual system may explain continued function in these organs when apparently severed from external neural connections (Owman and Sjöberg 1972). The arrangement may also account for the counterbalanced effect of the parasympathetic and sympathetic components in certain areas, such as the bladder neck and urogenital diaphragm (Boyd et al. 1960).

Evidence of parasympathetic innervation of the internal genitalia developed into the theory that contraction of the internal genitalia is a parasympathetic phenomenon (Potts 1957; Retief 1950). Histological and histochemical studies, however, demonstrate a greater concentration of α-adrenergic than cholinergic receptors at the vesicourethral junction, ductus deferens, prostate, and seminal vesicles (Semens and Langworthy 1938; Sjöstrand 1965). In addition, stimulation studies of the human ductus deferens and seminal vesicles show that the motor nerves end in α-ad-

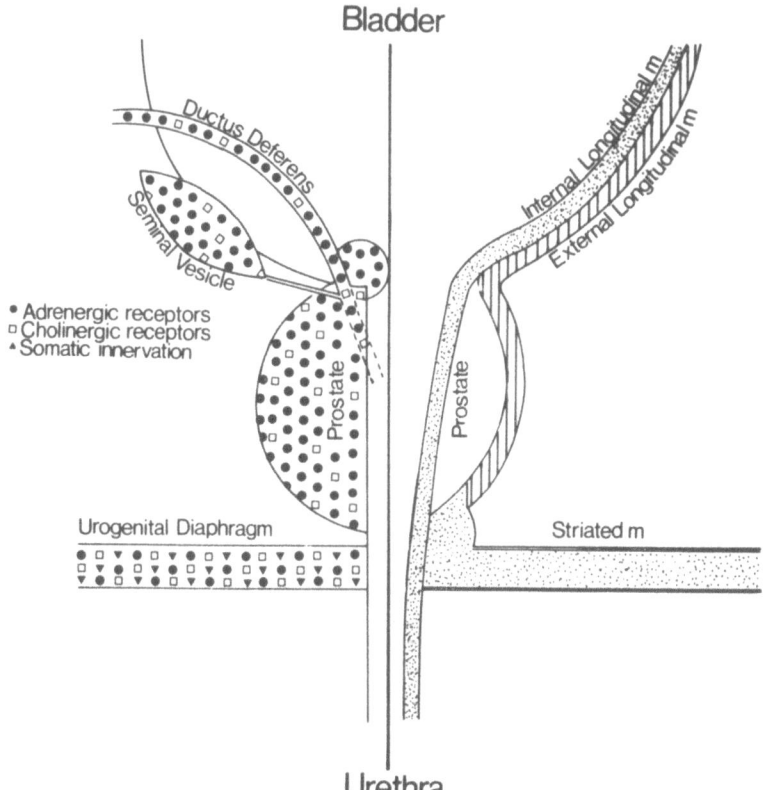

Fig. 1. Innervation of the male internal genitalia and urethra (*left*). Note the heavy concentration of adrenergic receptors, very pronounced at the bladder neck. Note the triple innervation of the urogenital diaphragm. Anatomy of the male urethra (*right*) (modified from Glezerman et al. 1976)

renergic receptors (McLeod et al. 1973). This suggests that sympathetic innervation predominates (Kleeman 1970). Functionally, sympathetic stimulation causes the bladder neck to close. Smooth muscle tissue at the bladder neck acts as an internal sphincter, preventing retrograde ejaculation and aiding in maintaining urinary continence (Kleeman 1970).

13.2 Physiology of Ejaculation

The mechanism of normal ejaculation comprises three stages which follow in rapid sequence, seminal emission into the posterior urethra, bladder neck closure, and antegrade ejaculation through the urethral meatus.

Afferent stimuli from the genitalia reach the cerebral cortex via the pudendal nerve (Kedia and Markland 1975). Psychic initiation of ejaculation can also occur (Munro et al. 1948). Efferent impulses travel through the anterolateral columns to both the thoracolumbar sympathetic outflow (T_{12}–L_3 sympathetic ganglia) and the sacral parasympathetic outflow through S_2–S_4 (Fig. 2). The thoracolumbar sympathetic outflow by the hypogastric nerve causes the ductus deferens to contract from the cauda epididymis to the ampulla of the vas. Almost simultaneously, the seminal vesicles and prostate contract and the bladder neck closes (Semens and Langworthy 1938). Contraction of the internal genitalia causes emission of seminal fluid into the posterior urethra.

Through the parasympathetic outflow of S_2, S_3, S_4, and the internal pudendal nerve, rhythmic contractions of the bulbocavernosus and ischiocavernosus muscles result in antegrade ejaculation of seminal fluid through the urethral meatus (Owman and Sjöberg 1972).

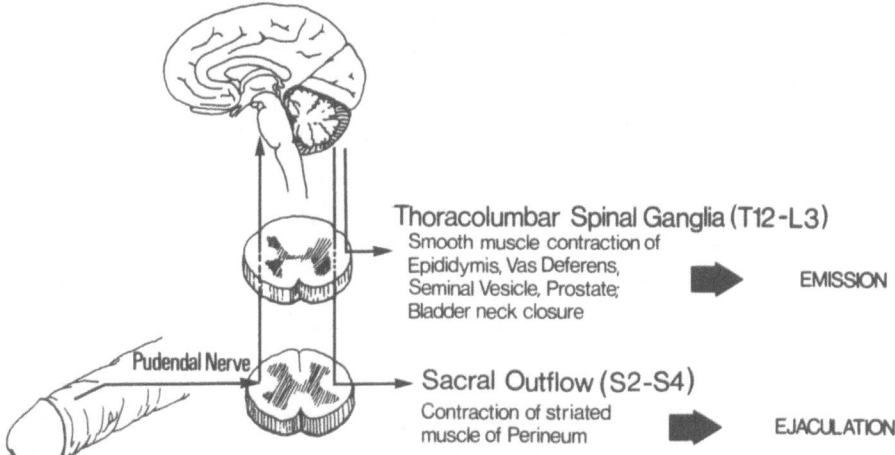

Fig. 2. Physiology of ejaculation (modified from Kedia et al. 1975)

13.3 Etiology of Retrograde Ejaculation

The causes of retrograde ejaculation are summarized in Table 1. The commonest cause of retrograde ejaculation is surgery of the bladder neck and prostate. This surgery is often performed later in life and usually does not affect fertility. Reiser (1961) found that retrograde ejaculation developed in 40% of patients who underwent transurethral prostatectomy, but in none who underwent open surgical prostatectomy: probably, transurethral surgery destroys more of the bladder neck and nerve endings. Ochsner et al. (1970) found that, among men who had open bladder neck surgery in childhood, retrograde ejaculation occurred in 33%. Koraitum and Al-Ghorab (1970), however, reported that it did not develop in men on whom anterior Y-V bladder neck plasty had been performed in adulthood, which reflected greater obstruction at the bladder neck in this group. Even so, while retrograde ejaculation frequently occurs after such operations, the complication is not inevitable if the posterior bladder neck is preserved or damaged as little as possible.

Lumbar sympathectomy may cause retrograde ejaculation. Whitelaw and Smithwick (1951) reported that a bilateral L_1 sympathectomy did not effect ejaculation, but that a bilateral sympathectomy which extended from L_1 to L_3 resulted in the loss of ejaculation in approximately 50% of patients. Rose (1953), in a group of patients with more extensive sympathectomies (T_9–L_3), noted that in 70% of such patients the ejaculatory dysfunction was failure of ejaculation: retrograde ejaculation was only demonstrated in 30%. It seems, therefore, that a limited sympathectomy may not produce any ejaculatory dysfunction. Sympathectomy of an intermediate extent often results in retrograde ejaculation, and extensive destruction of the sympathetic chain usually results in an ejaculatory disturbance which is often failure of ejaculation.

Table 1. Causes of retrograde ejaculation

Surgery of bladder neck and prostate	Medication
Sympathetic neuropathy	Major tranquilizers
	Antihypertensive drugs
Iatrogenic	
Surgery	*Noniatrogenic*
Lumbar sympathectomy	Diabetes mellitus
Retroperitoneal lymphadenectomy	Spinal cord trauma
Aortoiliac surgery	
Rectal surgery	Miscellaneous

Retroperitoneal lymphadenectomy is also well-recognized as a cause of ejaculatory dysfunction (Leiter and Brendler 1967). This procedure is particularly significant as it is often performed in younger men during their reproductive years. The disturbance results from destruction of the sympathetic nervous system, which is inseparably intertwined with the para-aortic lymph node chain. Bilateral lymph node dissection, which is performed in the staging or treatment of testicular tumors, results in extensive destruction of the sympathetic chain and usually causes failure of ejaculation (Kedia et al. 1975).

Aortoiliac surgery and abdominoperineal resection of the rectum cause sexual dysfunction which is usually due to injury of the presacral nerve. There was a 30% incidence of retrograde ejaculation found in patients who had extensive dissection of the aorta and common iliac vessels for aneurysmectomy (Weinstein and Machleder 1975). If a conscious effort is made to preserve the presacral nerve, antegrade ejaculation can be retained in 90% of patients following aneurysmectomy (Sabri and Cotton 1971). Goligher (1951) reported a 39% incidence of failure of ejaculation or retrograde ejaculation following abdominoperineal resection of the rectum. Schellen (1960) reiterated this, and stressed the importance of preserving the presacral nerve in excision of the rectum for nonmalignant disease – an operation often performed in younger people.

A temporary chemical sympathectomy may be caused by certain major tranquilizers and antihypertensive agents. Thioridazine (Mellaril, Sandoz Pharmaceuticals) (Kotin et al. 1976; Shader 1964), phenoxybenzamine (Dibenzyline, Smith

Kline + French Canada Ltd.) (Green and Berman 1954), guanethidine (Ismelin, CIBA Pharmaceuticals) (Schirger and Gifford 1962), and chlordiazipoxide (Librium, Hoffmann-La Roche Ltd.) (Hughes 1964) are reported to have this effect. This side effect is due to the specific α-adrenergic blocking action which these drugs possess. Most cause failure of ejaculation, but cases of retrograde ejaculation have been reported as well (Shader 1964).

Diabetes mellitus can produce retrograde ejaculation (Ellenberg and Weber 1966). The incidence of retrograde ejaculation in diabetes mellitus is low in comparison to the 50%–60% incidence of erectile difficulty in diabetic males (Wabrek 1979). The mechanism is probably a sympathetic neuropathy affecting bladder neck closure. Greene (Greene and Kelalis 1968; Greene et al. 1963) did sweat tests on a number of patients and demonstrated areas of anhydrosis in the lower extremities indicating a sympathetic nervous system dysfunction. Many diabetic males may have failure of ejaculation (Klebanow and MacLeod 1960), perhaps due to an abnormality of the smooth musculature of the internal genitalia.

Injury or disease affecting spinal cord function results in loss of ejaculation and retrograde ejaculation in a high percentage of cases (Talbot 1949). Munro et al. (1948) reported a 92% incidence of ejaculatory dysfunction in patients with spinal cord injuries which occurred between T_6 and L_3 and in patients with transections of the sacral cord segments or cauda equina.

Unusual causes of retrograde ejaculation have been reported. Keiserman et al. (1974) noted a type of partial retrograde ejaculation which consisted of antegrade ejaculation of a sperm-free, initial portion of semen and retrograde ejaculation of the remainder of sperm-containing semen. Sandler (1979) described a type of intermittent retrograde ejaculation which varied from aspermia to normal ejaculation. The etiology of both types of retrograde ejaculation was unexplained. Urethral stricture has been given as a cause of retrograde ejaculation in 10% of patients with aspermia (Girgis et al. 1968).

13.4 Diagnosis of Retrograde Ejaculation

Diagnosis of retrograde ejaculation generally can be made by finding spermatozoa in the postcoital urine of men who have absent or intermittent emission of an ejaculate. Kedia et al. (1975, reproduced by permission) outlined the following detailed schema, which permits delineation of retrograde ejaculation from the various types of ejaculatory failure:

1. *Preliminary urine examination.* A fructose test was done on a freshly voided specimen, as control, to rule out the abnormal presence of fructose before subsequent testing.
2. *Semen sample.* Patients were requested to masturbate and the seminal specimen was immediately examined for spermatozoa and fructose.
3. *Urinalysis after masturbation.* A voided urine sample immediately following masturbation was examined for spermatozoa and fructose to determine the possible presence of semen within the bladder caused by retrograde ejaculation.

4. *Examination of prostatic secretions.* The prostate was then massaged, examining the secretions for spermatozoa and fructose, to establish the presence or absence of spermatozoa secondary to ductus deferential peristalsis and seminal-vesicular contraction.
5. *Postprostatic massage urinalysis.* This was examined for spermatozoa and fructose to determine possible seminal vesicular secretions.

13.5 Treatment of Retrograde Ejaculation

Urine has a deleterious effect on sperm motility and viability. When normal spermatozoa were introduced into samples of varying osmolality and pH for different time periods, a decrease in spermatozoa motility of more than 50% was noted within 5 min of contact with urine (Crich and Jequier 1978). Urine was shown to be lethal

Table 2. Treatment of retrograde ejaculation

Retrieval of semen
Artificial insemination
Postejaculation-voiding insemination
Medication
α-Adrenergic stimulators
Anticholinergic drugs
Surgery
Miscellaneous

to spermatozoa if combined for longer periods of time. These effects were due to the low osmolality of the urine. The acidity of urine contributed as well, but control of this alone was insufficient to prevent a decrease in motility. Because of these findings, all forms of treatment have attempted to prevent or minimize contact of semen with urine to increase urine pH and osmolality.

Table 2 shows an outline of the various forms of treatment employed in retrograde ejaculation.

13.5.1 Retrieval of Semen

Retrieval of semen from the bladder and subsequent artificial insemination has been most widely used and successful treatment for retrograde ejaculation (Kragt and Schellen 1978). All retrieval methods have used fluid restriction to minimize urine output. In addition, several basic approaches have been employed.

13.5.1.1 Replacement of Bladder Urine with an Isotonic Alkaline Solution

After voiding, the bladder is irrigated with Ringer's glucose solution and a small volume (usually 2 ml) is left in the bladder. Following immediate masturbation, semen is retrieved by catheterization or voiding (Kapetanakis et al. 1978). The specimen is usually centrifuged, at 1500 rpm for 10 min (Glezerman et al. 1976) or 3400 rpm for 3–5 min (Bourne et al. 1971; Fuselier et al. 1976), and the sediment used for artificial insemination. On occasion, retrieved semen is simply left to stand for a short time and a small aliquot is used for artificial insemination (Walters and Kaufman 1959).

This method was first described by Hotchkiss and has been used successfully for more than 30 years (Hotchkiss et al. 1955). Many pregnancies have been reported (Bourne et al. 1971; Fuselier et al. 1976; Glezerman et al. 1976). Occasionally, alkalinization of the semen has not been adequate for good sperm motility. Supplementary oral alkalinization with sodium bicarbonate has been used with success (Bourne et al. 1971; Walters and Kaufman 1959). The number of inseminations required for conception has varied from 1 to as many as 16 (Hotchkiss et al. 1955). The multiple catheterizations required in some cases did cause troublesome urinary tract infections (Kapetanakis et al. 1978).

13.5.1.2 Systemic Alkalinization of the Urine

Systemic alkalinization of the urine with sodium bicarbonate (300 mg three times daily to 1 g four times daily) is used to achieve a urine pH in excess of 7.5. Semen is retrieved by voiding following masturbation. More than 50 pregnancies have been reported by this method (Glezerman et al. 1976; Kragt and Schellen 1978). Although catheterization is avoided, it is uncertain whether sufficient alkalinization of the urine can be routinely achieved in large numbers of patients.

13.5.1.3 Washing of Semen in Nutrient Alkaline Solution

Following masturbation, voided semen is washed with an alkaline nutrient solution (Eagle's solution). Glezerman et al. (1976) washed voided semen with 15 ml Eagle's solution and centrifuged it for 10 min at 1500 rpm. This was repeated and the semen used to achieve a successful pregnancy in one patient. This approach avoids catheterization, but requires quick retrieval of semen to minimize time and contact with the urine.

In patients with erratic ovulation, Kapetanakis et al. (1978) froze retrieved semen and stored it for subsequent artificial insemination. This avoids unnecessary catheterization in situations where prolonged courses of artificial insemination will probably be required.

Schram (1976) described a technique of immediate postejaculation voiding directly into the vagina. The wife was instructed to lie in the Trendelenburg position for 10–15 min following voiding. This was used with fluid restriction and resulted in one pregnancy. Marmar et al. (1977) reported three pregnancies using this technique in combination with oral alkalinization of the husbands urine. In addition, they recommended bicarbonate douching when the vagina was extremely acidic. Pregnancies occurred from the second to the fifth menstrual cycle. Despite some initial resistance, this method is apparently well-accepted by patients. It does avoid instrumentation and can be used immediately postcoitus.

While a variety of underlying pathological conditions have been treated by retrieval techniques, their greatest application is in patients with mechanical disruption of the bladder neck, since other forms of treatment have usually failed totally.

13.5.2 Medication

Medication has been used to improve smooth muscle function at the bladder neck in patients with retrograde ejaculation due to a neurogenic dysfunction. This has usually been due to a sympathetic neuropathy. The mode of action of the drug is usually to increase sympathetic or decrease parasympathetic activity at the bladder neck (Kragt and Schellen 1978; Stockamp et al. 1974).

Table 3 summarizes drugs used in treatment of retrograde ejaculation. The most experience has been with sympathomimetic medication which produces α-adrenergic stimulation. Stewart and Bergant (1974) used phenylpropanolamine one capsule twice daily and achieved antegrade ejaculation in a diabetic. Stockamp et

Table 3. Drugs used in the treatment of retrograde ejaculation

---

α-Adrenergic stimulators
Phenylpropanoloamine (Ornade, Smith Kline of French Canada Ltd.)
Midodrin (Gutron, Chemie Linz AG, Austria)
Oxedrine (Synephrine, Boehringer Ingelheim)

Anticholinergic drugs
Brompheniramine (Dimetane, A. H. Robins Canada Inc.)

---

al. (1974), using 60 mg i.v. oxedrine, produced antegrade ejaculation in six patients with bladder neck incompetence from retroperitoneal lymph node dissection. Jonas et al. (1979) used midodrine oral 5 mg three times daily for 10 days in nine patients who had a previous retroperitoneal lymph node dissection. None of the patients have produced antegrade ejaculation. He subsequently used 25–30 mg i.v. oxedrine as a single dose in 12 patients following retroperitoneal surgery. Seven of the 12 patients produced antegrade ejaculation.

Anticholinergic medication, which decreases parasympathetic activity and relatively increases sympathetic tone in the bladder neck can have similar effects. Andraloro and Dube (1975) used brompheniramine (8 mg) twice daily in a diabetic and achieved antegrade ejaculation.

Antegrade ejaculation is easily produced by oral medication in patients with minimal sympathetic dysfunction. In patients with more pronounced sympathetic disruption, parenteral administration of medication produces antegrade ejaculation in many patients. To date, however, there have been no reported pregnancies using medication of this type (Marmar et al. 1977). The only pregnancy involving a technique of this kind was in a diabetic given phenylpropanoloamine to produce antegrade ejaculation. The semen obtained was then used for artificial insemination (Thiagarajah et al. 1978). Perhaps continued use of this type of medication, employing different drug combinations and dosage schedules, will produce sufficient antegrade ejaculation to achieve pregnancy.

13.5.3 Surgery

Surgical reconstruction of the bladder neck to produce competence of this area during ejaculation has been used (Abrahams et al. 1975) (Fig. 3).

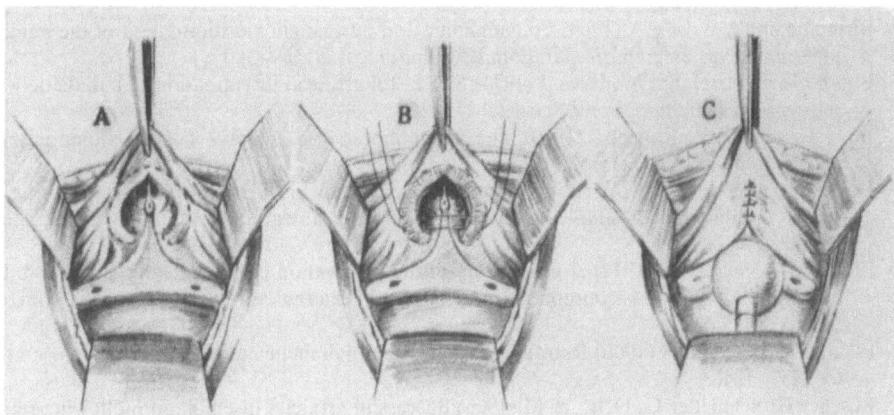

Fig. 3A. View of urethrovesical junction from within bladder reveals limits of incision. **B** Exposed muscle of bladder neck illustrates placement of sutures to reconstruct internal vesical sphincter. **C** Appearance of reconstructed internal vesical sphincter with no. 16 Foley catheter in place. (Abrahams et al. 1975, reproduced by permission)

Originally, two patients who had Y-V plasties of the bladder neck as children were described. Both of these patients achieved antegrade ejaculation with one reported pregnancy. K. Waterhouse (1979, personal communication) has now operated on a total of seven patients, all of whom had Y-V plasties as children. Six of these achieved antegrade ejaculation. The procedure seems successful in this small group of patients and should perhaps be reserved for use in these situations.

13.5.4 Miscellaneous

An innovative technique has recently been reported in two patients with retrograde ejaculation of uncertain etiology (Crich and Jequier 1978). Antegrade ejaculation was achieved by masturbation in the standing position with a full bladder, but no pregnancies have been reported.

13.6 Conclusions

Retrograde ejaculation has many causes. Its clinical presentation is often subtle and may easily be missed. Retrieval techniques have been and will continue to be the most successful form of treatment. In the future, new drugs or drug combinations which increase bladder neck competence may be successful in achieving pregnancies for patients with minimal neuromuscular bladder neck dysfunction.

13.7 References

Abrahams J, Solish G, Boorjian P, Waterhouse K (1975) The surgical correction of retrograde ejaculation. J Urol 114:888–890

Androloro V, Dube A (1975) Treatment of retrograde ejaculation with brompheniramine. Urology 5:520–522

Birmingham A, Wilson A (1963) Preganglionic and postganglionic stimulation of the guinea-pig isolated vas deferens preparation. Br J Pharmacol 21:569–580

Bourne R, Kretzschmar W, Esser J (1971) Successful artificial insemination in a diabetic with retrograde ejaculation. Fertil Steril 22:275–277

Boyd H, Chang V, Rand M (1960) The anticholinesterase activity of some antiadrenaline agents. Br J Pharmacol 15:525–531

Crich J, Jequier A (1978) Infertility in men with retrograde ejaculation: the action of urine on sperm motility and a simple method for achieving antegrade ejaculation. Fertil Steril 30:572–576

Elbadawi A, Schenk E (1974) A new theory of the innervation of bladder musculature. 4. Innervation of the vesicourethral junction and external urethral sphincter. J Urol 111:613–615

Ellenberg M, Weber H (1966) Retrograde ejaculation in diabetic neuropathy. Ann Intern Med 65:1237–1246

Fuselier H, Schneider G, Ochsner M (1976) Successful artificial insemination following retrograde ejaculation. Fertil Steril 27:1214–1215

Girgis S, Etriby A, El-Hefnawy H, Kahil S (1968) Aspermia: a survey of 49 cases. Fertil Steril 19:580–588

Glezerman M, Lunenfeld B, Potashnik G, Oelsner G, Beer R (1976) Retrograde ejaculation: pathophysiologic aspects and report of two successfully treated cases. Fertil Steril 27:796–800

Goligher J (1951) Sexual function after excision of the rectum. Proc R Soc Med 44:824–827

Green M, Berman S (1954) Failure of ejaculation produced by dibenzyline. Conn Med 18:30–33

Greene L, Kelalis P (1968) Retrograde ejaculation of semen due to diabetic neuropathy. J Urol 98:693–696

Greene L, Kelalis P, Weeks R (1963) Retrograde ejaculation of semen due to diabetic neuropathy. Fertil Steril 14:617–625

Hotchkiss R, Pinto A, Kleegman S (1955) Artificial insemination with semen recovered from the bladder. Fertil Steril 6:37–40

Hughes J (1964) Failure to ejaculate with chlordiazepoxide. Am J Psychiatry 121:610–611

Hutch J, Rambo O (1967) A new theory of the anatomy of the internal urinary sphincter and the theory of micturition. III. Anatomy of the urethra. J Urol 97:696–704

Jonas D, Linzbach P, Weber W (1979) The use of Midodrin in the treatment of ejaculation disorders following retroperitoneal lymphadenectomy. Eur Urol 5:184–187

Kapetanakis E, Rao R, Dmowski W, Scommegna A (1978) Conception following insemination with a freeze-preserved retrograds ejaculate. Fertil Steril 29:360–363

Kedia K, Markland C (1975) The effect of pharmacological agents on ejaculation. J Urol 114:569–573

Kedia K, Markland C, Fraley E (1975) Sexual function following high retroperitoneal lymphadenectomy. J Urol 114:237–239

Keiserman W, Dubin L, Amelar R (1974) A new type of retrograde ejaculation: report of three cases. Fertil Steril 25:1071–1072

Klebanow D, MacLeod J (1960) Semen quality and certain disturbances of reproduction in diabetic men. Fertil Steril 11:255–261

Kleeman F (1970) The physiology of the internal urinary sphincter. J Urol 104:549–554

Koraitum M, Al-Ghorab M (1970) Norman ejaculation after Y-V urethrocystoplasty. Br J Urol 42:464–465

Kotin J, Wilbert D, Verberg D, Soldinger S (1976) Thioridazine and sexual dysfunction. Am J Psychiatry 133:82–85

Kragt F, Schellen A (1978) Clinical report about some cases with retrograde ejaculation. Andrologia 10:380–384

Leiter E, Brendler H (1967) Loss of ejaculation following bilateral retroperitoneal lymphadenectomy. J Urol 98:375–378

Marmar J, Praiss D, De Benedictis T (1977) Post-coital voiding insemination. Technique for patients with retrograde ejaculation and infertility. Urology 9:288–290

McLeod D, Reynolds D, Demaree G (1973) Some pharmacologic characteristics of the human vas deferens. Invest Urol 10:338–341

Munro D, Horne H, Paull D (1948) The effect of injury of the spinal cord and cauda equina on the sexual potency of men. N Engl J Med 239:905–911

Ochsner M, Burns E, Henry H (1970) Incidence of retrograde ejaculation following bladder neck revision as a child. J Urol 104:596–597

Owman C, Sjöberg N-O (1972) The importance of short adrenergic neurons in the seminal emission mechanism of rat, guinea-pig and man. J Reprod Fertil 28:379–387

Potts I (1957) The mechanism of ejaculation. Med J Aust 1:495–497

Reiser C (1961) The etiology of retrograde ejaculation and a method of insemination. Fertil Steril 12:488–492

Retief P (1950) Physiology of micturition and ejaculation. S Afr Med J 24:509–512

Richardson K (1962) The fine structure of autonomic nerve endings in smooth muscle of rat vas deferens. J Anat 96:427–442

Rose S (1953) An investigation into sterility after lumbar ganglionectomy. Br Med J 1:247–250

Sabri S, Cotton L (1971) Sexual function following aortoiliac reconstruction. Lancet 2:1218–1219

Sandler B (1979) Idiopathic retrograde ejaculation. Fertil Steril 32:474–475

Schellen T (1960) A case of retrograde ejaculation caused by a colon operation. Fertil Steril 11:187–190

Schirger A, Gifford R (1962) Guanethidine: a new antihypertensive agent. Experience in the treatment of 36 patients with severe hypertension. Proc Staff Meet Mayo Clin 37:100–108

Schram J (1976) Retrograde ejaculation: a new approach to therapy. Fertil Steril 27:1216–1218

Semens J, Langworthy O (1938) Observations on the neurophysiology of sexual function in the male cat. J Urol 40:836–846

Shader R (1964) Sexual dysfunction associated with thioridazine hydrochloride. JAMA 188:1007–1009

Sjöstrand N (1965) The adrenergic innervation of the vas deferens and the accessory male genital glands. An experimental and comparative study of its anatomical and functional organization in some mammals, including the presence of adrenaline and chromaffin cells in these organs. Acta Physiol Scand [Suppl 257] 65:1–82

Stewart B, Bergant J (1974) Correction of retrograde ejaculation by sympathomimetic medication: Preliminary report. Fertil Steril 25:1073–1074

Stockamp K, Schreiter F, Altwein J (1974) Alpha-adrenergic drugs in retrograde ejaculation. Fertil Steril 25:817–820

Talbot H (1949) A report on the sexual function in paraplegics. J Urol 61:265–270

Thiagarajah S, Vaughan E, Kitchin J (1978) Retrograde ejaculation: successful pregnancy following combined sympathomimetic medication and insemination. Fertil Steril 30:96–97

Wabrek A (1979) Sexual dysfunction associated with diabetes mellitus. J Fam Pract 8:735–740

Walters D, Kaufman M (1959) Sterility due to retrograde ejaculation of semen: report of pregnancy achieved by autoinsemination. Am J Obstet Gynecol 78:274–275

Weinstein M, Machleder H (1975) Sexual function after aorto-iliac surgery. Ann Surg 181:787–790

Whitelaw G, Smithwick R (1951) Some secondary effects of sympathectomy with particular reference to disturbance of sexual function. N Engl J Med 245:121–130

14 Sexual Dysfunction in the Male

G. Kockott

14.1 Definition

Although widely used, the term "impotence" is rather vague. Other equally nonspecific terms are "male sexual functional disorders" and "male sexual inadequacy". All of these terms encompass a wide variety of dysfunctions that need to be further differentiated. In agreement with Schmidt and Arentewicz (1978), male sexual dysfunctions are defined here as disturbances in sexual behavior and sexual feeling in males as evidenced by impaired or atypical genitophysiological reactions or the complete absence of such reactions. There are two ways of describing them in more detail operationally: (1) in terms of the kind of sexual dysfunction that can occur during the different phases of sexual interaction (definition in terms of content); (2) in terms of the frequency of the dysfunction, the circumstances under which it occurs, and how long the problem has existed (definition in terms of form).

14.1.1 Kinds of Sexual Dysfunction

Sexual dysfunctions may occur during any of the five phases of sexual interaction, which are sexual approach (initiation of sexual contact), sexual stimulation (body contact, petting), intromission and preorgasmic coitus, orgasm, and postorgasmic period. The sexual dysfunctions that can occur in each phase are described in Sects. 1.1.1–1.1.5.

14.1.1.1 Sexual Approach

The most common problem at this stage is diminished interest in sex or the complete lack of such interest, with the result that little or no attempt is made to initiate sexual contact. Aversive feelings about sex may even develop. These *libido disturbances* can be caused by organic or psychiatric disorders and or by any other sexual dysfunction that results in failure to achieve a satisfactory sexual relationship.

14.1.1.2 Sexual Stimulation

Erectile disorders are the most common problem at this stage. There are two forms of erectile disorders. *Erectile impotence* is defined as the inability of the male to attain or maintain an erection sufficient for intercourse (LoPiccolo and LoPiccolo

1978). It is usually of psychogenic origin, but can sometimes be caused by organic disorders. In *priapism*, there is a relatively continuous erection that can become painful. It is usually of organic origin.

14.1.1.3 Intromission and Preorgasmic Coitus

Psychogenic erectile impotence, which usually is at its critical phase at the time of intromission, has already been mentioned. Painful coitus (dyspareunia) is a rather common symptom of female sexual inadequacy, but is also found in men. It is usually due to an organic disorder (e.g., phimosis, penile trauma), but in rare cases it is of psychogenic origin (e.g., phobic reaction when the glans penis is touched).

14.1.1.4 Orgasm

The various ejaculatory problems occur during this stage. They can be divided roughly into disturbances in which the timing of the ejaculatory process is disturbed and those in which the ejaculatory process itself is disturbed. Using a classification that is parallel to that for sexual dysfunctions in the female, disturbances of the first kind can be defined as *male orgasmic dysfunctions* since there is no disturbance of the ejaculatory process itself (Vogt 1980). Orgasm and ejaculation may occur prematurely, may be delayed, or may even be absent even though there is no erectile dysfunction. It is difficult to define *premature ejaculation (premature orgasm)* precisely (except in cases when the patient ejaculates before intromission), because there is no sharp line between undisturbed and disturbed sexual behavior. In the author's opinion, the crucial aspect of prematurity is the absence of a feeling of control over the ejaculatory process. Premature ejaculation may, therefore, be defined as ejaculation in which the male feels that he has no control or almost no control over the ejaculatory process. With very few exceptions, premature ejaculation does not appear to be of organic origin.

Delayed ejaculation (delayed orgasm), which is also called *retarded ejaculation* (Kaplan 1974), poses similar diagnostic problems. Here, again, there is no sharp line between undisturbed and disturbed ejaculatory behavior. In the extreme form of delayed ejaculation, namely in absent orgasm and ejaculation, which is also called ejaculatory incompetence (Masters and Johnson 1970) or anejaculation (Geboes et al. 1975), the diagnosis is easy. In most cases these dysfunctions are of psychogenic origin.

In the other group of ejaculatory disturbances, the ejaculatory process itself is disordered. It is easy to differentiate between delayed or absent ejaculation and retrograde ejaculation. In the latter, the man reaches orgasm at the desired time but with no visible ejaculation. Rather, ejaculation takes place in a retrograde manner into the bladder, which can be proven by an examination of the urine. Retrograde ejaculation is of organic origin. Other ejaculatory disturbances, both relatively rare, are spermatorrhea, where there is frequent dribbling of semen without orgasm, and anejaculation in spite of normal orgasm (ejaculatio deficiens). These disturbances may be due to both psychogenic and organic (e.g., spinal injury) factors.

14.1.1.5 Postorgasmic Period

Difficulties at this stage are not sexual dysfunctions in the strict sense, but rather problems of attitude toward sexual contact, coitus, etc. Persons with such problems often feel unhappy or irritated following orgasm. These problems are of little relevance to the present subject, however, unless they are the result of problems in another phase.

In summary, *erectile impotence and premature ejaculation are the most common forms of sexual dysfunction in men.*

14.1.2 Circumstances of Occurrence

All forms of psychogenic sexual dysfunction in men can occur either *primarily*, i.e., the dysfunction has existed since the very first sexual contact, or *secondarily*, i.e., the dysfunction began after at least one undisturbed sexual contact. The dysfunctions may occur *initially* only, i.e., at the beginning of a "sexual career" or a new partnership, or they may be *partner-dependent*. They may occur only during coital activity, but not during masturbation (*coital* form of dysfunction). And they may also be *situational*, e.g., if there is the possibility of being interrupted by others. Such formal information should be added to the term used to designate a particular dysfunction (e.g. primary erectile impotence, situational premature ejaculation).

14.2 Interviewing Technique and Differential Diagnosis Between "Organic" and "Psychogenic" Male Sexual Dysfunction

14.2.1 Interviewing Technique

Many patients still find it quite difficult to talk about their sexual problems even with a physician. In order to obtain the information necessary for a thorough diagnostic evaluation the physician should make sure that the following conditions prevail during the interview with the patient:

1. The patient should be able to speak with his physician alone and without interruption.
2. The patient should have the feeling that his problem is being taken seriously.
3. The patient should be allowed to discuss his problem in his own words. The physician may prefer to use somewhat different language, but terms should be avoided that the patient will not understand.
4. The patient may need some time until he can formulate his problem clearly. Therefore, the physician should consider making a special appointment to discuss the patient's sexual problem.
5. The physician himself should feel comfortable discussing the topic.

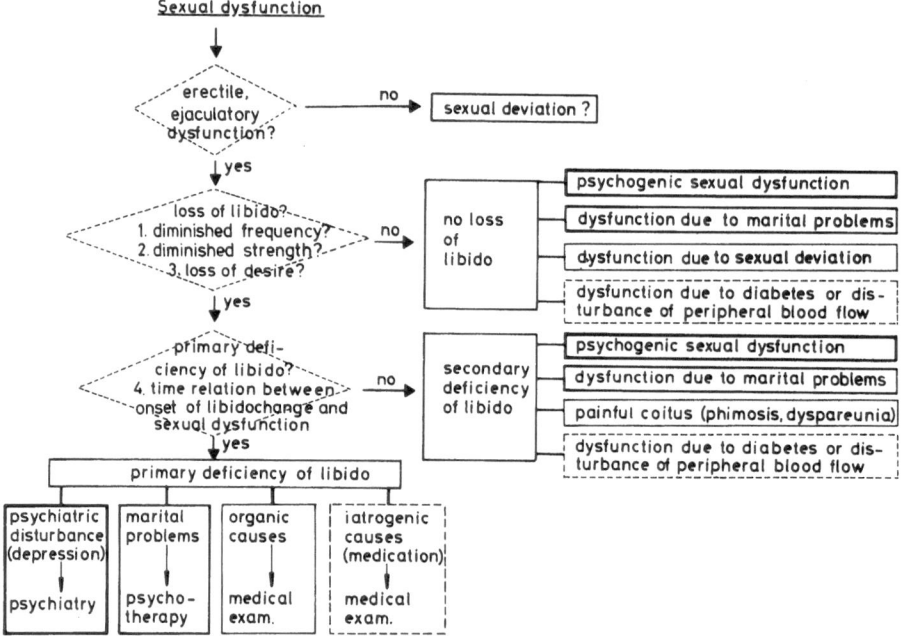

Fig. 1. Decision map for the diagnosis of sexual dysfunction. The heavier the line around the dysfunction, the more common that dysfunction is relative to the others listed

14.2.2 Differential Diagnosis

Although male sexual dysfunctions can be of organic origin, psychogenic causes are much more frequent. Most authors are of the opinion that about 80%–90% of male sexual dysfunctions fall into the latter category. In arriving at a diagnosis, it is useful to know whether the patient has a history of diminished libido or of a specific type of libidinal dysfunction. Libido is defined here as the delightful longing for some form of sexual activity that might lead to orgasm. Figure 1 shows, in the form of a decision map, how to determine whether there is a libidinal disturbance. The following three questions will lead to the necessary information:

1. How often is the longing for sexual activity experienced? There is no clear boundary between disturbed and undisturbed libido strength. But if the patient says he feels this longing about once a month, this should suggest libido deficiency.
2. How strong does the patient himself consider his desire for sexual activity to be in comparison to others of his age?
3. Has the patient noticed any change in his interest in sex recently?

If a libido deficiency has been established on the basis of the responses to these three questions, then a fourth question becomes necessary:

4. What is the relationship between the onset of libido dysfunction and the onset of functional symptoms (e.g., erectile impotence)? The answer will indicate whether there is a primary deficiency (libido loss first) or a secondary deficiency (functional symptoms first). If there is a secondary change in libido strength or none at all,

the sexual dysfunction is usually psychogenic. In general, organically caused sexual disorders are preceded by libido loss. But there are a number of exceptions to this rule which will be discussed in the section on etiology.

The differentiation between an organic and a psychogenic sexual dysfunction is often very difficult and sometimes even impossible. Sexual problems may simply coexist with organic illness by chance. Often both organic and psychic factors play a role in a sexual problem. Many of the secondary sexual dysfunctions seem to develop as a result of a transient organic disorder (e.g., a brief illness with general fatigue) and are then maintained by psychic factors, mainly performance anxiety that leads to sexual avoidance behavior. Current knowledge what specific factors influence sexual functioning and how they do this is still far from complete. Therefore, it is more appropriate to talk about sexual dysfunctions as being predominantly of psychogenic or predominantly of organic origin. The reader should keep this in mind when, for reasons of simplicity, the terms organic and psychogenic dysfunctions are used.

14.3 Etiology

14.3.1 Organic Sexual Dysfunctions

As already mentioned, sexual dysfunctions are usually due to a combination of several different factors, and even dysfunctions that are primarily of somatic origin are not beyond psychodynamic considerations. For example, diabetics who develop diabetes-related erectile impotence also often develop sexual anxieties (Kockott et al. 1980). In addition to treatment of their diabetes, these patients may very well need psychotherapeutic support or sexual counseling for their sexual anxieties.

It is relatively rare that male sexual dysfunctions are of organic origin. The most common organic causes are shown in Table 1 and described briefly below. A detailed discussion is not appropriate here because of infrequency.

14.3.1.1 Libido Disturbances

As already mentioned, in most cases of somatically caused male sexual dysfunctions the main symptom is primary libido deficiency. Any severe somatic illness can cause libido loss as part of general fatigue. A number of somatic disorders cause libido loss by disrupting the normal metabolism of the sex hormones. This is the case in thyroid and kidney disorders. Patients under dialysis seem to suffer especially often from libido disturbances. Patients with liver disease, in particular with cirrhosis of the liver, frequently develop a libido deficiency that leads to erectile impotence. Chronic alcoholism seems to influence the libido not only indirectly via liver disease, but also directly by acting on testosterone production. Both forms of hypogonadism cause impairment of libido. If the androgen deficiency existed prior to puberty, then there can be complete absence of libido, of which the patient may not be aware (Labhart 1978). Patients with Klinefelter's syndrome usually begin to be aware of libido deficiency only in the post-adolescent years. Libido disturbances frequently accompany acute or chronic organic brain syndromes, mainly in the form of

Table 1. Effects of physical illness on male sexuality

Libido disturbances

General ill health
Infections

All-encompassing illness
Malignancies

Disorders that affect metabolism of the sex hormones
    Thyroid dysfunctions
        Hypothyroidism
        Hyperthyroidism
    Renal diseases
        Chronic nephritis - - - dialysis
    Liver diseases
        Chronic hepatitis
        Cirrhosis
    Hypogonadism, primary and secondary
        Klinefelter's syndrome
        Disturbances of the pituitary

Damage to the brain
    Tumor
    Trauma   } Temporal or
    Cardiovascular accident } frontal lobe
    Temporal lobe epilepsy

Chronic alcoholism

Drugs
    Sedatives
    Psychopharmacological agents
    Antihypertensives
    Antiepileptics
    Estrogens
    Antiandrogens

Erectile disturbances

Any local genital disease that affects intromission mechanically
    Penile injury
    Large inguinal hernia
    Hydrocele
    Induration penis plastica
    Acute genital inflammations (gonorrhoea, herpes simplex genitalis, balanitis, orchitis, epididymitis, etc.)
    Condylomata acuminata gigantea
    Cancer of the penis

Neurological disorders with damage to the lower neurological apparatus
    Amyotrophic lateral sclerosis
    Tabes dorsalis
    Spinal cord injury
    Multiple sclerosis

Vascular diseases
    Diseases of the aorta and iliac arteries
        Leriche syndrome
  Thrombosis of veins or arteries of penis

Diabetes mellitus

Table 1 (continued)

Ejaculatory disturbances

  Premature ejaculation
  Conditions that cause irritation during the sexual response
      Urethritis
      Prostatitis

  Delayed or absent ejaculation
  Drugs that also influence libido
  Surgical conditions
      Lumbar sympathectomy
      Abdominal aortic surgery
  Spinal cord injuries
  Local genital trauma
      Rupture of the urethra

Retrograde ejaculation

---

libido deficiency as part of a general impairment of mental activity. In the case of trauma to the forebrain, interest in sexual activity appears to be increased as a result of lack of inhibition (e.g., increased impulsiveness, loss of moral and ethical standards). Patients with temporal lobe epilepsy seem to be prone to development of libido deficiency. A number of drugs cause libido impairment. All sedatives and most psychopharmacological agents taken in high dosage can produce this side effect. Many antihypertensive and antiepileptic drugs may also cause libido deficiency. But it is not quite clear whether the medication is the only reason why the libido disturbances develop or whether the underlying illness contributes to the sexual difficulties as well. Estrogen therapy in males (e.g., for carcinoma of the prostate) will also lead to an impairment of libido.

In old age there is a physiological decrease in libibo due to a decrease in androgen production after the age of 60 (Pirke and Doerr 1973, 1975; Nieschlag et al. 1973; Pirke et al. 1977), and sociocultural factors, such as moral and religious views and to interpersonal factors.

14.3.1.2 Erectile Impotence

An impairment or loss of libido always seems eventually to lead to erectile impotence. But there are some somatic disturbances that cause erectile impotence without libido deficiency or with only secondary libido impairment. These disorders do not influence the libido primarily as do the disorders described in Sect. 3.1.1. Rather, they influence the genitals themselves (e.g., trauma), the nerves (e.g., multiple sclerosis, diabetes mellitus), or blood vessels (e.g., disturbance of peripheral blood flow, diabetes mellitus) of the genitalia. The most common form of organically caused erectile impotence is that due to diabetes. Of 175 randomly selected male diabetic outpatients who were studied by Kolodny et al. (1974), 85 (49%) were impotent. Typically the onset of erectile impotence is gradual, usually developing over a period of 6 months to 1 year. The patients suffer from "prevailing erectile impotence" (experienced during all kinds of sexual activity), as opposed to the "situational erectile impotence" (experienced during contact with a partner only) found in patients with a psychogenic erectile disturbance (Kockott et al. 1980). There seems to be no definite correlation between the occurrence of erectile impotence and the duration or mode of treatment of diabetes either with insulin or with oral agents, but there is a greater incidence of peripheral neuropathy in the diabetics with sexual dysfunctions than in those without such dysfunctions (Kolodny et al. 1974). Plasma testosterone levels are within normal limits (Faerman et al. 1972; Kolodny et al. 1974; Neubauer et al. 1972). Diabetes-related disturbances of the neuronal pathways (Neubauer and Schöffling 1977) and the blood vessels of the genitalia (Raboch 1977; Ruzbarsky and Michal 1977) are being considered as etiological factors. Neurological disorders that involve damage to the lower neurological apparatus, such as multiple sclerosis, spinal cord injury, or amyotrophic lateral sclerosis, may cause erectile impotence of the "prevailing" type. Vascular diseases, especially of the iliac arteries or the penile veins and arteries, also lead to this type of erectile impotence, as do local genital disorders, such as penile injury with damage to the corpora cavernosa.

14.3.1.3 Ejaculatory Disturbances

A somatic disorder is almost never the primary cause of premature ejaculation. However, conditions that cause irritation during the sexual response, such as urethritis or prostatitis, may be contributing factors.

Ejaculation can be delayed by a number of drugs. All drugs that decrease libido also lead to delayed or absent ejaculation. Such drugs include psychopharmacological agents (e.g., thioridazine, chlorpromazine), antihypertensives (e.g., guanethidine, α-methyldopa), barbiturates and antiandrogens (e.g., cyproterone acetate, estrogens). The α-adrenergic blocking agents (e.g., phenoxybenzamine) seem to cause delay of ejaculation with little influence on sexual interest. Phenoxybenzamine is currently used widely for treatment of pheochromocytoma, vascular diseases, and in lower motor neuron lesions of the bladder. The undesired side effect of delayed ejaculation caused by all these drugs seems to be reversible even if the medication is taken for longer than 1 year (Haider 1966). Surgical conditions (e.g., lumbar sympathectomy) and spinal cord injuries may also cause retarded ejaculation.

Retrograde ejaculation appears to be exclusively of somatic origin. This form of ejaculatory disturbance is discussed elsewhere in this book.

14.3.2 Psychogenic Sexual Dysfunctions

The vast majority of sexual dysfunctions in men are, primarily, due to psychogenic factors. Erectile problems that are initially without concomitant libido disturbances are one of the most frequent forms of psychogenic sexual dysfunction. Typically they occur only during partner contact, with spontaneous erections at night and in the morning usually remaining undisturbed. Erections are also undisturbed during masturbation, except where the patient masturbates not because of sexual urgency but to see whether he is still able to have an erection. Men with erectile problems frequently masturbate for this reason. As previously mentioned, ejaculatory problems are almost exclusively psychogenic, especially premature ejaculation.

Such psychogenic sexual dysfunctions may be due to lack of information, to misinformation about sexuality, or they may be situational: they may also be the expression of a partner problem or they may be understood in terms of the patient's life history. Therapy may consist of sexual counseling, partner therapy, or psychotherapy with special emphasis on the sexual dysfunction, with the choice of therapy dependent on why the dysfunction has developed. Further discussion of the psychogenic factors that may be involved is included in Sect. 14.4.

Primary libidinal disturbances of psychogenic origin are rare. If they are psychogenic, the causal factor is frequently depression, with the libidinal disturbance being part of general apathy. However, in such cases other symptoms of depression are also seen, in particular sleep and eating problems. Here it is the depression that must be in the foreground of treatment. Psychogenic primary libido disturbances can also be the expression on the sexual level of partner problems in other areas.

14.4 Therapy

14.4.1 Therapy of Organic Sexual Dysfunctions

Treatment must be directed primarily toward the underlying somatic illness. This is especially true for disorders that affect the metabolism of the sex hormones. For adequate sexual functioning, a certain level of plasma testosterone is necessary (Horton and Tait 1966; Gandy and Peterson 1968; Young and Kent 1968).

Many drugs can cause impotence. If impotence occurs, a decision must be made whether it is crucial for the health of the patient to continue with the medication that diminishes sexual drive or whether a different drug can be used. In hypertensive patients sexual dysfunctions may be due to antihypertensive drugs (primary libido loss) or to changes in the vessels of the penis (erectile impotence, but no primary libido loss). New microsurgery techniques are now being developed to manage the latter conditions better (Michal et al. 1979).

Some somatic conditions produce sexual dysfunctions that appear to be irreversible. This seems to be the case especially for diabetes-related impotence and for erectile impotence due to disorders of the lower neurological apparatus (e.g., paraplegia, amyotrophic lateral sclerosis). Sexual counseling is very important for patients with these conditions. The main points stressed in such counseling would usually be that sexual interaction is much more than having coitus with the penis inserted into the vagina and that there are many other forms of sexual interaction that are enjoyable. In some cases of irreversible erectile impotence a penile prothesis might be considered. But this should always be the method of last resort and should be tried only if the patient's partner gives her consent ahead of time. Otherwise she may have a strong reaction, resulting in such severe partner problems that partner therapy may then be necessary.

14.4.2 Therapy of Psychogenic Sexual Dysfunctions

14.4.2.1 Sexual Counseling

Sexual dysfunctions that are the result of inadequate sex education, unfavorable living arrangements, minor conflicts with the partner, or inhibitions about expressing sexual wishes to the partner can often be treated successfully by means of sexual counseling. Situations for which sexual counseling is appropriate include the following examples: some men do not know that after ejaculation there is a refractory period in which it is impossible to have another full erection; a surprisingly large number of people are misinformed about current patterns of sexual behavior, particularly, the frequency of sexual relations is often greatly overestimated; on the other hand, the range of sexual activity is frequently underestimated, e.g., genital-oral positions are often considered abnormal although they are now relatively common; if a young couple shares an apartment with one set of parents, the couple may find it very disturbing to know that the parents are quite well-informed about their sexual activity, and this may lead to a great deal of inhibition regarding sex on the part of both partners; frequently one partner is unable to tell the other about a desire for a particular kind or frequency of sexual activity, afraid that his partner will consider his ideas "perverse" and will turn him down. This is particularly true if he is in doubt about the "normality" of his desires himself. Many people are also unaware of the physiological changes relating to sexual behavior that come with age, such as delayed erections and reduced frequency of ejaculatory urgency.

It is frequently possible in the course of a few counseling sessions with both partners together to clarify and resolve such problems and thus resolve the sexual problem. The family physician who knows the couple and their background would appear to be particularly well-suited to providing this kind of counseling. In the beginning he may be only a facilitator, encouraging the couple to discuss the problem by preventing the dialogue from deteriorating into a pointless argument. Or the physician may help one partner to talk about things he would otherwise not risk mentioning. If the physician wants to act as a sex educator it is, of course, essential that he first make sure he is well-informed himself.

14.4.2.2 Partner Therapy

The sexual sphere may be affected by tensions in the general relationship simply because it is one of the areas of communication in the relationship. Frequently a problem in the general relationship is completely displaced to the sexual sphere. In addition, the sexual inhibitions of one partner have an effect on the other partner, since arousal often does not develop at the same pace in the man and woman but rather the level of arousal of one influences the level of arousal of the other.

Since partnership and sexual problems are so closely intertwined it is often difficult to decide whether a sexual problem is secondary to difficulties in the partnership or the reverse. A decision has to be made as to which facets of the relationship are most disturbed so that therapy can be directed to the most urgent complex of problems. If a partner problem can be demonstrated to be in the foreground, then treatment of the sexual disorder will be successful only if the overall relationship can be improved. Communication therapy (e.g., Watzlawick et al. 1967) would be appropriate here. A detailed discussion is beyond the scope of this discussion. In brief, this therapy is comprised of three main steps: (1) improvement in the partners' ability to communicate with each other; (2) realization by the partners that a change is necessary (cognitive restructuring, change in motivation); (3) active learning of new behavioral patterns (behavior modification).

Active learning of new behaviors is necessary because recognition of a communication problem will not by itself produce change. But behavioral changes lead to changes in feelings and thus to changes in the partners' perception and understanding of each other. These new behavior patterns must be learned.

14.4.2.3 Psychoanalysis

Psychoanalysts regard sexual dysfunctions as defense mechanisms against sex-related anxiety that is the result of early experience with the sexual drive and of the kind of early parent-child relationship.

According to this view, sexual dysfunctions in adults can be defensive reactions to anxieties related to experiences in the oral, anal, and phallic phases of psychosexual development in Freud's sense. From the theoretical concept of psychoanalysis, there are very few publications on the treatment of male sexual dysfunctions. If there is impotence, the psychoanalyst sees it as a symptom of an underlying neurosis with conflicts in the unconscious. It is not the impotence (a symptom) that he treats, but rather the personality disorder or neurotic disturbance that he has postulated. To the author's knowledge there is only one study (Obler 1975) in which psychoanalytic treatment (psychoanalytically oriented group psychotherapy) is compared with more direct approaches to sexual problems such as behavior therapy or the Masters and Johnson (1970) approach (see Sect. 14.4.2.4.1). Nevertheless, the overall impression of practicing psychotherapists is that the more direct psychotherapeutic approach is more effective than psychoanalysis.

14.4.2.4 Behavior Therapy

14.4.2.4.1 Therapy Concept and Format

In most male sexual dysfunctions, performance anxiety plays a very prominent role as a causative and/or maintaining factor. This is true whether or not other conflicts are also involved. Because of the fear of failure, sexual contacts are usually avoided: Thus, the dysfunction has a phobic element.

A treatment form first described in detail by Masters and Johnson (1970) is in current use and has proven extremely effective in, among other things, reducing sexual performance anxiety. This therapy can be described as behavior therapy-oriented psychotherapy tailored to the treatment of sexual problems. Behavior therapy is a new form of psychotherapy that makes use of research findings on the psychology of learning for the treatment of emotional problems in humans. In the underlying theoretical model, behavior problems are seen as inappropriate behavior that has been learned. Prior to therapy the behavior therapist determines the factors that have led to the development of the behavior problem and cause it to be maintained (behavioral analysis). Then the therapist tries to change the disturbed behavior by changing the maintaining factors. In therapy, according to Masters and Johnson,

Table 2. Studies on behavior therapy of sexual dysfunctions with follow-up data. The data on treatment effectiveness in the different papers are presented in many different forms. Therefore, they have been combined into the two categories "successful" (improvement, marked improvement, cure) and "unsuccessful" (unimproved, got worse, failure)

Reference	No. of patients	Diagnosis	Initial results	Follow-up		
				No. of patients	Duration	Results
Semans (1956)	12	Premature ejaculation	Successful	8	15 months	Successful
Wolpe (1958)	8	"Impotence"	Successful	3	6 months–1 year	Successful
Friedman (1968)	19	Erectile impotence, premature ejaculation, delayed ejaculation	18 successful, 1 unsuccessful	4	6 months	2 successful, 2 relapse
				13	12 months	12 successful, 1 relapse
Friedman and Lipsedge (1971)	19	"Impotence"		19	6 months–5 years	14 successful, 5 unsuccessful
Masters and Johnson (1970)	245	Erectile impotence	176 successful 69 unsuccessful	176	5 years	19.4% unsuccessful
	186	Premature ejaculation	182 successful 4 unsuccessful			
	17	Delayed ejaculation	14 successful 3 unsuccessful			
Meyer et al. (1975)	7	Erectile impotence, ejaculatory disturbances, orgasmic dysfunctions	7 successful	6	7 months (average)	5 successful, 1 unsuccessful
Ansari (1976)	21	Erectile impotence	15 successful 6 unsuccessful	21	8 months	7 successful, 14 unsuccessful

Kockott 1976, Behavior therapy for sexual inadequancy: Conclusions from a controlled study. Paper presented at the 6th annual conference of the European Association of Behavior Therapy, Greece. Unpublished work	32	Erectile impotence, premature ejaculation	24 successful 8 unsuccessful	20 20	1–3 years	15 successful, 5 unsuccessful
Mathews et al. (1976)	18	Erectile impotence, premature ejaculation	Group comparison on different parameters; successful throughout	18	4 months	successful
Yulis (1976)	37	Premature ejaculation	33 successful, 4 unsuccessful	37	6 months	33 successful, 4 unsuccessful
Auerbach and Kilmann (1977)	16	Secondary erectile impotence	16 successful	16	3 months	Successful
Golden et al. (1978)	15	Premature ejaculation	15 successful	15	2 months	Successful

which is always carried out with both partners participating, performance anxiety as the major factor in the maintenance of the man's sexual dysfunction is dealt with first.

The first step is to instruct the partners not to have intercourse. This alone has the effect of making the relationship more relaxed and affection can again be experienced without anxiety. Under the protection of this prohibitive instruction the behavioral chain is then rebuilt step by step. The therapist gives the couple suggestions and instructions for specific things they are to practice at home (such as sensate focus and the "squeeze technique"). Parallel to this, the problems in the partnership are discussed. Based on the concept that sexual arousal and anxiety are incompatible, the partners are instructed to continue sexual activity only as long as they find it pleasant and not accompanied by anxiety. The prerequisite is the cooperation of the male patient's sexual partner. She is requested never to pressure the patient into a stage in which he feels ill at ease. The procedure in detail is as follows: the exercises begin with what is called "sensate focus". The partners are relaxed and unclothed. In the therapy session beforehand it has been agreed which partner will begin to touch and stimulate the body of the other and to provide the partner with pleasant sexual feelings. At this time the genital area is expressly excluded. Through openness to sensory experiences and undisturbed by goal-oriented activity, the couple can gradually develop satisfactory erotic interactions. Additional areas of the body are gradually included in the sensate focus exercise until foreplay in the usual sense is possible without anxiety. Depending on what type of sexual dysfunction the man has, additional special techniques are then used, e.g., in the case of erectile impotence, the "manual and coital teasing technique" and in the case of premature ejaculation the "squeeze technique" (Masters and Johnson 1970).

14.4.2.4.2 Initial Results

Masters and Johnson conducted an intensive, quasi-inpatient treatment program with sessions every day for 2 weeks. Most other authors conducted therapy on an outpatient basis at weekly intervals for 15–20 weeks. All authors report good to excellent results, with overall rates of therapeutic success of 70%–80%. However, the criteria for success vary widely and are often not defined very carefully. The Masters and Johnson (1970) statistics are of particular interest because of the large number of cases involved (448 men). But even these authors do not define success and failure very clearly. Nevertheless, the data indicate that patients with premature ejaculation respond particularly well to this form of therapy (97.8% success), whereas patients with primary erectile dysfunctions are the most difficult to treat effectively (59.4% success). These conclusions are in agreement with the author's own observations. Primary erectile problems are not maintained via sexual inhibitions and behavioral deficits in the sexual area alone. It is the author's impression that strong maternal ties, general problems with social interaction, and fear of commitment often also play a large role. In such cases psychotherapy addressed primarily to the sexual symptoms cannot always be adequate therapy.

Up to now there have been only a few studies in which different forms of therapy have been compared for effectiveness (Kockott et al. 1975; Mathews et al. 1976; Obler 1973, 1975). In the studies reported, behavior therapy was found to be superior to conventional therapy with drugs and general advice and also to psy-choanalytically oriented group psychotherapy.

14.4.2.4.3 Follow-up Studies

Table 2 lists all follow-up studies with more than a few subjects reported in the English-language literature. Follow-up was from 2 months to 5 years. Again the reports from Masters and Johnson (1970) are of particular interest. These reports include the largest number of patients (176) with the longest follow-up (up to 5 years). The initial therapy results in patients with premature ejaculation and with primary erectile problems were maintained, but there was treatment reversal in a number of subjects with secondary erectile disturbances, with a drop from an initial success rate of 75% to a follow-up rate of 71%. Overall treatment effectiveness at 5-year follow-up was still 80%, however. Other authors report similarly good results. Both the present author and other therapists (J. H. J. Bancroft 1979, personal communication; D. Wilchfort 1970, personal communication) have even had patients who reported additional improvement during the follow-up period.

Recently a number of authors (Auerbach and Kilmann 1977; Golden et al. 1978; Kockott 1979) have carried out the behavior therapy approach described above in groups, i.e., the discussion part of the therapy in groups with the "exercises" done at home as in therapy with individual couples. The results so far are as good as in individual therapy.

For some patients the additional group dynamics effect seems to be especially helpful. Additional studies are necessary to determine the patient groups for which individual and group therapy are best suited.

14.4.2.4.4 Conclusions

Behavior therapy in the treatment of psychogenic sexual dysfunctions in the male is undoubtedly effective. Of paramount importance to success, however, is the diagnosis. If the sexual dysfunction is the expression of major problems in the general relationship, it cannot be treated adequately with a therapy oriented to sexual problems. In such cases partner therapy is indicated. On the other hand, the majority of sexual dysfunctions are probably amenable to treatment with the form of behavior therapy as described here, if therapy is tailored to the individual situation on the basis of the behavioral analysis. Behavior therapy of sexual dysfunctions does not fulfill impossible wishes, however. The patient who tries to solve all of this problems through overemphasis on sexual activity will be disappointed. But still, the re-establishment of good sexual functioning generally does lead to much-improved feelings of self-esteem, which especially in men are strongly affected by sexual dysfunction.

14.5 Effect of Psychological Factors on the Production and Action of Spermatozoa

Psychogenic sexual dysfunctions in the male may be the indirect cause of infertility. This is because they frequently preclude coital activity sufficient for impregnation. It now appears that psychological factors may also have a direct influence on the production and action of spermatozoa. There are insufficient numbers of studies substantiating this view, but there are a few which do suggest it.

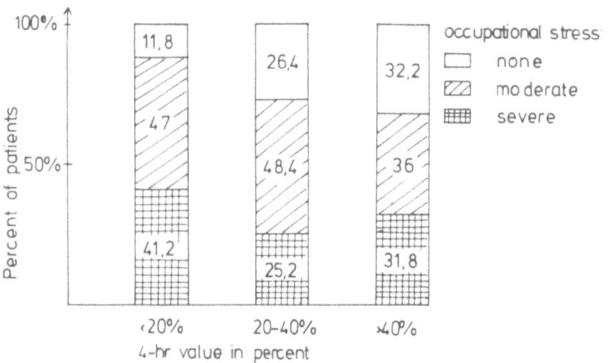

Fig. 2. Degree of motility in percent (4-h value) and relationship to occupational stress (n = 444 initial spermiograms and questionnaires) (Lübke and Stauber 1980)

Stieve (1952) describes a man who had raped four women within three weeks. The man was executed 41 days after the last rape. A histological examination of his testes showed Sertoli's cells and spermatogonias only. In Stieve's view the only possible explanation for why spermatogenesis ceased is that this was due to the fear and the emotional tension associated with the death sentence. The pregnancies of two of the four raped women and the post mortem examination of the other two women whom the man murdered after the rape seem to suggest that at the time of these rapes the man has been fertile.

According to Vogt (1980), if spermiograms made at short intervals show widely varying values for sperm count/ml, total sperm count or total volume of seminal discharge, this is evidence that emotional factors must be involved. He feels that psychogenic factors must be disturbing seminal transport, rather than that spermiogenesis is disturbed. Although spermatogenesis takes 72–76 days (Heller and Clermont (1973), widely varying sperm counts can be found to occur normally when counts are made at short intervals.

Lübke and Stauber (1980) have observed wide fluctuations in the parameters of sperm count, sperm motility, and sperm morphology especially often in neurotic patients. Furthermore, they have demonstrated a relationship between occupational stress and the degree of sperm motility (Fig. 2). A significantly larger percentage of the men with severe infertility problems than of those with only slight infertility problems indicated on a questionnaire that they were subject to moderate or severe occupational stress.

Changes in sperm quality due to stress are usually reversible after the stressful situation has been dealt with (Stieve 1952; Borelli 1960; Lübke and Stauber 1980).

Lübke, Stauber and Vogt mention a number of other possible psychological factors: ambivalence about having children; disturbances in the partner relationship; uncomfortable feelings about sexuality; and disorders of personality development. These authors recommend psychological guidance as the treatment of choice for patients with such problems. It has even been observed that when a couple with a fertility problem decides to seek advice jointly, this by itself is often enough to enable pregnancy to occur (Vogt 1980; Lübke and Stauber 1980). The mechanism at work here is unknown, however.

It may be that the influence of psychological factors on the production and action of spermatozoa is much greater than has been assumed. Studies testing this hypothesis are urgently needed.

14.6 References

Ansari JMA (1976) Impotence: Prognosis (a controlled study). Br J Psychiatry 128:194–198

Auerbach RM, Kilmann PR (1977) The effects of group systematic desensitization on secondary erectile failure. Behav Ther 8:330–339

Borelli S (1960) Die psychogenen Fertilitäts- und Sexualstörungen beim Manne. In: Schuermann H, Doepfmer R (Hrsg) Fertilitätsstörungen beim Manne. Springer, Berlin Göttingen Heidelberg (Handbuch der Haut- und Geschlechtskrankheiten, Ergänzungswerk Bd VI/3, S 641–735)

Faerman I, Vilar O, Rivarola MA, Rosner JM, Jadzinsky MN, Fox D, Perez L, Coret A, Bernstein-Hahn L, Saraceni D (1972) Impotence and diabetes. Diabetes 21:23–30

Friedman D (1968) The treatment of impotence by brietal relaxation therapy. Behav Res Ther 6:257–262

Friedman DE, Lipsedge MS (1971) Treatment of phobic anxiety and psychogenic impotence by systematic desensitization employing methohexitone-induced relaxation. Br J Psychiatry 118:87–90

Gandy HM, Peterson RE (1968) Measurement of testosterone and 17-ketosteroids in plasma by the double isotope dilution derivative technique. J Clin Endocrinol 28:949–977

Geboes K, Steeno O, de Moor P (1975) Primary anejaculation: diagnosis and therapy. Fertil Steril 20:1018–1020

Golden JS, Price S, Heinrich AG, Lobitz WC (1978) Group versus couple treatment of sexual dysfunctions. Arch Sex Behav 7:593–602

Haider J (1966) Thioridazine and sexual dysfunctions. Int J Neuropsychiatry 2:255–257

Heller CG, Clermont Y (1973) Spermatogenesis in man: An estimate of its duration. Science 140:184–186

Horton R, Tait JF (1966) In vivo studies of steroid dynamics – androstendione and testosterone. In: Vermeulen A, Exley D (eds) Androgens in normal and pathological conditions. Proceedings of the 2nd Symposium. Steroid Hormones. Excerpta Medica, Amsterdam, p 199

Kaplan HS (1974) The new sex therapy. Brunner & Mazel, New York; Bailliere Tindall, London

Kockott G (1979) Behavior therapy in groups of patients without partners and couples suffering from sexual dysfunctions. Paper presented at the 5th annual meeting of the International Academy of Sex Research, Prague (Abstr), p 10

Kockott G, Dittmar F, Nusselt L (1975) Systematic desensitization of erectile impotence: a controlled study. Arch Sex Behav 4:493–500

Kockott G, Feil W, Revenstorff D, Aldenhoff J, Besinger U (1980) Symptomatology and psychological aspects of male sexual inadequacy: results of an experimental study. Arch Sex Behav 9:457

Kolodny RC, Kahn CB, Goldstein HH, Barnett DM (1974) Sexual dysfunction in diabetic men. Diabetes 23:306–309

Labhart A (1978) Klinik der inneren Sekretion, 3rd ed, Springer, Berlin Heidelberg New York

LoPiccolo J, LoPiccolo L (1978) Handbook of sex therapy. Plenum, New York London

Lübke F, Stauber M (1980) Die sterile Ehe aus gynäkologischer Sicht. In: Kaden R (Hrsg) Allgemeine Pathologie der Sexualfunktionen. Deutscher Ärzte-Verlag, Köln, S 127–268

Masters WH, Johnson VE (1970) Human sexual inadequacy. Churchill, London

Mathews A, Bancroft J, Whitehead A, Hackmann A, Julier D, Bancroft J, Gath D, Shaw P (1976) The behavioral treatment of sexual inadequacy: a comparative study. Behav Res Ther 14:427–436

Meyer JK, Schmidt CW jr, Lucas MJ, Smith E (1975) Short-term treatment of sexual problems: interim report. Am J Psychiatry 132:172–176

Michal V, Pospichal J, Ruzbarský V, Lachman M (1979) Vasculogenic impotence. Paper presented at the 5th annual meeting of the International Academy of Sex Research, Prague (Abstr), p 16

Neubauer M, Schöffling K (1977) Sexualstörungen bei diabetischen Männern. In: Oberdisse K (Hrsg) Diabetes mellitus B. Springer, Berlin Heidelberg New York (Handbuch der inneren Medizin, Bd VII/2B, S 465)

Neubauer M, Demisch K, Schöffling K (1972) Diabetische Sexualstörungen. Sexualmedizin 1:242–247

Nieschlag E, Kleyn HK, Wiegelmann W, Solbach HG, Krüskemper HL (1973) Lebensalter und endokrine Funktion des Testes des erwachsenen Mannes. Dtsch Med Wochenschr 98:1281–1284

Obler M (1973) Systematic desensitization in sexual disorders. J Behav Ther Exp Psychiatry 4:93–101

Obler M (1975) Multivariate approaches to psychotherapy with sexual dysfunctions. Consult Psychol 5:55–60

Pirke KM, Doerr P (1973) Age-related changes and interrelationship between plasma testosterone, oestradiol and testostroerone-binding globulin in normal adult males. Acta Endocrinol 74:792–800

Pirke KM, Doerr P (1975) Age-related changes in free plasma testosterone, dihydrotestosterone and oestradiol. Acta Endocrinol 80:171–178

Pirke KM, Doerr P, Sintermann R, Vogt HJ (1977) Age-dependence of testosterone precursors in plasma of normal adult males. Acta Endocrinol 86:415–429

Raboch J (1977) Impotenz durch Hochdruck und Diabetes. Selecta 11:1056–1057

Schmidt G, Arentewicz G (1978) Sexuelle Funktionsstörungen. In: Ponratz LJ (Hrsg) Klinische Psychologie. Hogrefe, Göttingen (Handbuch der Psychologie, Bd VIII/2, S 2269)

Semans JH (1956) Premature ejaculation: A new approach. South Med J 49:353–357

Stieve H (1952) Der Einfluß des Nervensystems auf Bau und Tätigkeit der Geschlechtsorgane des Menschen. Thieme, Stuttgart

Vogt HJ (1980) Andrologie. In: Eicher W (Hrsg) Sexualmedizin in der Praxis. Gustav Fischer, Stuttgart, S 117–201

Watzlawick P, Beavin JH, Jackson DD (1967) Pragmatics of human communication interactional patterns, pathologies, and paradoxes. Norton, New York

Wolpe J (1958) Psychotherapy by reciprocal inhibition. Stanford University Press, Stanford

Young HH, Kent JR (1968) Plasma testosterone levels in patients with prostatic carcinoma before and after treatment. J Urol (Baltimore) 99:788–793

Yulis S (1976) Generalization of therapeutic gain in the treatment of premature ejaculation. Behav Ther 7:355–358

III. Surgical Treatment

15 Varicocele: Its Role in Male Infertility

H. Fenster and M. McLoughlin

The relationship between infertility and presence of a varicocele has been argued by many investigators over the last century (Tulloch 1952; Russell 1954; Ivanissevich 1960; MacLeod 1965; Amelar et al. 1977). A varicocele was first documented by Celsus in the first century A.D. when he described the condition and reported that "the testicle of varicocele is smaller than the unaffected side". He also described a surgical procedure for the treatment of varicocele (Hotchkiss 1970). The first cause and effect association between a varicocele and infertility was described by Barfield before the turn of the century, but it was not until 1952 when Tulloch reported a case of varicocele ligation with resultant pregnancy that the association was verified. Since then, numerous series have suggested that the presence of a varicocele could result in lower fertility rates (Scott and Young 1962; Brown et al. 1968; Dubin and Amelar 1977). Most investigators have accepted the relationship between varicocele and male subfertility, but recent challenges suggest that we re-evaluate the entire subject (Rodriguez-Rigau et al. 1978).

The incidence of varicocele is greater in subfertile males than in the general population (Russell 1954). In reviewing incidental varicoceles found in the general population, approximately 60% were associated with semen abnormalities (Johnson et al. 1970). These data, plus reports that surgical management of varicocele results in pregnancy in up to 53% of patients, support the concept that varicocele and male infertility are associated. But the fact that not all men with varicocele are infertile and surgical management does not improve fertility in 100% of cases has prompted some doubt as to the role of surgery in this problem. It is also difficult to explain why a unilateral anatomical abnormality (varicocele) can cause bilateral testicular dysfunction and subfertility. Finally, it has been suggested that varicocelectomy is a "sham" operation and there may be other ways to treat the condition (Rodriguez-Rigau et al. 1978).

These points will be reviewed and discussed here.

15.1 Definition and Classification

Varicocele was defined in 1550 by Pare as a "compact pack of vessels filled with melancholic blood". A modern definition of varicocele is a dilatation of veins of the spermatic cord. The pampiniform plexus represents the veins of the spermatic cord, the name being derived from its resemblence to a vine (pampinustendril) (Ham 1965). The veins wrap themselves around the vas deferens in a fashion similar to tendrils of a plant winding around other structures for support. The veins ascend in three longitudinal groups: the anterior or spermatic group (varicocele); the middle or vasal group; the posterior or cremasteric group (Palomo 1949). As the veins ascend from the scrotum they decrease in number and increase in size and enter the deep inguinal ring as the internal spermatic vein. There are cross-communications between the right and left pampiniform plexuses above the external inguinal ring. These anastomoses exist at several levels, including the pubic bone, inguinal canal, and above the internal inguinal ring (Etriby et al. 1975).

Varicocele occurs on the left side in as many as 98% of varicocele patients (Amelar and Dubin 1975). The anatomical explanation for this occurrence is based on the following facts: the left internal spermatic vein joins the left renal vein at right angles, whereas the right vein joins the vena cava obliquely and outflow may consequently be decreased on the left side; in patients with a right varicocele the right spermatic vein enters the vena cava at right angles strengthening this argument (Amelar and Dubin 1975); the left testis lies lower than the right, resulting in the total length of the pampiniform plexus being greater on the left side; the valve at the orifice of the left internal spermatic vein may be blocked by various structures including the left colon and superior mesenteric artery, thus resulting in obstruction and venous varicosities.

Varicoceles may be classified according to etiology, stages of development, and size. The origin of the varicocele may be idiopathic and associated with infertility or secondary to renal vein obstruction, as seen with tumors. According to the stage classification, in the development of the varicocele the primary defect lies in the internal spermatic vein in stage I, whereas in stage II a secondary varicosity develops in the cremasteric system (Hendry 1976). Finally, the size and, therefore, physical findings of the varicocele can also be used. This classification ranges between the nonpalpable or subclinical varicocele and the large abnormality easily palpated by the patient himself.

15.2 Pathogenesis and Etiology

Varicoceles are a dilatation of veins of the pampiniform plexus which may result from loss of valve action or valve agenesis at the orifice of the internal spermatic vein at its entry into the renal vein (Ivanissevich 1960). This allows blood from the renal vein to reflux freely into the internal spermatic vein with subsequent retrograde flow into the pampiniform plexus. The veins then dilate and become varicose, producing the clinical picture of varicocele (Amelar and Dubin 1975). Although this mechanism explains the pathophysiology of varicocele formation and has been demonstrated by venogram studies, it does not explain the mechanism by which a varicocele causes infertility. In order to explain the manner in which the presence of a varicocele may lead to male infertility, some of the major theories to explain the observed association will be examined.

15.2.1 Metabolites

Since a varicocele may be caused by retrograde flow of blood down the internal spermatic vein and there is a mixing of blood on both sides, metabolites may be refluxed down the vein, producing adverse effects on both testes. Blood from the renal and/or adrenal veins may contain toxic substances, perhaps an adrenal steroid with an inhibiting influence on sperm production (Amelar et al. 1977). The original concept of toxic metabolites refluxing down the internal spermatic vein is credited to MacLeod (1965), who suggested that adrenocortical hormones in the venous blood of the pampiniform plexus might damage the testes. Further work in this area has shown that measurements of venous levels of various adrenal hormones in patients undergoing vein ligation for varicocele show no differences between the spermatic vein and other veins in the body (Charney and Baum 1968; Agger 1971).

Comhaire and Vermeulen (1974) measured catecholamine concentrations and found these to be higher in the spermatic vein of varicocele patients undergoing surgery for infertility, compared to a control group of patients operated on for other reasons. They concluded that catecholamines in the pampiniform plexus could lead to chronic testicular vasoconstriction and impaired spermatogenesis.

Dierschke et al. (1975) studied hormonal concentrating mechanisms involving the local transfer of testosterone between the spermatic artery and veins in the rhesus monkey and suggested that this may have an influence. It was proposed that there is transfer of testosterone from veins to arteries with a high concentration in the testis. High levels of androgen can maintain spermatogenesis in men (Steinberger et al. 1973), therefore, Grayhack (1976) has suggested that interruption of venous return might allow pharmacologic concentration of testosterone in the testes, thus influencing spermatogenesis. In this respect, perhaps varicocele causes infertility because of lack of a metabolite, i.e., testosterone or a metabolite interfering with testosterone action.

The data on the role of metabolites in causing infertility in the varicocele patient is controversial and inconclusive at this time. Certainly not all levels of known adrenal metabolites have been measured and one can only suggest that it is quite possible that retrograde passage of metabolites may affect spermatogenesis.

15.2.2 Heat

Another major mechanism proposed has been the effect of heat on the testes. Crew (1921) proposed that differences in abdominal and scrotal temperatures could adversely affect sperm production. The concept that the scrotum is a temperature regulator for the testes and the theory that a varicocele can cause increased scrotal temperature, and so impair spermatogenesis, has been put forth by a number of investigators (Moore and Quick 1924; Hanley 1956). Hanley and Harrison (1962) suggested that stasis of blood in the pampiniform plexus led to increased heat in the scrotum with an inhibiting effect on the testes. Zorgniotti and MacLeod (1973) were able to correlate increased intrascrotal temperature and impaired testicular function in varicocele patients.

Kay et al. (1979) created an artificial varicocele by partial ligation of the left renal vein in the rhesus monkey and demonstrated a 1 °C increase in the temperature of testes of monkeys with this varicocele. This work supports previous evidence that heat plays an active part in the pathogenesis of infertility by varicocele formation.

Agger (1971), using needle-thermometer puncture techniques, demonstrated a decrease in temperature in the left testis after varicocele ligation, accompanied by improved postoperative sperm counts. A comparison of scrotal thermography with left renal vein venography showed a significant correlation with subclinical varicocele, abnormal semen analysis, unilateral decreased testicular firmness, abnormal thermograms, and reflux into the left internal spermatic vein on by venography (Comhaire et al. 1976). Using contact scrotal thermography, Lewis and Harrison (1979) studied postoperative failures and subclinical varicocele to demonstrate changes in temperature: early results in these patients showed a correlation between varicocele and increased scrotal temperatures, and suggested both the value of this form of evaluation and the relationship between heat and varicocele. These papers suggest that heat changes secondary to the presence of a varicocele may play a very important role in the cause of infertility.

15.2.3 Hormonal Factors

Measurement of circulating levels of LH, FSH, and testosterone is common practice in the evaluation of the subfertile male, especially in the differentiation of hypogonadotropic disease from primary testicular failure (de Kretser et al. 1974; Ruder et al. 1974).

One might ask, however, if there are hormonal differences between patients with and without varicoceles. Swerdloff and Walsh (1975) found no abnormalities in serum LH, FSH, testosterone, and estradiol in patients with varicoceles. Hudson and McKay (1979) found that men with varicoceles and sperm counts less than 10×10^6/ml had increased LH and FSH responses to gonadotropin-releasing hormone (LHRH) when compared to groups of men with or without varicoceles. This suggests that patients with severe oligozoospermia and varicocele have a pantesticular defect in spermatogenesis and androgen production.

15.2.4 Abnormal Gases

Abnormal perfusion of gases, such as carbon dioxide and oxygen, may impair spermatogenesis (Glezerman et al. 1976). More work is required to substantiate this theory.

15.2.5 Epididymal Factors

There could be an effect of varicocele on the epididymis resulting from retrograde flow in the pampiniform plexus, which could impair maturation of spermatozoa in the epididymis and lead to motility disturbances (Glezerman et al. 1976). Many factors in the epididymis determine motility and maturation, including blood supply, adequate levels of tissue androgens, electrolyte composition of the epididymis, and spermatozoon-induced activity (Fenster and McLoughlin 1979). Perhaps occult epididymal obstruction allows for some epididymal dysfunction and, in combination with varicocele, causes impaired spermatogenesis and subfertility. Many of these factors may interact and impair fertility in the presence of a varicocele. The number and combination of these factors involved could explain why all patients with varicocele are not infertile.

15.3 Diagnosis

The first approach to the diagnosis of varicocele is the medical history and physical examination. Only occasionally will the patient have an abnormal feeling or heaviness in the left scrotum or have palpated the veins himself. Usually, the presence of a varicocele is readily diagnosed on physical examination with examination in both standing and recumbent positions. Classically, the idiopathic varicocele will disappear in the lying position due to venous decompression into the renal vein, whereas the varicocele secondary to tumor invasion of the renal vein will remain because of an anatomical block. This observation, however, may not hold true for large varicoceles. Scrotal palpation of a typical varicocele has been likened to a "bag of worms." Small varicoceles can be demonstrated by having the patient stand while performing Valsalva's maneuver. Care should be taken in examing both sides, since 14% of patients with infertility may have bilateral varicoceles (Amelar et al. 1977). Physical examination will fail to demonstrate the subclinical varicocele.

The presence of a varicocele does not necessarily imply a relationship to infertility. MacLeod (1965) described what he considered to be the classical semen analysis in patients with infertility and varicocele. A triad, known as the "stress pattern" was described, consisting of oligozoospermia, impairment of sperm motility, and increase of immature and tapering sperm forms. Evidence suggests that when this pattern is present in patients with varicoceles a good result from internal spermatic vein ligation can be expected (MacLeod 1966). The presence of a varicocele with associated unilateral small testis suggests that the varicocele and infertility are related in that patient and that surgical treatment has a good chance of success (Lipshultz and Corriere 1977).

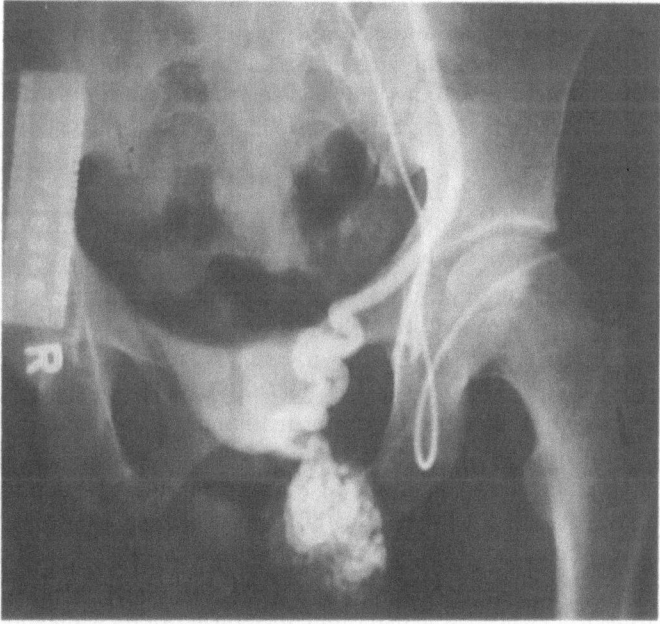

Fig. 1. Venographic demonstration of varicocele

Testicular biopsies performed in patients with varicocele classically show germinal cell hypoplasia and premature sloughing of immature sperm forms within the lumen of the seminiferous tubules (Dubin and Hotchkiss 1969; McFadden and Meham 1978). In addition, orchipathia and varicocele may be found with focal Leydig cell hyperplasia and hyaline sclerosis of testicular blood vessels (Hornstein 1964). Nevertheless at present testicular biopsy is not indicated in the patient with varicocele (McFadden and Mehan 1978).

Patients with a subclinical varicocele may be difficult to diagnose as it cannot be palpated on physical examination. In addition, in examining the patient in whom varicocelectomy has failed, it may be difficult to separate a recurrence of a varicocele from residual dilated veins. Contact scrotal thermography (Lewis and Harrison 1979) and Doppler ultrasound (Greenberg et al. 1977) have been used in the diagnosis.

The definitive test for the diagnosis of varicocele is the presence of internal spermatic vein reflux on venogram (Fig. 1). The study is performed by selective catheterization of the left renal vein, attempting to demonstrate reflux of contrast material down the left internal spermatic vein. Indications at present are quite limited and include subclinical varicocele and suspected postoperative varicocele in a patient who remains infertile with a palpable fullness in the scrotum. Hopefully, contact scrotal thermography and Doppler ultrasound will replace venography as a diagnostic aid.

15.4 Indications for Treatment

Surgical treatment of varicocele is indicated in selected patients with infertility and in others with local symptomatology.

The present indication for the surgical management of a varicocele in the treatment of male subfertility is the actual presence of a varicocele in association with a stress pattern seen on at least two semen analyses. The female partner should have no serious underlying condition contributing to infertility and attempts at pregnancy should have taken place for at least 1 year. In difficult cases, scrotal thermograms, Doppler ultrasound, or venography may be of value in determining the presence of the subclinical varicocele in a patient with a classical stress pattern found by semen analysis. The question of therapy for a male presenting subfertility and stress pattern and no varicocele detected on physical examination has been addressed (Fogh-Anderson et al. 1975): A series of subfertile patients without clinical varicocele were treated with varicocelectomy, producing a pregnancy rate of 32%. Since the size of a varicocele is not important in producing infertility (Amelar et al. 1977), in certain patients with a small amount of reflux into the internal spermatic vein, a clinical varicocele may not be apparent but the primary defect may be present. Although, at this time, ligation of the internal spermatic vein cannot be recommended when a stress pattern in the absence of varicocele is present, surgery might be considered in patients who also show a positive scrotal thermogram or Doppler ultrasound and the presence of a unilateral small testes. Further clinical trials will be needed to determine the efficacy of these diagnostic techniques.

15.5 Management

15.5.1 Surgical

The classical approach to the treatment of varicocele related to infertility has been surgical, with the recent introduction of adjunctive medical therapy. The surgery of varicocele dates back to Celsus who, in the first century A.D., ligated and cauterized the veins (Hotchkiss 1970).

The transcrotal approach is a well-described technique with exposure and ligation of both the cremasteric and internal spermatic veins (Hanley 1955). Care is taken not to injure the vas deferens and spermatic artery. Complications include secondary hydrocele, orchialgia, scrotal swelling and hematoma formation, and testicular atrophy. Because of our increased understanding of varicocele and improved surgical techniques, enthusiasm for this approach has diminished but not disappeared (Hanley 1955).

In 1918, a new operation for the treatment of varicocele was reported (Ivanissevich and Gregokini 1918). The spermatic vein was ligated lateral to the epigastric vessels where it is often a large single vessel. The approach was inguinal and the technique of high ligation of the spermatic vein became popularized. Modifications have been introduced using an inguinal incision over the internal inguinal ring with exposure of the spermatic cord (Amelar et al. 1977). A Penrose drain is placed under the cord, and the veins dissected from the cord, ligated, and partially excised at the internal ring. The wound is then closed in layers. Again, care must be taken to prevent injury to the vas deferens and internal spermatic artery. Hendry (1976) also utilizes an inguinal approach and ligates both the internal spermatic, as well as the cremasteric veins.

A popular operation performed today is high ligation of the spermatic veins above the inguinal canal. We recommend this procedure, based on knowledge of the anatomy and pathophysiology of varicocele as described. The higher the incision (scrotum, inguinal area, suprainguinal area) the larger and fewer the veins and, thus, the easier the procedure. Because of cross-communication between veins of the pampiniform plexus, high ligation above the internal inguinal ring will allow for correction of all possible sites of anastamosis. If the adverse effect of varicocele is retrograde flow in the spermatic vein rather than the varicocele itself, then the treatment should be directed at venous reflux. The ideal surgical treatment that follows from this concept would be to singly tie off the internal spermatic vein(s), rather than to excise the varicocele. From the technical viewpoint, high ligation is an easier and safer procedure than other forms of varicocelectomy and is associated with a low complication rate. Consequently we recommend the high ligation procedure.

In one series of 40 patients the spermatic vessels were exposed 2 cm above the internal inguinal ring and both vein and artery were ligated without incidence of testicular atrophy (Palomo 1949). Ivanissevich (1960) reported a modification of his original technique in which the inguinal canal was not entered.

Presently, we perform a high ligation of the internal spermatic vein (Fig. 2). The procedure is performed under general anesthesia and both the abdomen and genitalia are prepared. A small transverse skin incision is made 1 cm above and lateral to the left anterior superior iliac spine. The muscle layers are split, rather than cut,

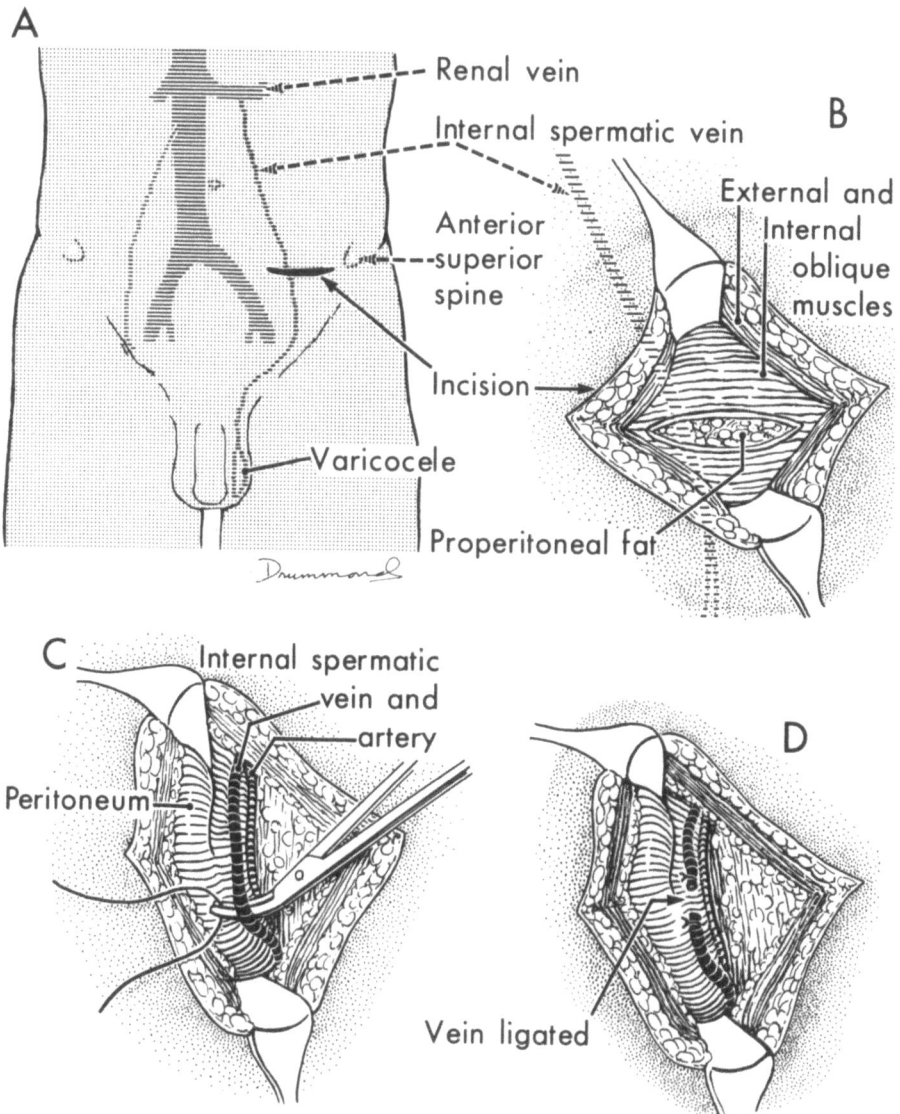

Fig. 2. High ligation of internal spermatic vein

in the direction of their fibers and the peritoneum exposed and retracted medically by two thin retractors. The spermatic vessels lie along the peritoneal reflection as the veins course from deep in the retroperitoneum to a more superficial level at the internal inguinal ring. The vas deferens and ureter are not exposed and not subject to injury. We then utilize a maneuver, originally described by Salema (1938), to aid in identifying all spermatic vessels. The patient is placed in reversed Trendelenburg's position and the scrotum is then tugged upon. This positioning has the effect of filling the veins and allowing easier visualization. The tugging maneuver causes the vessels to indent the peritoneum and also aids in visualizing all veins.

The position is then switched to Trendelenburg's and the scrotum manually compressed. This empties the dilated scrotal and spermatic veins. The artery is identified and carefully isolated from the vein. The veins are ligated with 2-0 silk sutures and a segment sent for histological identification. Occasionally, there are two veins and both must be ligated for the procedure to be successful. Following the vein ligation the Salema maneuver is then repeated. If complete separation of the veins has been accomplished there is no "to-and-fro" motion of the peritoneum except for the spermatic artery. We have found the Salema maneuver helpful in this respect. The wound is then closed in layers without drains. Complications of this procedure are few and include recurrence of varicocele, hydrocele formation, and wound hematoma in fewer than 1% of cases.

15.5.2 Medical

Increased numbers of pregnancies have been reported with the use of human chorionic gonadotropin (hCG), 4000 IU twice weekly for 10 weeks, in men with pretreatment sperm counts less than 10 million/ml after having undergone varicocelectomy (Amelar et al. 1977). Chehval and Mehan (1979), using a different dose schedule of hCG, achieved a similar response. hCG stimulates the production of testosterone by Leydig's cells. Whether this has a beneficial effect in oligozoospermia is unknown. Weiss et al. (1978), using testicular tissue incubated with radiolabelled precursors, showed that patients with varicocele and sperm counts of less than 10 million/ml had a suppression of in vitro testosterone formation and androgen biosynthesis secondary to Leydig's cell dysfunction.

These concepts of endocrine dysfunction and clinical response rate to hCG suggest that certain patients with varicocele and low sperm counts have Leydig's cell dysfunction. hCG administration might increase Leydig's cell activity and stimulate the seminiferous tubules. Although the above work is interesting, it remains controversial and there is still insufficient evidence to show that hCG is a useful adjunct to treatment in such men after varicocelectomy.

15.6 Results

Reported results on varicocelectomy for male infertility show semen parameter improvement of 55%–58% and pregnancy rates of 30%–55% (Hanley and Harrison 1962; Brown et al. 1968; Stewart 1974; Amelar et al. 1977). Dubin and Amelar (1977) reported on 986 patients with varicoceles undergoing surgical correction over a 12-year period. Semen quality improved in 70%, and 53% of wives became pregnant. In the future the use of hCG in related patients with low sperm counts and possible Leydig's cell dysfunction may be a valuable adjunct, but requires further experimental and clinical studies. Varicocelectomy results in changes in both semen and testicular biopsies (Johnson and Agger 1978; Glezerman et al. 1976). Improvement in sperm motility occurs first, followed by improvement in morphology, and finally sperm count (Glezerman et al. 1976). Reports of pre- and postoperative testes biopsies have shown improvement in the seminiferous epithelium following surgery (Johnson and Agger 1978).

Weiss et al. (1978) reported on 455 infertile couples which included 108 males with varicocele. These patients were divided into two groups according to therapy. The incidence of pregnancy in the group treated with surgery compared to the group treated without surgery was the same; 46% and 51%, respectively. The patients who had surgery usually showed improvement in semen analysis, whereas the others did not. In the nonsurgery group, the female partners were treated with a variety of techniques. These studies emphasize the fact that certain males with varicoceles and borderline subfertility may be able to cause conception in the female if, in the latter, underlying problems of subfertility are corrected. Perhaps some of these females have subclinical disease but, their treatment allows the fertility potential of the couple to increase to a level allowing conception. At present, in the management of male subfertility, best results occur with varicocelectomy and this continues to be the treatment of choice (Amelar et al. 1977; Cockett et al. 1979; Greenberg et al. 1977; Stewart 1974).

15.7 Discussion and Conclusions

The evidence presented supports the concept that there is an association between varicocele and male infertility. Although the mechanism is still not certain, it appears that internal spermatic vein reflux may lead to increased testicular heat, reflux of metabolites, epididymal dysfunction, and possibly interaction of other factors causing testicular abnormalities and decreased spermatogenesis. All men with varicocele are not infertile, as fertility depends on many factors. It is possible that the number and interaction of these various factors determine which males with varicoceles show abnormal semen analyses and subfertility. Although varicocele is usually a unilateral abnormality, cross-communications exist between the right and left pampiniform plexuses and can explain the systemic effect and bilateral testicular dysfunction. The evidence reported supports the proposal that varicocelectomy or high ligation is not a sham operation, but the most effective form of treatment for male infertility available today. Although some evidence has been discussed suggesting that certain patients with varicocele and abnormal semen analysis can cause conception in selected, treated female partners, this is still controversial and speculative and requires more clinical trials. At present, varicocelectomy is the recommended treatment of choice. Medical treatment with hCG may be of value but this remains unproven. Finally, surgical management does not improve fertility in all patients. There are probably a number of reasons for this, including improper selection of patients, incomplete surgery, and recurrence of reflux, and other male and female factors causing infertility that are not yet identified.

Although we have just begun to unravel the varicocele mystery, the experimental and clinical evidence to date does suggest that varicocele plays a very important role in male subfertility, and that surgical and possibly medical treatment can be of substantial value to these patients.

15.8 References

Agger P (1971) Scrotal and testicular temperature: Its relation to sperm count before and after operation for varicocele. Fertil Steril 22:286–297

Amelar RD, Dubin L (1975) Infertility in the male. In: Karafin L, Kendall AR (eds) Urology, vol II. Harper & Row, Hagerstown, New York London, pp 19–20

Amelar RD, Dubin L, Walsh PC (1977) Male infertility, Saunders, Philadelphia London Toronto, pp 57–68

Brown JS, Dubin L, Hotchkiss RS (1967) The varicocele as related to fertility. Fertil Steril 18:46–56

Brown JS, MacLeod J, Hotchkiss RS (1968) Results of varicocelectomy in subfertile men. In: Amelar RD, Dubin L, Walsh PC (eds) Male infertility. Saunders, Philadelphia London Toronto, pp 58–89

Charney CW, Baum S (1968) Varicocele and infertility. JAMA 204:1165

Chehval MJ, Mehan DJ (1978) Chorionic gonadotrophins in the treatment of the subfertile male. Fertil Steril 31:666–668

Cockett ATK, Urry RL, Doughtery KA (1979) The varicocele and semen characteristics. J Urol 121:435–436

Comhaire F, Vermeulen A (1974) Varicocele sterility: Cortisol and catecholamines. Fertil Steril 25:88–95

Comhaire F, Monteyne R, Kunnen M (1976) The value of scrotal thermography as compared with selective retrograde venography of the internal spermatic vein for the diagnosis of "subclinical" varicocele. Fertil Steril 27:694–698

Crew FAE (1921) A suggestion as to the cause of the aspermatic condition of the imperfectly descended testes. J Anat 56–98

Dierschke DJ, Walsh SW, Mapletoft RJ, Robinson JA, Ainther OJ (1975) Functional anatomy of the testicular vascular pedicle in the rhesus monkey: Evidence for a local testosterone-concentrating mechanism. Proc Soc Exp Biol Med 148:236–242

Dubin L, Amelar RD (1977) Varicocelectomy: 986 cases in a 12-year study. Urology 10:446–449

Dubin L, Amelar RD (1978) Varicocele. In: Howards SS, Lipshultz LI (eds) The urologic clinics of North America: Male infertility. Saunders, Philadelphia London New York, pp 563–572

Etriby AA, Ibrahim AS, Mahoud K, Elhaggar S (1975) Subfertility and varicocele. 1. Venogram demonstration of anastomosis sites in subfertile men. Fertil Steril 26:1013–1017

Fenster HN, McLoughlin MG (to be published) Epididymovasostomy for epididymal obstruction. In: Lipshultz LL, Corriere JW, Hafez ESE (eds) Surgery of the male reproductive organs. Martinus Nijhoff, The Hague Netherlands

Fogh-Anderson P, Nieldon NC, Rebbe H, Stokemann G (1975) The effect on fertility of ligation of the left spermatic vein in men without clinical signs of varicocele. Acta Obstet Gynecol Scand 54:29–32

Glezerman M, Rakowszczyk M, Lunderfeld B, Beer R, Goldman B (1976) Varicocele in oligospermic patients: Pathophysiology and results after ligation and division of the internal spermatic vein. J Urol 115:562–565

Grayhack JT (1976) Editorial comments. Year book of urology. Year Book Medical Publishers, Chicago, pp 351–352

Greenberg SH, Lipshultz LI, Morganroth J, Wein AJ (1977) The use of the Doppler stethoscope in the evaluation of varicoceles. J Urol 117:296–298

Ham AW (1965) Histology. Lippincott, Philadelphia Montreal, pp 964–965

Hanley HG (1955) The surgery of male subfertility. Ann R Coll Surg Engl 17:159–183

Hanley HG (1956) Surgical correction of errors of testicular temperature regulations. Proceedings of the IInd World Congress on Fertility and Sterility

Hanley HG, Harrison RG (1962) Nature and surgical correction of varicocele. Br J Surg 50:64–67

Hendry WF (1976) Male subfertility. In: Hendry WF (ed) Recent advances in urology. Churchill Livingstone, Edinburgh London New York, pp 232–244

Hornstein D (1964) Zur Klinik und Histopathologie des männlichen primären Hypogonadismus. III. Mitteilung, Hodenparenchymschäden durch Varicocelen. Arch Klin Exp Dermatol 218:347–383

Hotchkiss RS (1970) Infertility in the male. In: Campbell MF, Harrison JH (eds) Urology. Saunders, Philadelphia London Toronto, pp 674–675

Hudson RW, McKay DE (1979) The response of men with varicoceles to gonadotrophin-releasing hormone (Abstr). Fertil Steril [Suppl] 32:248–249

Ivanissevich O (1960) Left varicocele due to reflux, experience with 4470 operative cases in 42 years. J Int Coll Surg 24:742–755

Ivanissevich O, Gregokini H (1918) A new operation for the cure of varicocele. Sem Med 61:17

Johnson D, Pohl D, Rivera-Correa H (1970) Varicocele: An innocuous condition? South Med J 63:34–36

Johnson SG, Agger P (1978) Quantitative evaluation of testicular biopsies before and after operation for varicocele. Fertil Steril 29:58–63

Kay R, Alexander NJ, Baugham WL (1979) Induced varicoceles in rhesus monkeys. Fertil Steril 31:195–199

Lewis RW, Harrison RM (1979) Contact scrotal thermography: Application to problems of infertility. J Urol 122:40–42

Lipshultz LI, Corriere JN (1977) Progressive testicular atrophy in the varicocele patient. J Urol 117:175–176

MacLeod J (1965) Seminal cytology in the presence of varicocele. Fertil Steril 16:735–757

MacLeod J (1969) Further observations on the role of varicocele in human male infertility. Fertil Steril 20:545–563

McFadden MR, Mehan DJ (1978) Testicular biopsies in 101 cases of varicocele. J Urol 119:372–374

Moore CR, Quick WJ (1924) The scrotum as a temperature regulator for the testes. Am J Physiol 68:70–79

Palomo A (1949) Radical cure of varicocele by a new technique: Preliminary report. J Urol 61:604–607

Rodriguez-Rigau LJ, Smith KD, Steinberger E (1978) Relationship of varicocele to sperm output and fertility of male partners in infertile couples. J Urol 120:691–694

Russell JK (1954) Varicocele in groups of fertile and subfertile men. Br Med J 1:1231–1233

Salema O (1938) Slipping manipulation in Ivanissevichs' operation. Sem Med 45:142

Scott LS, Young D (1962) Varicocele. Fertil Steril 13:325–334

Steinberger E, Root A, Ficher M, Smith KD (1973) Role of androgens in initiation of spermatogenesis in man. J Clin Endocrinol Metab 37:746–751

Stewart B (1974) Varicocele in infertility: Incidence and results of surgical therapy. J Urol 112:222–223

Swerloff RS, Walsh P (1975) Pituitary gonadal hormones in patients with varicocele. Fertil Steril 26:1006–1012

Tulloch WS (1952) Consideration of sterility: Subfertility in the male. Edinburgh Med J 59:29

Weiss DB, Rodriguez-Rigau LJ, Smith KD, Steinberger E (1978) Leydig cell function in oligospermic men with varicocele. J Urol 120:427–430

Zorgniotti AW (1975) The spermatozoa count: A short history. Urology 5:672–673

Zorgniotti AW, MacLeod J (1973) Studies in temperature, human semen quality and varicocele. Fertil Steril 24:854–863

16 Obstruction in the Male Reproductive Tract

L. V. Wagenknecht

The male is the causative factor in about 50% of childless marriages (Dubin and Amelar 1971). The reasons for male infertility or subfertility are, in decreasing order, varicoceles, testicular failure, insufficient semen volume, endocrine and sexual problems, vasal obstruction, cryptorchism, etc. Following an interview with the couple and a thorough physical examination of the male, the analysis of the ejaculate gives preliminary information. Azoospermia is the principle indication of an obstruction of the reproductive tract. Other causes of azoospermia are retrograde ejaculation, neurogenic disorders, or defective or absent spermatogenesis. Azoospermia due to *primary testicular pathology* is often associated with an elevated FSH level: Klinefelter's Syndrome, bilateral mumps orchitis, torsion or trauma of both testicles, or radiation injury; however, with maturation arrest azoospermia may be accompanied by a normal FSH (Amelar et al. 1971). Cryptorchism leads to infertility in 37%–100% of cases, depending on the effectiveness of hCG therapy or the patient's age at time of surgery (Schirren 1971).

Retrograde ejaculation of semen into the bladder can result from surgery on the prostate and bladder neck or from lesions of the sympathetic nerve supply of the internal bladder sphincter (amputation of the rectum, total cystectomy, radical prostatectomy, injury of the spinal cord, radiation treatment for prostate cancer, α-adrenergic blocking agents). Retrograde ejaculation is discussed at length elsewhere.

Neurogenic disorders might lead to failure of seminal emission by impairment of contractility of the vas deferens and the seminal vesicles (Kedia et al. 1975). This seems to be the causative factor for azoospermia after lymph node dissection for testicular tumor, following treatment with sympatholytic drugs or in diabetic neuropathy.

In order to differentiate between obstruction and other causes of azoospermia, the patient's history (mumps, testicular trauma, epididymitis, transurethral resection, etc.) and the physical examination (size and location of the testicles, induration of the epididymis, absent vas deferens) provide important clues for diagnosis. Laboratory examinations include LH, FSH, and testosterone in the blood serum, which are normal in vasal occlusion. FSH is elevated when there is seminiferous tubular insufficiency. With a deficiency of Leydig cell function LH also rises. Testicular biopsy is the single most important investigation. In comparison with other causes of azoospermia, obstruction of the male reproductive system is frequently encountered (Dubin and Amelar 1971). The causes of obstruction and recent advances in microsurgical techniques applied to male infertility (epididymovasostomy, vasovasostomy, and alloplastic spermatocele) will be discussed here.

The necessity of employing microsurgery on the male reproductive tract is based upon the fact that, in handling delicate structures, the surgeon is more limited by his eyes than by his hands. Microsurgery requires instruments which differ in construction and handling from ordinary surgical utensils. At times, the sutures used are hardly visible with the naked eye. In our center, magnifying glasses were used exclusively until 1975, and subsequently high magnification loops with head lamps and operation microscopes (OP-Mi 6 and 7, Zeiss) have been employed (Wagenknecht et al. 1980). The following factors account for improved results of reconstructive procedures: a better understanding of the pathophysiology of obstructive phenomena, microdissection under optimal lighting and magnification, the availability of nonreactive suture material, and the general advancement of surgical techniques.

16.1 Causes of Obstruction of the Male Reproductive Tract

Patients with azoospermia and normal FSH levels frequently have epididymo-vasal obstruction. In order to exclude primary testicular pathology, a biopsy is done. In the case of an obstructive lesion, spermatogenesis is usually normal. Testicular biopsy often reveals an accumulation of cellular material within the lumen of a high number of tubules. If a vas deferens can be palpated and if the seminal fructose level in the ejaculate is normal, the problem is usually epididymo-vasal obstruction. These patients should undergo scrotal exploration in an attempt to correct the obstruction. Vasography as a diagnostic procedure before surgery is not indicated, since this might in itself lead to secondary obstruction of the vas. Severe oligozoospermia can also be caused by partial vasal obstruction due to inflammatory epididymo-vasal strictures.

The term *excretory azoospermia* is applied to a stenosis or aplasia of the vas deferens and/or parts of the epididymis without impairment of testicular function. The causes of excretory azoospermia are as follows: (1) specific or nonspecific inflammation of the epididymis or of the vas deferens, (2) obstruction of the vas caused by vasography, (3) hypoplasia or aplasia of the vas deferens or of parts of the epididymis, (4) voluntary vasectomy, (5) unrecognized ligation or section of the vas during herniotomy.

During a period of 12 years, 30,000 males were examined in the Andrology Unit, University of Hamburg, for impaired fertility. About 1000 of them were found to have excretory azoospermia (3%). Of these men, 509 were admitted to the Urology Clinic of this center for surgery.

16.1.1 Obstruction After Inflammation

Inflammatory occlusion is generally limited to the junction of the lower vas and the cauda of the epididymis. However, vasal stenosis might include the whole convoluted segment and relatively extended part of the straight portion. Of our 453 patients with excretory azoospermia explored at the time of attempted epididymovasostomy, 52% showed inflammatory occlusion at the epididymo-vasal junction.

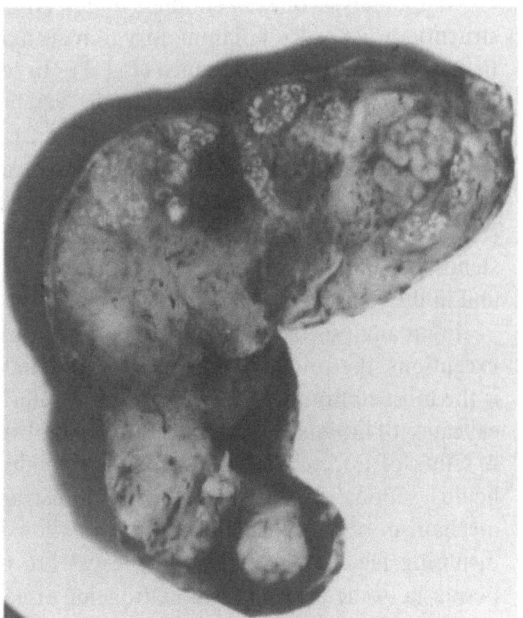

Fig. 1. Section through an epididymis showing extensive fibrous tissue formation (homogenous areas) in the cauda and in the corpus, four indentations on the convex border after repeated peroperative incisions, and convoluted tubular structures. Only one clearly dilated tubular cone appears in the epididymal caput, which is covered by an adynamic tubular conglomeration and sclerotic tissue (courtesy of Prof. A. F. Holstein, Institute of Anatomy, University of Hamburg, FRG)

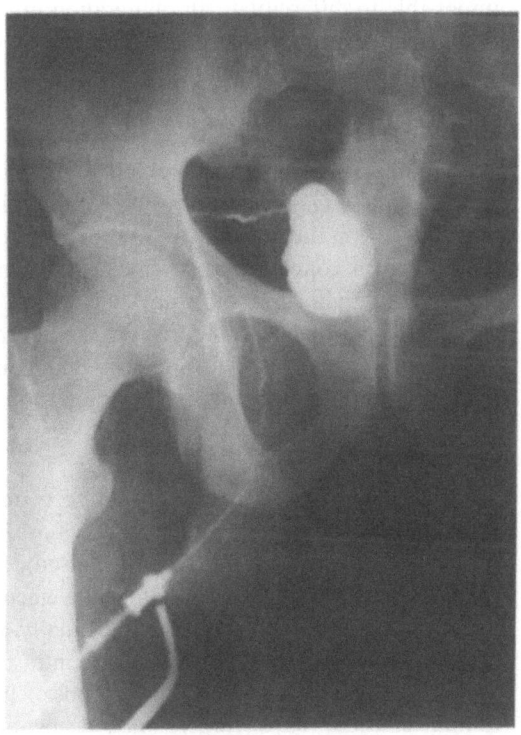

Fig. 2. Vasography on the right side demonstrates preurethral dilation of the vas deferens

In an analysis of 1294 childless males, Amelar and Dubin (1978) found vasal obstruction in 7.4%. An inflammatory fibrosis may involve not only the cauda, but also the corpus of the epididymis (Fig. 1). In comparison to the above-mentioned lesions, preurethral obstructions of the vas between its ampullary section and the colliculus seminalis are relatively rare (Fig. 2). Their causes are valvular obstruction, enlargement of the utriculus prostaticus, interampullary muscle, and sphincter spermaticus (Sachse 1965). Inflammation of the seminal vesicles and the prostate (tuberculosis, gonorrhea, unspecific bacteriuria) can also result in a preurethral stenosis of the seminal pathway. Genital tuberculosis occurs mainly in the prostate and in the seminal vesicles.

In an analysis of 325 cases with epididymal tuberculosis the cauda was, with few exceptions, the principle part involved (Steinhauser and Wurster 1975). Gonorrhea is the most common cause of obstructive infertility. The important pathophysiological cause of inflammation and subsequent obstruction of the male reproductive tract is reflux of infected or sterile urine (Altenähr et al. 1979). Each lesion of the colliculus seminalis, as by transurethral instrumentation, can destroy the valvular mechanism of the ejaculatory duct and allow for urinary reflux (Sachse 1966). Predisposing factors for reflux into the vas are urethritis, urethral valves, benign hyperplasia of the prostate, and neurogenic diseases. The inflammatory process within the epididymis, vas deferens, seminal vesicles, and prostate follows the same course of hyperemia, edema, epithelial desquamation, plasma exudation, and infiltration of the tissue by leukocytes. In an analysis of 235 surgical samples obtained over a period of 1 year from patients with suspected tumor, epididymitis was diagnosed in 25% and epididymal sclerosis was seen in a further 25% (Altenähr et al. 1979). It is impossible to differentiate an obliteration of the vas caused by systemic inflammation from one or multiple stenoses initiated by vasography.

16.1.2 Obstruction After Vasography

Vasography should be done exclusively during surgical exploration for excretory azoospermia (Fig. 3) and not as a separate diagnostic investigation. Manipulation with a needle in the duct may in itself lead to secondary obstruction. In addition, the injection of a concentrated, sticky contrast medium might induce an obstructive process. Superinfection following transcutaneous vasographies may also be a cause of secondary occlusion of the vas. We saw several patients with a multiplicity of long obstructions of the vas following transcutaneous vasographies. Some years ago, this fact led us to the conclusion that even intraoperative vasography might be detrimental. For some years, we therefore employed catheterization and injection of saline into the vas exclusively to prove patency.

The availability of new hydrophilic contrast mediums again encouraged intraoperative vasography. This is a necessary requirement, as illustrated in Fig. 2: during the operation a splint easily passed 20 cm upwards into the vas (probably rolled up in a preurethral dilation of the ejaculatory duct) and 20 ml saline was injected into that sac with no resistance. Finally, vasography clarified the situation.

In order to examine the effect of contrast mediums of different concentration and composition, experiments in 9 groups of 10 rats each were done. In comparison to three control groups (surgery only, vas ligation only, saline injection), six contrast

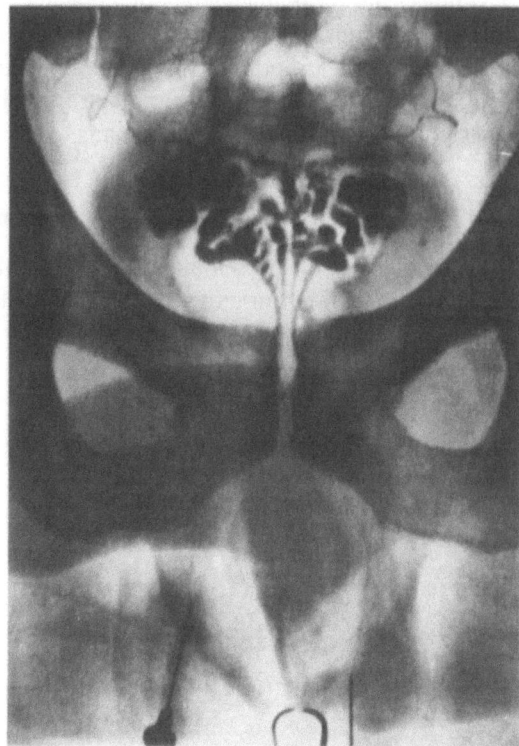

Fig. 3. Intraoperative vasography simultaneously performed on both sides shows patency of both vasa and visualization of the seminal vesicles

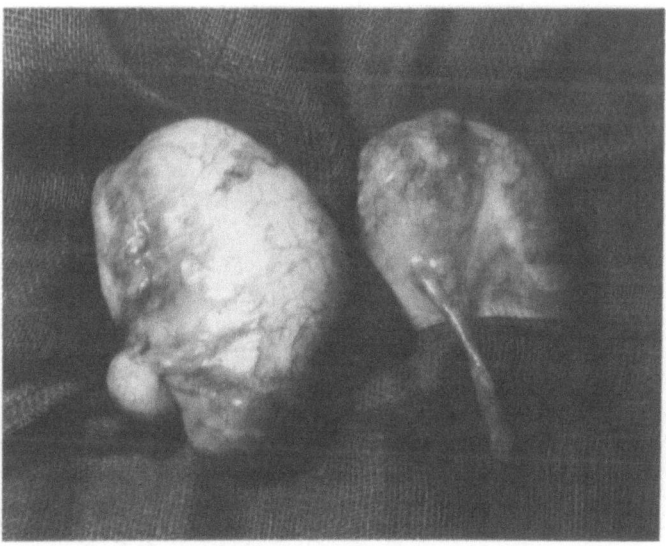

Fig. 4. Flaccid epididymal caput with neighboring venous conglomerations separated from a rudimentary round corpus, with missing cauda and vas deferens on the right side. Adynamic caput with a tail-like rudimentary structure of epididymal corpus-cauda on the left side

mediums caused varying degrees of damage to the vas deferens (Wagenknecht et al. 1982a), including irritation of the epithelium, inflammation, cellular infiltration, fibrosis of the wall, septum formation within the vas, fenestration, and actual obliteration. According to these experiments, onyl hydrophilic contrast mediums of low concentration should be used in humans.

16.1.3 Aplasia or Hypoplasia of the Vas Deferens

Aplasia of parts of the seminal pathway combined with normal spermatogenesis (Fig. 5) is not a rare cause of azoospermia (Vickers 1975; Wagenknecht et al. 1980), although the frequency of vas aplasia is poorly defined and the selection of the pa-

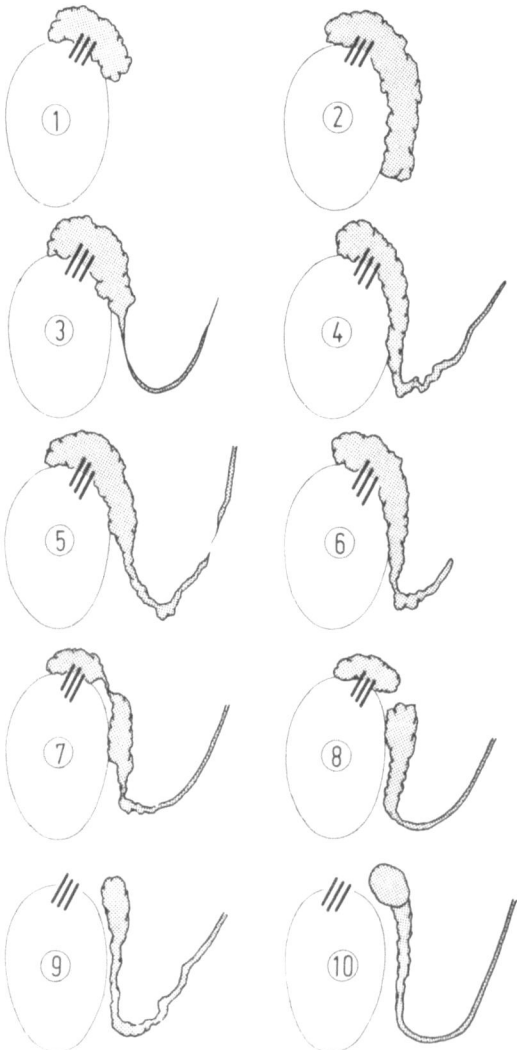

Fig. 5. Different forms of aplasia of the vas deferens and epididymis (see Sect. 1.3)

tient populations is relative to each report. Amelar and Dubin (1975) found bilateral congenital absence of the vas in 2% of infertile patients. In our series of 453 attempted epididymovasostomies, reconstruction of the seminal pathway was impossible in 127 cases (28%) because of epididymo-vasal aplasia or extensive obstruction: partial aplasia of the vas and/or of the epididymis was found in 82% of these cases. This high number is explained by the fact that our center receives scores of infertility problems from throughout West Germany.

The testicles and ductuli efferentes (which correspond later to the head of the epididymis) develop from the genital fold. The corpus and cauda of the epididymis, vas deferens, and seminal vesicle originate from the wolffian duct. This embryonal development explains that, in the majority of these cases, a normal testicle and epididymal caput are found. The upper remnant of the epididymis might show total or partial cystic degeneration. The most frequent form of seminal aplasia is a completely missing vas deferens on both sides with partial aplasia of the epididymis (Fig. 5, nos. 1–3). This occurred in 70% of our cases (Wagenknecht et al. 1982 b). In 15 patients complete unilateral vas aplasia was seen and the opposite side showed partial vas aplasia (Fig. 5, nos. 4–6), a missing part (Fig. 5, no. 5), or a normal patent vas in few cases (Fig. 5, nos. 7 and 8). Occasionally we saw a remnant caudal vas or a missing junction between vas and epididymis (Fig. 5, nos. 9 and 10). In all cases with total vas aplasia, fructose values and ejaculate volume were below normal. Since the seminal vesicles are the main location of fructose production, the concomitant aplasia of the seminal vesicles may be concluded.

Typical operative findings in cases of vas aplasia are as follows: hydatids of Morgagni or spermatoceles are more frequent than in other cases; venous conglomerations take the place of the missing epididymal structures; a cap of fat tissue distal to the epididymal caput or an extensive body of fat around the remaining part of the epididymis is frequently encountered.

16.1.4 Obstruction After Vasectomy

Vasectomy is a simple and safe method of birth control with few risks (Amelar et al. 1977; Klosterhalfen 1976). Vasectomy must still be considered a permanent form of sterilization even though up to 50% of patients with vasal patency after vasovasotomy become fertile.

The preferred method of vasectomy includes resection of 0.5–1 cm of the vas for histologic verification, short electrocoagulation of the vasal endothelium, fascies cover of the lower end of the vas, and U-shaped ligation of the upper end. This technique should be employed both in elective and prophylactic vasectomy. Postoperative complications are hematoma, infection, and painful irritation.

Formation of a spermatic granuloma frequently occurs at the cut end of the vas days to years after vasectomy. Sperm granuloma are considered by Silber (1979 b) as a kind of pressure relief and a favorable prognosis for future vasectomy reversal. Others found that the amount of sperm extravasation and the size of sperm granulomas correlate with the level of sperm autoantibodies found in about 60% of vasectomized men (Amelar and Dubin 1978); however, data on the development of sperm-agglutinating and sperm-immobilizing antibodies after vasectomy show great discrepancy. No exact correlation can be drawn so far between antibody levels and subfertility. The occurrence of sperm granulomas can be reduced if the cut ends of the vas are fulgurized rather than ligated (Schmidt 1966, 1978). The presence of sperm granuloma increases the chances of spontaneous recanalization after vasectomy (Schmidt 1966). Recanalization can be prevented by covering the distal end with the sheath of the vas. Psychological complications, such as decreased sexual desire or impotence, are avoidable if husband and wife are informed preoperatively about the technical details of vasectomy and are reassured that spermatogenesis continues and reanastomosis of the vas is possible.

16.1.5 Obstruction After Herniotomy

A further cause of obliteration of the vas might occur during herniotomy by inadvertently severing or ligating the vas deferens (Klosterhalfen and Wagenknecht 1972, 1977). Inguinal wound infection or extensive scar formation might also obstruct the vas. It usually remains undiagnosed because it is unilateral; however, when bilateral, the patient presents azoospermia. At the time of infant herniotomy, it is often not appreciated how tiny and delicate the vas deferens is, or recognized how closely it adheres to the sac of the hernia. Herniotomy can inadvertently include resection of the vas. Bilateral herniotomies in babies or small children seem to be especially prone to this complication. If one considers that in some institutions as many as 15% of infant hernia sacs may be found to contain a vas deferens, bilateral infant herniotomy may conceivably sterilize as many as 2% (Silber 1979a). This finding is particularly disturbing, since a number of pediatric surgeons advocate bilateral inguinal herniotomy in cases with unilaterally detected hernias.

Vasovasostomy for ligation of the vas subsequent to herniotomy is more difficult than after voluntary vasectomy. The vas' ends are entrapped in partially extensive scar tissue and the anatomical situation might be obscure. Some times the vas is ligated, sectioned, or obliterated at several points and resection of the nonusable part is necessary. A vasovasostomy without tension might only be possible by mobilization of the vas from the lateral pelvic wall and by partial testicular elevation. The wall of the vas, severed by herniotomy, might be so fragile that a rupture may occur during intraoperative vasography.

Silber (1979b) proposed an autotransplant of the vascularized vas from the opposite side if the vas of the better testicle is partially resected or nonusable.

16.2 Therapy and Results

16.2.1 Epididymovasostomy

It is generally accepted that optimal preconditions for epididymal microdissection and epididymovasostomy include optical enlargement (Fig. 6 a), special instruments (Fig. 6 b), nonreactive suture material, and microsurgical training. Since inflammatory occlusion is generally limited to the lower vas and to the cauda of the epididymis, it allows reanastomosis between the intact parts. Epididymovasostomy might also be indicated after vasectomy if an unconventional vasectomy renders the lower part of the vas nonusable, or the rise in pressure after vasectomy caused a rupture of

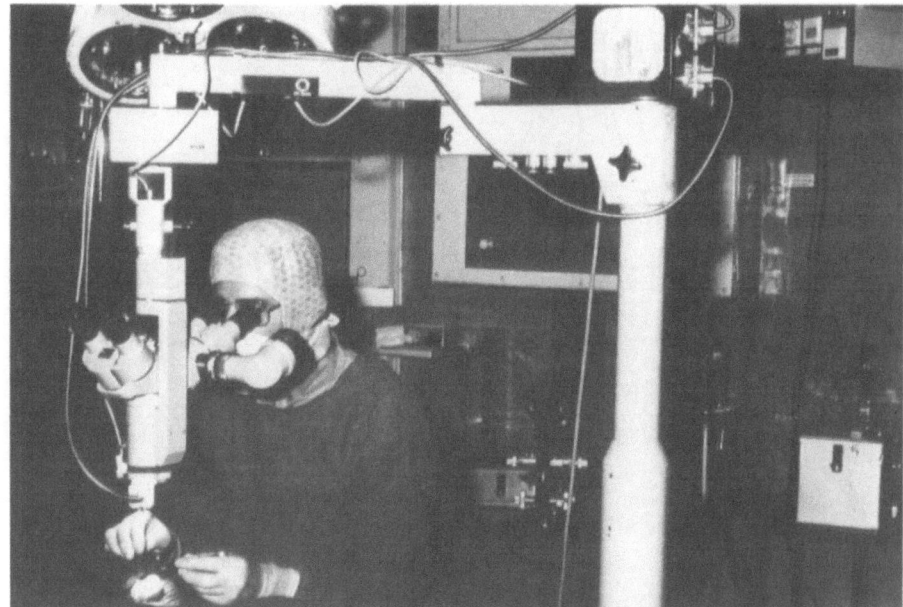

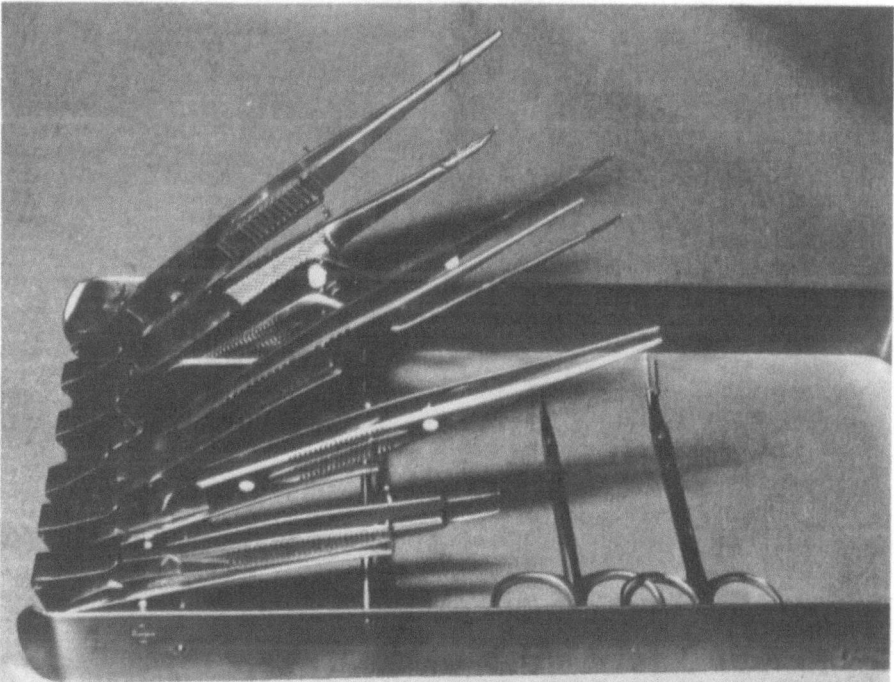

Fig. 6 a Surgical microscope (OP-Mi 7, Zeiss) and conventional light microscope installed for surgery on the male genital tract. **b** Microsurgical instruments: straight and angulated forceps with surgical and anatomical tips; straight and curved needle holders; and scissors

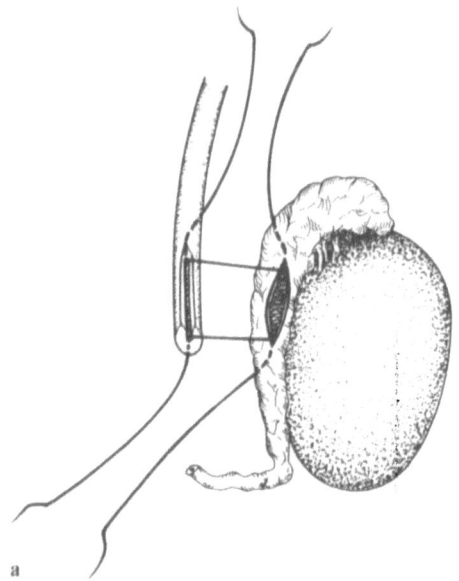

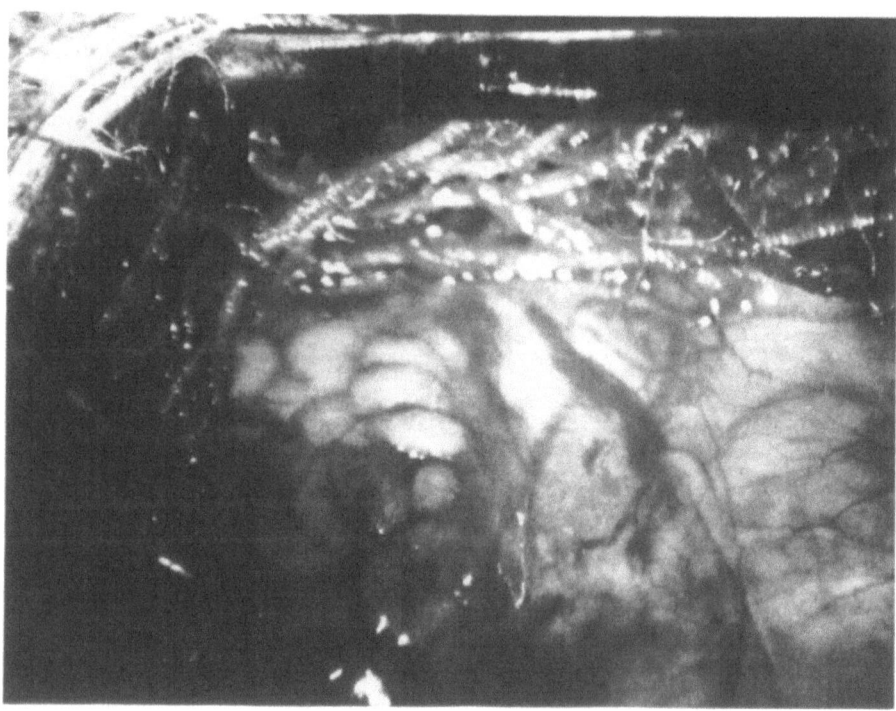

Fig. 7 a–d. Epididymovasostomy. **a** Diagram of an anastomosis between the incised vas deferens and the epididymal corpus. **b** Following a 5-mm excision of the epididymal tunica, the dilated canaliculus is exposed (×40). The fine structure of capillaries is clearly visible between two forceps. **c** A separate suture (8×0 Prolene) grasps the incised vas and the tunica of the epididymis (×25). **d** Completed anastomosis between epididymis and vas deferens

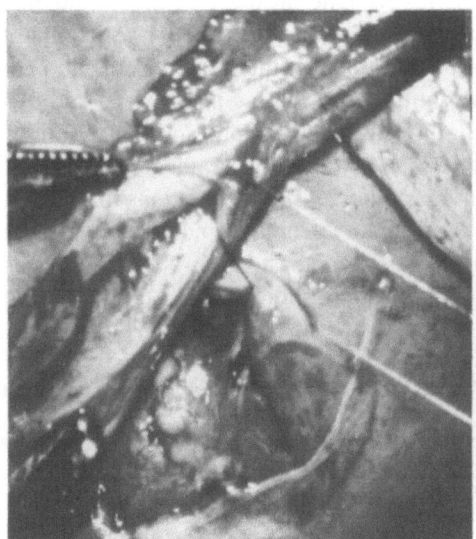
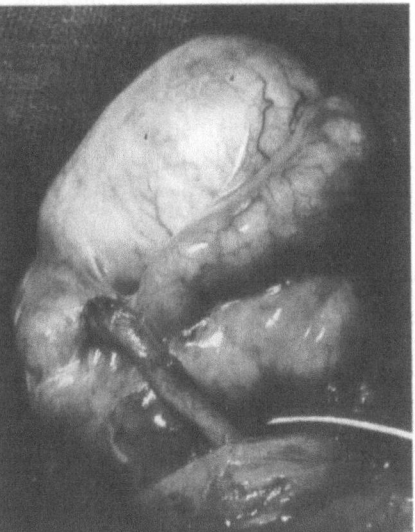

c   d

the epididymal tubule (Silber 1979 b). During recent years, the following technique
was employed: the testicles were exposed via a scrotal-midline incision of 2–3 cm.
Following section of the normal vas deferens and verification of its patency (Fig. 3),
the end of the vas was spatulated 0.5–1 cm (Fig. 7 a, c). The tunica of the epididymis
was removed over the lowest dilated area of the epididymis which is closest to the
cauda (Fig. 7 b). Hemostasis was done with bipolar microcoagulation. At the incised
angle pointing toward the testicle mere compression of bleeding vessels was preferred. One or two "meanders" of the exposed epididymal canaliculus (Fig. 7 b) were
incised in an oval-shaped fashion. The outflowing yellowish-white secretion was
sampled on a slide and examined immediately under the conventional light microscope. The number and the motility of spermatozoa were determined. If the swab
showed azoospermia another epididymal incision, closer to the testicle was chosen.
Bluish areas or white sclerotic tissue were unfavorable conditions, since they were
the result of severe epididymal destruction. They must be removed carefully under
the surgical microscope. While dissecting these areas, progressively healthy tubules
were opened and the outflowing secretion were often contained a surprising number
of progressively motile spermatozoa. An anastomosis of the vas with the tunica of the
epididymis was done with 8×0 Prolene (Eticon). The crucial angle next to the testicle was anastomosed with two to three separate sutures (Fig. 7 c) and both sides
with continuous suture. No permanent splint was used to bridge the anastomosis.
The last knot of the watertight suture was done over an introduced mammography
cannula. Via the latter, α-chymotrypsin was injected into the reanastomosis. This
was done to flush out blood coagula, test the watertight anastomoses for leaks, and
minimize edema. Following completion of the anastomosis (Fig. 7 d) the scrotal
contents were repositioned, the wound was closed, and a suspensory was applied for
10 days. Recently we adopted a one-layer side-to-end epididymovasotomy where
3–5 mm of the tunica over the lowest dilated epididymal canal is removed under the

surgical microscope using magnification 15–30. One meander of the epididymal canal is opened longitudinally. Four separate sutures (8 × 0 Prolene) grasp 2 mm of the tunica, 1 mm of the central tubular opening, 1 mm of the vasal mucosa and penetrate the vasal wall to emerge at the adventitia of the vas 3–4 mm from its end. After these four important sutures are positioned and tied, four additional sutures between the epididymal tunic and the vasal adventitia close the remaining interspaces of this side-to-end, watertight anastomosis. These operations are not included in our statistics. Scrotal exploration with an attempted epididymovasostomy was done in 453 patients (Table 1). In 326 cases, an anastomosis between the epididymis and the vas was possible. Following bilateral epididymovasostomy, patency

Table 1. Results of epididymovasostomies from 1964 to 1980 in the Department of Urology, University of Hamburg

Epididymovasotomy	No. of cases	No. available for follow-up	No. with patency (%)	No. of children
Bilateral	234	180	85 (47%)	28
Unilateral	85	55	17 (32%)	7
Crossed	7	6	0	
Total	326	241	102 (42%)	35
Surgical correction impossible	127	–	–	–

of the vas was obtained in 47% of cases, which contrasted with a 32% patency of unilateral anastomoses. In seven cases a crossed anastomosis was done because of a total obstruction of the epididymis on one side, and the vas on the other side: Follow-up of six of the latter patients failed to demonstrate patency. Reconstructive procedures might be long and difficult if situations are encountered as in Fig. 8. In the first case, a correction was impossible on one side because of the stenosis of the vas after herniotomy, vasographies, and inflammation combined with a total sclerosis of the epididymis; the other side showed extensive inflammatory obstruction which could be bridged (Fig. 8a). In another case (Fig. 8b), epididymovasostomy was possible on the right side following testicular elevation; on the other side it had to be combined with vasovasostomy for postherniotomy obstruction of the vas. It was particularly satisfying that these men became fertile and fathered healthy children.

At times several incisions of the epididymal tubule from the cauda to the caput and immediate microscopic examination of the outflowing secretion show no spermatozoa. Histologic examination of the removed epididymis might, nevertheless, demonstrate dilated tubular regions which may be found in a deeper layer or bordering the testicle (Fig. 1). In the latter situation (closer than 0.5 cm to the testicle) an epididymovasostomy is not promising, since spermatozoa remain immature and mainly immobile. Following an anastomosis of the vas to the epididymal caput 6–10 mm from its upper extremity, some of our patients fathered children.

Several techniques have been described as shortcuts between the epididymis and the vas deferens. These procedures may be divided into three major groups.

Firstly, the vas is cut and buried into the caput of the epididymis (Hanley 1955). Because 9–15 ductuli efferentes, originating from the rete testis, form efferent cones within the caput, the theoretical chances are very good that by a wide incision of the caput and anastomosis to the vas patency will be obtained. However, due to the lack of maturation of spermatozoa the fertility rate is low.

Secondly, a latero-lateral anastomosis is performed between the epididymal tunica and the vas deferens (Bayle 1960; Schoysman 1976). Like the Hanley technique, this procedure functions like a fistula.

Thirdly, a direct end-to-end anastomosis of a dilated epididymal tubule to the vas has been proposed (Silber 1979a). This appears to be the most logical and in-

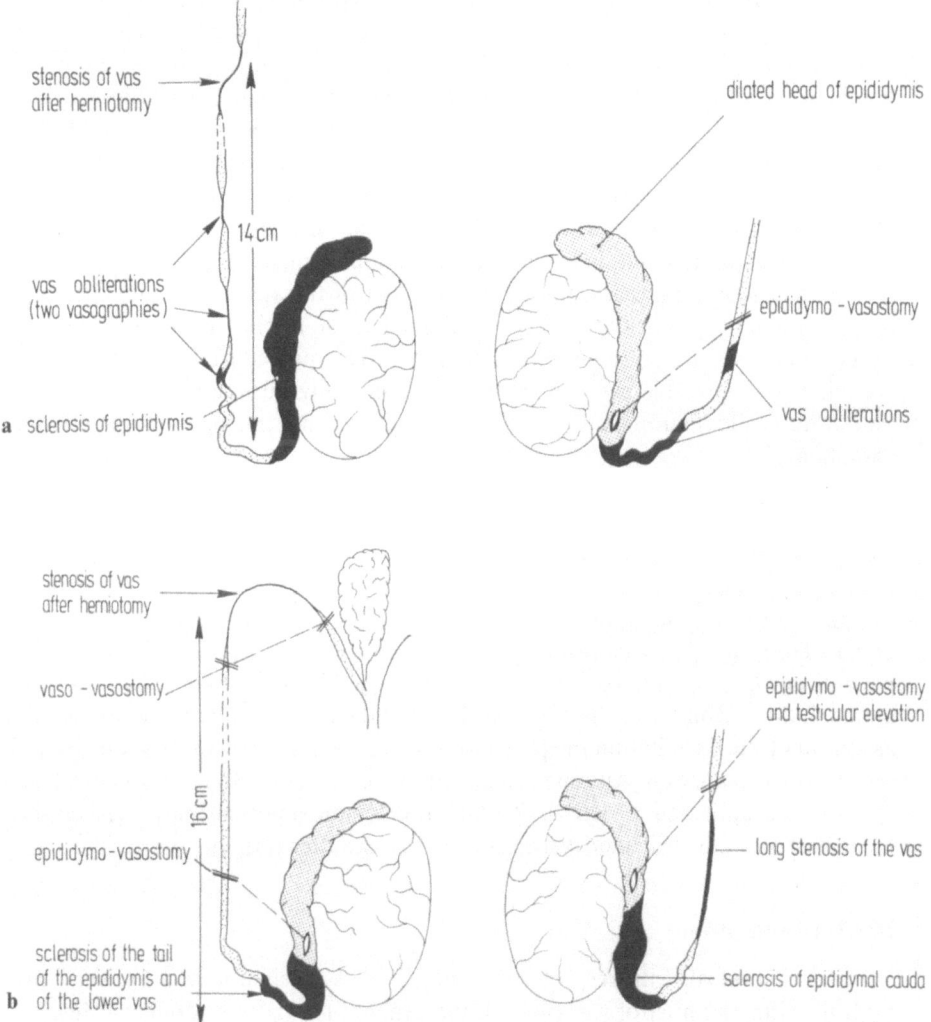

Fig. 8a,b. Difficulties encountered during surgical correction for obstructive infertility. **a** Various stenoses of the vas deferens and of the epididymis following inflammation, vasographies, and herniotomy. **b** Necessary double vas anastomosis on the right side and testicular elevation for epididymovasotomy on the left

genious concept, since the continuity of the seminal pathway is reconstructed in two layers under direct vision and it is not left to chance that the sperm flow from the grossly incised epididymis establishes a permanent fistula into the vas. In the lowest dilated area "the epididymis is sectioned transversely with large scissors, like a sausage" (S. J. Silber, personal communication). The many-sectioned lumina of the epididymal canal all secrete fluid at first during this immediate decompression. After a while, sperm oozes out of only one tubular section and this is directly anastomosed to the mucosa of the vas using four to six interrupted 10×0 nylon sutures; the outer muscularis sheath of the vas is fixed to the epididymal tunica with separate sutures $6-8 \times 0$ (Silber 1979 a).

Some time ago we tried this procedure, but we encountered several difficulties. It seemed difficult to decide which of the sectioned tubular sections would be the only important opening for reanastomosis with the vas. Especially when there was little or no sperm flow, watery secretion, and the constant irrigation of the epididymal section necessary for microscopic vision, it seemed hazardous to pick one of the sectioned epididymal meanders for reanastomosis with the vas. Furthermore, the use of 10×0 polyphilic Vicryl (Eticon) tore the fragile epididymal canaliculus: The latter problem can be eliminated with the use of monophilic Vicryl $10-11 \times 0$. There is also a mismatch of the diameter of both structures as well as in the size of the lumina and, inversely, in the outside diameter of vas and epididymis. It appeared unsafe to anastomose the outer half of the vasal wall with the epididymal section itself. For this reason we adopted a side-to-end epididymovasostomy using a one-layered suture, as described above. This procedure is easy to perform and eliminates possible difficulties in finding the only important tubular section. Since one epididymal meander is opened longitudinally, this opening matches the vasal lumen.

Following the realization that maturation of spermatozoa increases proportionally to the length of the passage through the epididymis, the anastomosis is done over the lowest dilated part of the epididymis.

The first semen analysis is not advised before 2 months post-surgery. The patient's eagerness to learn the result is the reason why samples are frequently examined earlier. The result of vasovasostomy is best judged after 6 to 12 months. We have seen patients in whom spermatozoa appeared in the ejaculate 8–10 months after surgery, although the reason for this is not clear. None of the theoretical considerations, such as immunological inhibition of spermatogenesis or paralysis of vasal nerves, offer a satisfactory explanation. Although some authors have claimed that in some patients spermatozoa appeared as late as 2 years after epididymovasostomy, we consider the operation a failure if azoospermia persists 1 year after surgery.

16.2.2 Vasovasostomy

Vasectomy reversal, with respect to patency, is now possible in almost every case. With the rising number of vasectomies, the demand for vasovasostomies is increasing. For some countries the demand for reversal is documented; in India 106 per 1000 and in England 42 per 1000 vasectomies (Schmidt 1975). Vasoresection, currently performed at the upper scrotal area, generally leaves neighboring ends for vasovasostomy. A non-usable caudal segment of the vas requires epididymovasostomy. In exceptional cases, presenting a long defect of the vas, only an alloplastic spermatocele can permit percutaneous aspiration of spermatozoa from the reservoir for artificial insemination (Wagenknecht et al. 1975; Kelâmi et al. 1976; Schoysman 1968). The main reasons for vasovasostomy are remarriage, death of children, and improved economic situation.

The skin incision is chosen over the probable site of vasectomy as scrotal midline incision in cases of voluntary vasoresection or inguinal approach when the vas was severed during a former herniotomy. The healthy ends of the vas are freed and sectioned (Fig. 9). They are drawn together by a stay-suture through the adventitia and the vessels to allow for an anastomosis without traction. The patency of the vas is verified by vasography (Fig. 3) and the outflowing secretion from the lower end of the vas is microscopically examined. If spermatozoa are missing in this sample, a lower vas occlusion or an epididymal rupture due to the rise in pressure following vasectomy are possibilities (Elsässer 1974; Silber 1979 b; Schmidt 1966; Lee 1976, 1981). There is a disproportion of the lumina between the lower and upper end of the vas (Fig. 9 a).

Three surgical techniques have been used in our center. From 1967 to 1973 the adventitia of the vas was reanastomosed by separate, silver wire sutures with magnifying glasses (two times) and a splint was used to bridge the anastomosis for 10 days (Fig. 9 b). This procedure has been abandoned. From 1974 to the present, four to eight non-resorbable sutures through the entire wall are used without employing a splint (Fig. 9 c). The suture material is 8×0 Prolene with needles on both ends. The needle transverses the vas on each side, entering the mucosa 1 mm from its edge and emerging on the adventitia about 3 mm from its cut end. The sutures are placed first on the anterior half of the vas. Following rotation of one edge-suture to the opposite side, three to four sutures are placed on the other half. The sutures are tied instrumentally with firm approximation. If tied too tightly, they cut into the tissue and can tear the mucosa in particular. Some additional superficial sutures of the adventitia may be added in order to obtain a water-tight anastomosis. As an alternative method, we perform a modification of Silber's double-layer anastomosis under the surgical microscope: four separate resorbable sutures (10×0 Vicryl) grasp the inner half of the muscular wall and the endothelial lining of the vas (Fig. 9 d). The adventitia and the outer muscular layer are reapproached by separate sutures 8×0 Prolene.

Results of 112 vasovasotomies in 56 patients are shown in Table 2. Follow-up by semen analysis showed an overall patency of 76% with an average sperm density of 42 million/ml ejaculate and 63%–86% of motile spermatozoa of normal morphology. Of 34 patients showing patency, 18 fathered children (53%). With the improvement of optical visibility, suture material, and surgical technique the results improved considerably (Tables 2, 3). Since we did not obtain better results with Silber's double-layered technique in comparison to full thickness anastomosis of the vas (Table 2), we feel that the latter is adequate and best performed with magnification 4–15. If a vasovasostomy is not possible because of a nonusuable lower part of the vas or an epididymal rupture, microdissection and an epididymovasostomy are required. Sperm count and motility tend to improve continually over a period of 2 years following vasovasostomy. In case of persistent azoospermia after vasovasostomy, a reintervention can be done after at least 6 months.

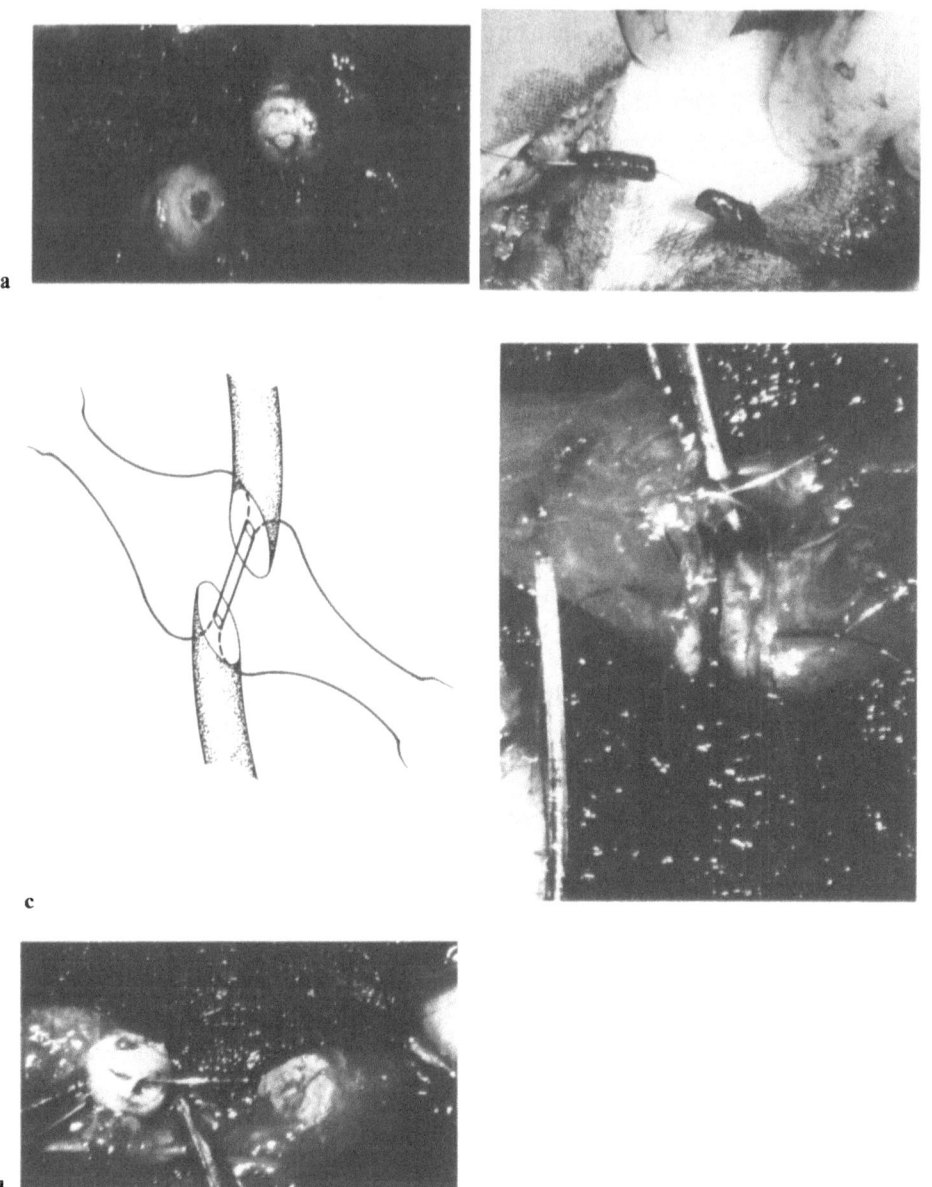

Fig. 9a–d. Vasovasostomy. **a** Unequal lumina of both ends of the vas. **b** Outdated technique over an inlying splint. **c** Preferred one-layer vas anastomosis employing four to eight separate non-resorbable sutures through the entire wall of both ends of the vas (diagram on the *left*, intraoperative situation on the *right*). **d** Double-layered technique (Silber 1977) beginning with four resorbable sutures for mucosal adaptation, followed by non-resorbable sutures for the outer layer

Table 2. Results of various techniques of vasovasostomy

Techniques of vasovasostomy	No. of cases	No. of follow-ups	Patency no. (%)	Children
Anastomosis of muscle wall (Silver wire) + splint + loops (two times)	28	17	11 (64%)	5
Anastomosis of entire wall (four to six sutures Prolene 6–8 × 0), no splint, loops (4.5 times)	16	16	14 (87%)	7
Double-layer technique (Silber 1978) (four sutures Vicryl 10 × 0, Prolene 8 × 0), no splint, surgical microscope	12	12	10 (83%)	6
Total	56	45	34 (76%)	18

Table 3. Results of vasovasostomies as indicated in the literature (first two series are retrospective analyses, the remaining are homogenous series)

Reference	No. of cases	Patency (%)	Pregnancy (%)
O'Connor (1948)	420	38	
Derrick et al. (1973)	1630	30	19.5
Dorsey (1973)	129	88.3	18
Amelar and Dubin (1975)	93	84	33
Schmidt (1975)	117	80	30
Lee (1976)	185	81	35
Silber (1979b)	42	71	

16.2.3 Alloplastic Spermatocele

In 28% of our scrotal explorations for excretory azoospermia, surgical correction was impossible because of a long stenosis or aplasia of the vas deferens (Table 1).

Until now there was no promising treatment for these men. It might, however, be possible to create a sperm reservoir and aspirate spermatozoa, which can then be used for insemination. The prototype of an artificial spermatocele is a normally occurring spermatocele which is found in 0.5%–1% of surgically explored men. Schoysman (1968) proposed the use of venous transplants upon the epididymis for creation of an artificial spermatocele (Fig. 10). Unfortunately, this graft showed early obliteration in 65 cases which were operated upon by Schoysman and other investigators (Schoysman and Drouart 1972; Klosterhalfen and Wagenknecht 1972; Vickers 1975; Schoysman 1976; Ludvik 1977). In 16 of our own cases, saphenous vein grafts were implanted upon the caput or the corpus of the epididymis (Fig. 10b). All showed shrinkage and fibrous obliteration within days to weeks after operation (Klosterhalfen and Wagenknecht 1972).

Since 1973, a cup-shaped silicone prosthesis with a Dacron fixation border has been successfully used as an artificial spermatocele in rats and bulls (Wagenknecht

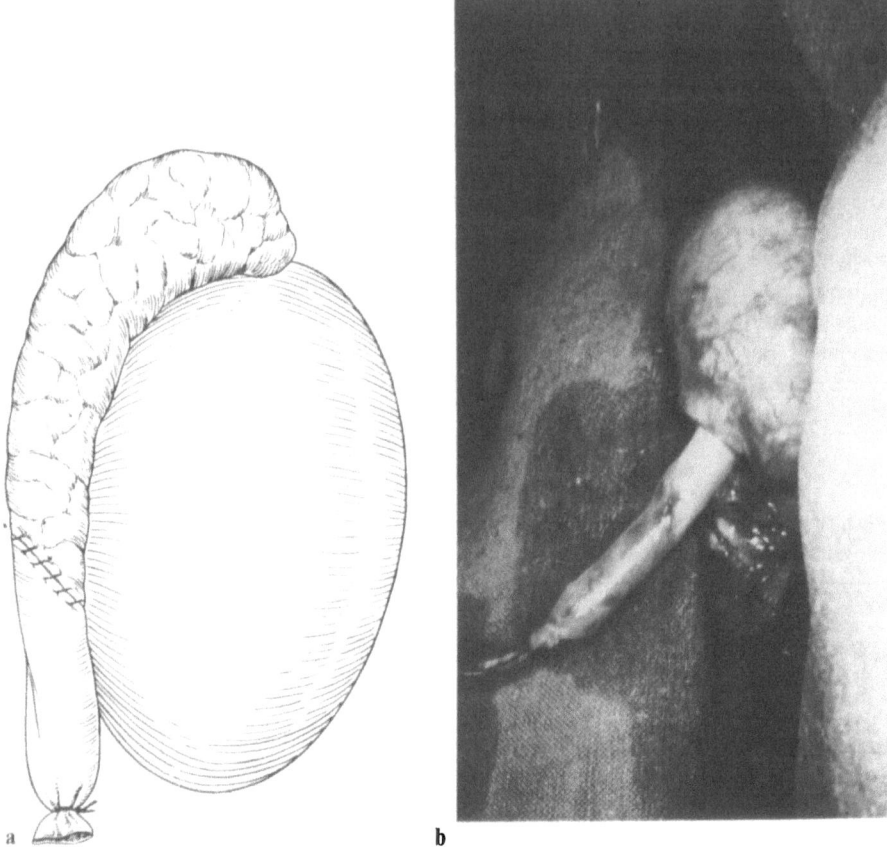

Fig. 10 a, b. Artificial spermatocele using venous transplant: **a** diagram; **b** intraoperative situation

et al. 1975, 1976, 1980). Following percutaneous aspirations of the contents of this prosthesis in bulls, 50% of inseminated cows became pregnant and delivered healthy calves.

Preparatory efforts for implantation of an alloplastic spermatocele involved the Departments of Andrology, Urology, and Gynecology. The operation was scheduled 5–10 days prior to ovulation of the patient's spouse.

Gynecological examinations of the wives showed luteal insufficiency in all but one case, treated by clomiphene for 1–3 months.

We implanted 30 cup-shaped silicone prostheses ($20 \times 8 \times 8$ mm, Ruesch, Waiblingen-Stuttgart, distributed by Link, Barkenhausenweg 10, 2000 Hamburg 63, FRG) upon the middle or upper part of the epididymis in 16 patients (Wagenknecht et al. 1980). Indication for this alloplastic graft was agenesis of the vas with partial aplasia of the epididymis in 12 patients and long stenosis of the vas in four cases (Fig. 11).

The surgical technique is similar to the one used for epididymovasotomy: following preparation of the implantation site, about 1 cm of the tunica of the epididymis is removed without damaging the underlying canaliculus (Fig. 11 b). Hemostasis is accomplished with bipolar microcoagulation or by mere compression of the vessel. The Dacron-felt border of the prosthesis is sutured with the tunica at the angle next to the testicle with three separate stitches 6–8×0 Prolene and at the circumference with continuous sutures. The outer border of the graft is fixed with a second suture to obtain a watertight anastomosis. The prosthesis is filled with α-chymotrypsin to minimize edema (Fig. 11 c) and then replaced with the testicle into the scrotal sac. During a hospitalization of about 10 days, percutaneous punctures of the silicone prosthesis and aspiration of its contents are done at 2-day intervals and, thereafter, once a week for as long as it remains open (Fig. 11 d). Single aspirations showed 300,000–120 million spermatozoa and the aspirated volume varied between 0.4 and 1.4 ml. The aspirated fluid was reddish during the first two to four punctures of the prosthesis and thereafter became clear. In all cases the aspirated spermatozoa showed poor motility despite good sperm counts. The longest duration of postoperative aspirations with positive sperm counts has been 7 months (Fig. 12, Table 4). In all cases the prosthesis was easily palpable under the scrotal skin and percutaneous puncture of the graft did not pose any difficulty. However, all prostheses eventually became clotted. On the average, aspirations in these 16 patients were done for 3 months with positive sperm counts for 2 months (Table 5).

Around the time of ovulation, 58 inseminations via a cap were done in 16 females using 0.5–0.8 ml aspirated volume. These have not yet resulted in any lasting pregnancy. Between ovulations, the aspirated samples were deep-frozen in pellet form for later use. However, the aspirated spermatozoa are extremely fragile and

Table 4. Results of postoperative aspiration from an alloplastic spermatocele implanted in a patient with vasal aplasia. The total number of spermatozoa is calculated in relation to the aspirated volume which varied between 0.5 and 1.2 ml

Postoperative aspiration (days postoperatively)	Total sperm count in millions	
	Left side	Right side
6	17.0	7.0
8	7.0	12.0
10	5.0	69.0
15	47.1	15.9
20	90.2	23.9
23	95.5	24.3
25	3.7	55.6
27	0.9	3.7
30	0.3	1.7
43	22.1	0.3
85	16.8	60.5
112	3.7	47.2
114	2.8	52.8
133	–	22.1
146	–	29.0
151	–	24.0
209	–	17.0
210	–	–

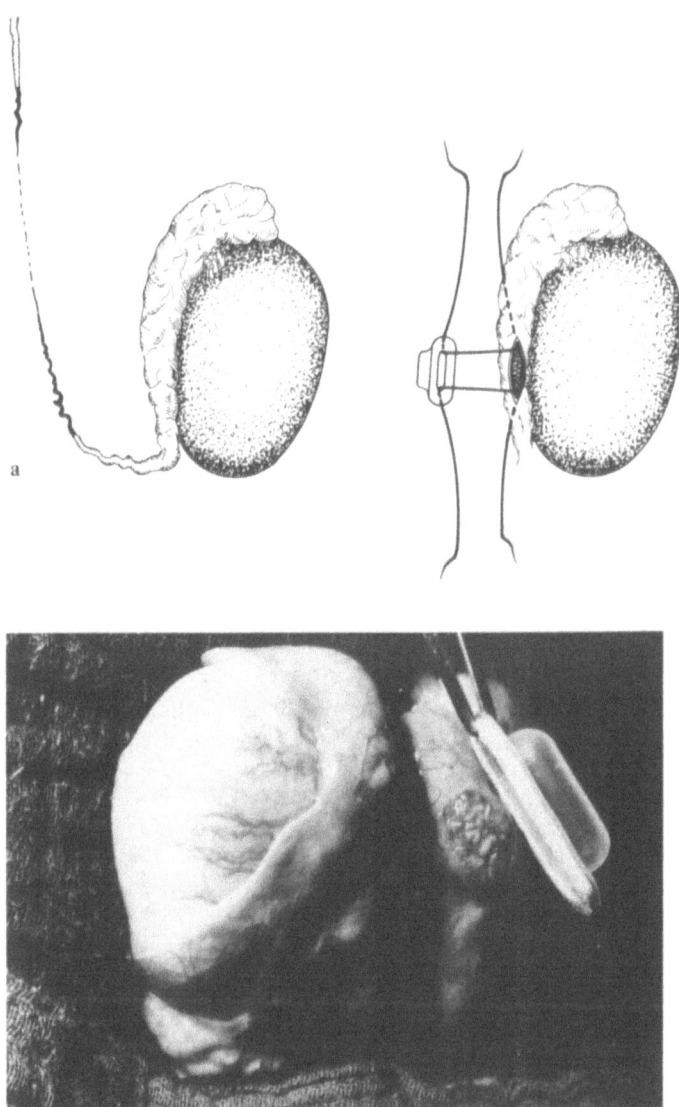

Fig. 11a–d. Artificial spermatocele using a silicone-Dacron prosthesis. **a** Diagram of the technique (*right*) applicable for cases with long stenosis of the vas (*left*). **b** Intraoperative preparation of implantations: oval-shaped epididymal tunica-defect over which a prosthesis is fitted (*right*); outflowing secretion following an incision of a tubule in the center of excised field (*left*). **c** Implanted prosthesis filled with α-chymotrypsin. **d** Percutaneous aspiration of the prosthesis

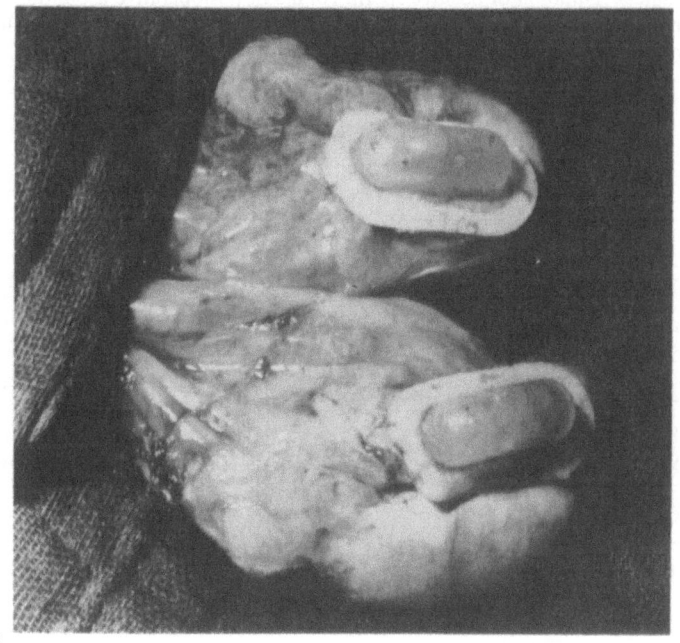

c

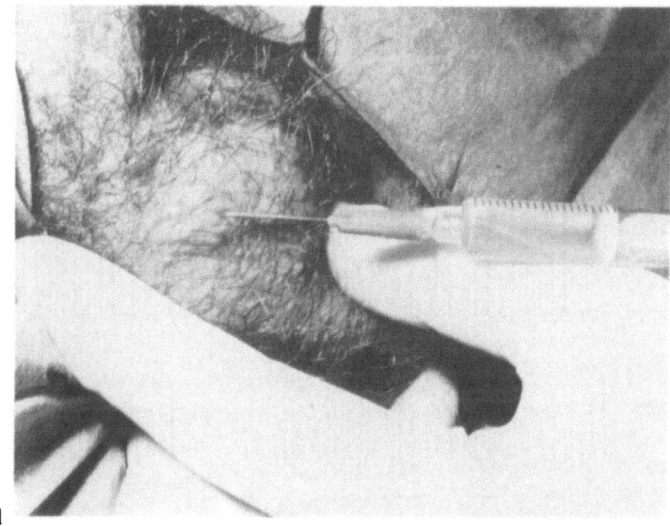

d

Table 5. Duration of positive sperm counts in postoperative aspirations from alloplastic spermatoceles in 16 patients. On the average, aspirations from the prosthesis were done for 3 months (follow-up) with positive results for 2 months

Case	Last positive sperm count (days after implantation)	Follow-up (days after implantation)	Particulars
1	32	54	
2	38	65	
3	59	77	
4	41	92	
5	13	13	Lost to follow-up
6	209	210	Positive sperm count for 7 months
7	33	53	
8	78	93	Epididymitis 1 month postoperatively
9	34	88	Maximum sperm count per aspiration 105 million/ml
10	36	73	Surgery performed in Hôpital Necker, Paris, France
11	33	85	Surgery performed in Hôpital Necker, Paris, France
12	67	82	
13	28	54	
14	93	152	Maximum sperm count per aspiration 162.5 million/ml
15	72	96	
16	18	33	Wound infection
Average	55	80	

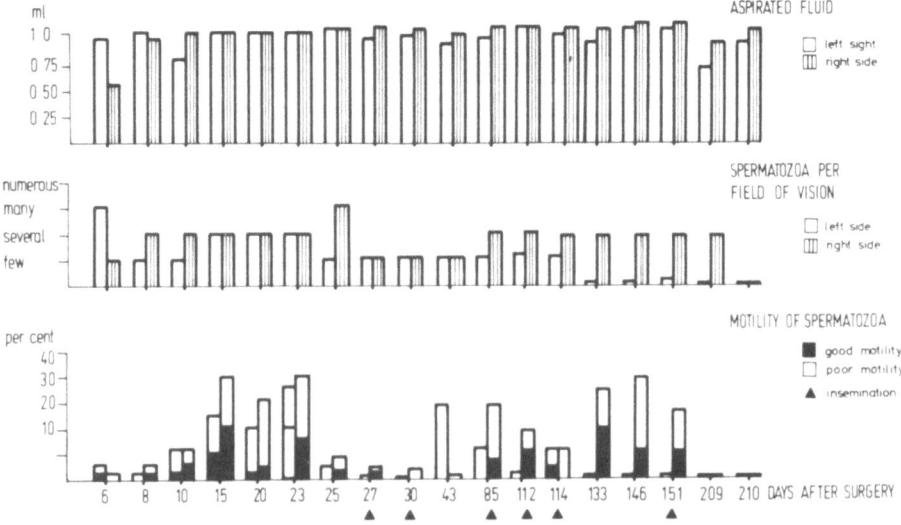

Fig. 12. Results of postoperative aspirations from an alloplastic spermatocele for 7 months after implantation

only 10%–20% showed progressive motility after thawing. There was no local in-flammatory reaction due to the implanted alloplastic material. The prostheses were explanted in four patients and were found to be covered by a thin layer of fibrous tissue. Within the Dacron fixation border, fibrous tissue formation and lymphatic lacunae were noted.

Recently, R. Schoysman (1980, personal communication) obtained one preg-nancy following insemination with the aspirated content from such a prosthesis. Us-ing a similar silicone-Dacron prosthesis in patients with vas aplasia A. Kelâmi and H. Sommerkamp (1980, personal communication) induced two childbirths.

16.3 Discussion and Conclusions

Obstruction of the reproductive tract is the cause of male infertility in 3%–10% of andrological patients (Schirren 1971; Amelar and Dubin 1978). In decreasing fre-quency, these obstructions are located on the epididymo-vasal junction, the lower vas, and the ejaculatory duct. Congenital aplasia of parts of the epididymis and the vas deferens is diagnosed in a high percentage of surgically explored cases. With the rising number of vasectomies for birth control, consultations for reversal are increas-ing. An azoospermic ejaculate and normal spermatogenesis are sufficient pa-rameters for surgical exploration and an attempt for reconstructive surgery. In-traoperative vasography should be done with hydrophilic contrast medium of low concentration (Wagenknecht et al. 1982 a). Epididymovasostomy should be done as close to the cauda as possible, based upon the fact that sperm maturation increases the longer the passage through the epididymis (Holstein 1969; Wagenknecht et al. 1976).

The incision of the epididymis should not extend more than few millimeters be-cause (1) the epididymis contains only *one* meandering canaliculus which will be sectioned more often the longer the incision, (2) only the exact and wide opening of the canaliculus closest to the testicle is important for sperm flow, and (3) the longer the incision the higher the danger of bleeding and activation of fibrous tissue forma-tion. For these reasons we now favor a direct one-layer epididymovasostomy. If this is done as a side-to-end anastomosis, one eliminates the possibility that the wrong tubule is anastomosed to the vas during end-to-end reconstructions. The fixation of the outer layer of the vas with the epididymal tunic guarantees an anastomosis without traction. Macroscopic appearance of abundant yellowish-white excretion following incision of the epididymis most often correlates microscopically with a positive sperm count and good motility of spermatozoa. The latter is not true for cases of aplasia or congenital obstruction (Wagenknecht et al., to be published b). With congenital obstruction of the vas the determination of the exact location for epididymal anastomosis is easy since the epididymal tubule comes to a blind end. Contrary to the situation after vasectomy, the rise in epididymal pressure in con-genital obstruction is of a different nature since we have never seen rupture or lesions related to that pressure. Pathophysiology, e.g., the mechanism of phago-cytosis, seems to be quite different in congenital obstruction and vasectomy. In con-genital obstruction, one generally finds spermatozoa with a varying proportion of normal and pathological forms and a varying proportion of normal and pathological forms and a varying percentage of progressive motility. The angle of the anasto-mosis next to the testicle is of prime importance, since if one meander of the ca-naliculus is severed or ligated by the suturing needle the patient will remain in-fertile. A splint is disadvantageous since it only bridges the less vulnerable vas and not the epididymal canaliculus: it impairs sperm flow, increases the risk of extrava-sation of spermatozoa, favors sperm granuloma, and infection. Following bilateral epididymovasostomy, patency was remarkably higher as compared to unilateral anastomoses. Results obtained by Hanley (1955), Bayle (1960) and Schoysman (1976) are based upon favorable conditions of inflammatory vasal occlusion and epididymovasostomy performed on both sides. In our unselected series of 326 epididymovasostomies, inflammatory obstruction with its better prognosis was found in only 52% of cases.

Amelar and Dubin (1975) reported on 22 cases with azoospermia due to epididymal obstruction: In 15, the cause was inflammation and, in seven, it was congenital. Of the 15 cases with inflammatory obstruction, patency was achieved in eight, but only four (25%) showed good quality semen. Surgery failed in all seven cases with a congenital defect. Hanley (1955) reported only one pregnancy following 83 epididymovasostomies for congenital obstruction. In a report of substantial ex-perience, Schoysman (1976) divided his epididymovasostomies into two series: "In a first group of patients of 72 operations with a follow-up of 5 years there were 38 patencies and 10 pregnancies. A second group of 148 operations with 4 years follow-up gave 43% of patencies and 17 pregnancies."

Reports on this kind of surgery are hard to compare for the following reasons: (1) no adequate and precise records on how and exactly where the anastomosis was performed; (2) many technical variations within small series; (3) wide variety of lesions within the group of epididymal blocks; (4) more technical modifications de-scribed than hard data given. The extent of the surgeon's experience, the impor-tance of microdissection and microsutures, better lighting and magnification, and the variation in needles and suture material can hardly be judged with relation to such results.

Vasectomy reversal is now feasible in almost every case. However, each patient undergoing vasectomy must be informed that pregnancy after vasovasostomy only follows patency in about 50% of cases. It is well-recognized that the longer the in-terval between vasectomy and reversal the poorer the results (Amelar and Dubin 1975; Schmidt 1978; Silber 1979 b). As pointed out by Silber (1978), 91% of patients in whom reversal was done within 10 years after vasectomy developed normal sperm counts, while only 35% achieved this when the reversal was performed more than 10 years after vasectomy. In our 56 patients, vasovasostomy was done 2–6 years after vasectomy.

Evaluation of the sperm granuloma seems to be controversial: on the one hand, the release of epididymal pressure appears to be positive (Silber 1978) and, on the other hand, the formation of sperm autoantibodies seems to be directly related to the amount of extravasation of sperm protein and to the size of the sperm granu-loma (White et al. 1975; Amelar et al. 1977). It has been experimentally demon-strated that sperm granulomata are responsible for a higher rate of stenoses at the site of the vas anastomosis or at the outlet of a splint (Belker 1979; Silber 1979 b). Silber (1978 b) argues that sperm granuloma following vasectomy should be considered as a favorable condition for vasovasostomy because it prevents pressure upon epididymo-vasal structures. This concept, although supported by correlated intraoperative findings and postoperative spermiograms, would deny any importance of autoantibody formation due to extravasation of sperm protein. It is hard to imagine that a short-term leak of spermatozoa might significantly reduce epididymal back-pressure over the years. One could argue, with respect to technical details of vasovasostomy, that a double-layer procedure with the objective of achieving a leak-proof anastomosis (in order to prevent sperm granuloma and autoantibody formation) no longer has any basis. Any reanastomosis, if not immediately patent (edema, more suture material, and knots incorporated within the tiny vas), would further impose detrimental pressure. Because of the above, and comparison of the results of Silber's double-layered anastomosis with a full-thickness procedure (Table 2), we are convinced that the most important factor in vasovasostomy is an effective approximation of the lumina by nonreactive suture material. The unassisted eye is simply not sufficient for placement of six to eight sutures in a 1–3 mm lumen like the vas, keeping them separate, equally spaced, and placed at the mucosal edge. Microsurgery with magnification 4–15 is, therefore, indispensable; however, even the best technique carries the inherent risk of stricture at the site of the anastomosis. Fortunately, a failure of vasovasostomy can be corrected in a second attempt.

In conclusion, the reasons for failure of epididymovasostomy and vasovasostomy is a function of the following: improper surgical technique; scar tissue formation caused by inadequate suture material, hemorrhage, sperm granuloma, infection, and splints; possible role of immobilizing and agglutinating antibodies found in up to 60% of cases with excretory azoospermia; an adynamic canaliculus, epididymal back-pressure, and excessive phagocytosis; no viable spermatozoa on the intraoperative swab; incomplete follow-up.

Additional experimental and clinical studies are necessary to define the relationship between sperm granuloma, autoantibody formation, and infertility after vasectomy reversal and epididymovasostomy. The questions of what sperm antibodies really mean and whether the known immunological facts are the most important ones still remain.

The epididymo-vasal pressure, with respect to the duration of obstruction, has to be examined further. As we know from clinical routine and urodynamic studies, a sudden ureteral occlusion leads to loss of kidney function within a few days. In order to avoid a similar (but more prolonged) effect upon the epididymis after vasectomy, pressure regulation of some sort might be desirable. Vasodynamic recordings and flow studies might give valuable information on the possible recovery of muscle contractility. Electron-microscopic examination of epididymal structures in vasal aplasia and at various intervals after vasectomy or epididymitis could result in a better understanding of pathophysiological mechanisms. By studying the effects of different surgical techniques, and by analyzing failures, we can improve results.

Until recently there was no chance for patients with vasal aplasia to have their own children. Following promising experimental studies with an alloplastic spermatocele, preliminary results in men show that a cup-shaped silicone-Dacron prosthesis may serve successfully as a temporary sperm reservoir. Up to 160 million spermatozoa were obtained by single percutaneous aspirations of this prosthesis. The longest time this graft has remained open to date is 7 months. Following implantation of 30 prostheses in 16 men the average duration of possible sperm aspiration was 2 months. The spermatozoa showed better morphology and motility the earlier they were obtained after surgery and the further caudal the prosthesis was implanted upon the epididymis. The short passage of spermatozoa through the remaining epididymal canaliculus may account for the reduced maturation and longevity of aspirated spermatozoa. The epididymal tubules are dilated and adynamic, thus, reducing the flow into the prosthesis. Timing the procedure aroung the sponse's time of ovulation seems to be of prime importance. We feel that intrauterine insemination, rather than injection of the aspirated material into a portio-cap (as done in this center) may increase chances for success. Schoysman (1980) induced one pregnancy following intrauterine insemination of the aspirated material from the described prosthesis. A. Kelâmi and H. Sommerkamp (1980, personal communication) reported two births following aspiration from a similar prosthesis implanted in two men with vas aplasia. The alloplastic spermatocele offers s last chance for cases with vas aplasia considered to be hopeless. Further indications are long stenoses of the vas and neurogenic impairment of ejaculation and erection in paraplegic patients.

16.4 References

Altenähr E, Paulsen M, Hasselbeck T (1979) Pathologie und pathologische Anatomie entzündlicher Erkrankungen der männlichen Adnexe. Verhandlungsbericht der Deutschen Gesellschaft für Urologie. Springer, Berlin Heidelberg New York, S 6–9

Amelar RD, Dubin L (1975) Commentary on epididymal vasostomy, vasovasostomy and testicular biopsy. In: Boedecker (ed) Current operative urology. Harper & Row, New York, pp 1181–1185

Amelar RD, Dubin L (1978) Neue Gesichtspunkte zur Ätiologie der männlichen Infertilität. Extr Urol 1:189–198

Amelar RD, Dubin L, Hotchkiss RS (1971) Restoration of fertility following unilateral orchiectomy and radiation therapy for testicular tumors. J Urol 106:714–717

Amelar RD, Dubin L, Walsh PC (1977) Male infertility. Saunders, Philadelphia

Ansbacher R (1973) Vasectomy: sperm antibodies. Fertil Steril 24:788–792

Barker JF (1941) Anastomosis of the vas deferens. W Va Med J 37:222–225

Bayle H (1960) Stérilité masculine: résultats opératoires du traitement des azoospermies excrétoires. Presse Med 68:760–765

Belker AM (1979) Urologic microsurgery: current perspectives. I. Vasovasotomy. Urology 14:325–327

Boreau J (1974) Images of the seminal tracts. Karger, Basel

Derrick FC, Yarbrough W, D'Agostino J (1973) Vasovasotomy: results of questionnaire of members of AUA. J Urol 110:556–557

Dorsey JW (1973) Surgical correction of post-vasectomy sterility. J Urol 110:554–555

Dubin L, Amelar RD (1971) Etiologic factors in 1294 consecutive cases of male infertility. Fertil Steril 22:469–472

Elsässer E (1974) Mögliche Störungen der männlichen Fertilität nach gelungener Rekanalisation der Samenwege. Ergebnisse von Tierversuchen. Proc Symp Exp Urol, S 40–41

Fernandes M, Shah KN, Draper JW (1968) Vasovasotomy: Improved microsurgical technique. J Urol 100:763–766

Hanley HG (1955) The surgery of male subfertility. Ann R Coll Surg Engl 17:159–163

Hanley HG, Hodges RD (1959) The epididymis in male sterility: A preliminary report of microdissection studies. J Urol 82:508–512

Holstein AF (1969) Morphologische Studien am Nebenhoden des Menschen. Thieme, Stuttgart

Kedia KR, Markland C, Fraley EE (1975) Sexual function following high retroperitoneal lymphadenectomy. J Urol 114:237–239

Kelâmi A, Roloff D, Prey K, Affeldt K, Seppelt G (1976) Alloplastic reservoir on epididymis: An experimental study on mini-pigs and beagle dogs. Proc Int Cong Andrology, CIDA, ECO, Barcelona, pp 162–163

Klosterhalfen H (1976) Die Sterilisation des Mannes. Muench Med Wochenschr 118:907–910

Klosterhalfen H, Wagenknecht LV (1972) Traitement chirurgical de l'infertilité de l'homme – analyse de 442 cas. Proc 66. Cong Franc Urol, Paris, pp 63–65

Klosterhalfen H, Wagenknecht LV (1977) Refertilisation nach Sterilisation beim Mann. Dtsch Aerztbl 74:1531–1534

Lee HY (1976) Clinical experiences of vasovasotomy in Korea. Proc Internat Cong Andrology, CIDA, ECO, Barcelona, pp 86–87

Lee HY (1981) Evaluation of vasovasotomy: Macroscopic vs microscopic anastomosis. J Kor Med Ass 24:243–249

Ludvik W (1977) Die artificielle Spermatocele. Acta Urol 8:193–195

Montie JE, Stewart BH (1974) Vasovasotomy: past, present and future. J Urol 112:111–113

O'Connor VJ (1948) Anastomosis of the vas deferens after purposeful division for sterility. J Urol 59:229–230

Phadke GM, Phadke AG (1967) Experiences in the reanastomosis of the vas deferens. J Urol 97:888–890

Sachse H (1965) Morphologie und Funktion des Samenwegsverschlusses. Med Klin 60:1925–1927

Sachse H (1966) Klinik des insuffizienten Samenwegsverschlusses. Med Klin 61:537–540

Schirren C (1982) Praktische Andrologie, 2. ed. Karger, Basel New York

Schmidt SS (1966) Techniques and complications of elective vasectomy: The role of spermatic granuloma in spontaneous recanalisation. Fertil Steril 17:467–469

Schmidt SS (1973) Prevention of failure in vasectomy. J Urol 109:296–297

Schmidt SS (1975) Vas anastomosis: a return to simplicity. Br J Urol 47:309–314

Schmidt SS (1978) Vasovasotomy. Urol Clin North Am 5:585–592

Scholtmeijer RJ, von Leenwaarden B (1977) Vasovasotomy: a modified technique. Eur Urol 3:124–127

Schoysman R (1968) La création d'une spermatocèle artificielle dans les agénésies du canal déférent. Bull Soc Belge Gynec Obstet 38:307–312

Schoysman R (1976) Exploration and treatment of obstructions and infections in the seminal duct and accessory genital glands – surgical procedures. Proc Internat Cong Andrology, CIDA, ECO, Barcelona, pp 62–64

Schoysman R, Drouart JM (1972) Progrès recent dans la chirurgie de la stérilité masculine et féminine. Acta Chir Belg 71:261–280

Silber SJ (1977) Perfect anatomical reconstruction of vas deferens with a new microscopic surgical technique. Fertil Steril 28:72–76

Silber SJ (1978 a) Vasectomy and its microsurgical reversal. Urol Clin North Am 5:573–579

Silber SJ (1978 b) Vasectomy and vasectomy reversal. Fertil Steril 2:125–140

Silber SJ (1979 a) Microsurgery. Williams & Wilkins, Baltimore

Silber SJ (1979 b) Epididymal extravasation following vasectomy as a cause for failure of vasectomy reversal. Fertil Steril 31:309–312

Steinhauser K, Wurster U (1975) Die Nebenhodentuberkulose im Wandel der Zeit. Urologe A 14:6–9

Vickers MA (1975) Creation and use of a scrotal sperm bank in aplesia of the vas deferens. J Urol 114:242–245

Wagenknecht LV, Holstein AF, Schirren C (1975) Tierexperimentelle Untersuchungen zur Bildung einer künstlichen Spermatocele. Andrologie 7:273–286

Wagenknecht LV, Weitze KF, Hoppe LP, Krause D, Holstein AF, Schirren C (1976) Alloplastic spermatocele for treatment of male infertility. Proc Internat Cong Andrology, CIDA, ECO, Barcelona, pp 160–162

Wagenknecht LV, Weitze, KF, Hoppe LP, Krause D, Schirren C, Peter KH, Rüsch R (1977) Further experiences with an alloplastic spermatocele: Experiments in bulls. Andrology 9:179–181

Wagenknecht LV, Leidenberger FA, Schütte B, Becker H, Schirren C (1978) Clinical experi-
ence with an alloplastic spermatocele. Andrologie 10:417–426
Wagenknecht LV, Klosterhalfen H, Schirren C (1980) Microsurgery in andrologic urology. I.
Refertilisation. J Microsurg 1:370–376
Wagenknecht LV, Becker H, Langendorff HM, Schäfer H (to be published a) Vasography:
clinical and experimental investigations. Andrologie
Wagenknecht LV, Lotzin CF, Holstein AF, Schirren C (to be published b) Vas deferens
aplasia: clinical and anatomical factures of 70 cases. Andrologie
White AG, Watson GS, Darg C, Edmond P (1975) Lymphocytotoxins in vasectomized men. J
Urol 114:240–2411

17 Hydrocele, Spermatocele, and Peyronie's Disease

A. Kelâmi

17.1 Hydrocele

17.1.1 Definition and Etiology

A hydrocele is produced by transudation or exudation of fluid between the testicular membranes. This condition is usually unilateral and can be seen at any age. Hydrocele fluid can be colorless, clear yellowish, cloudy, or pinkish red. The extension of the hydrocele depends upon the condition of the tunica vaginalis: (1) if the obliteration of the processus vaginalis is delayed or does not take place, then herniation of the intestinal segments into the scrotum and a hydrocele may occur; (2) if the obliteration is complete and there is accumulation of fluid around the testis, then a simple hydrocele exists; (3) if the obliteration occurs above the testis and below the peritoneal cavity, then the hydrocele is localized on the cord.

A hydrocele can be primary or secondary and its nature depends upon the condition of the scrotal contents. When no pathological conditions are present it is classified as a primary hydrocele and is the result of transudation in which the production of fluid outstrips its absorption. The reason for this is not known. When pathological conditions are present it is classified as a secondary hydrocele and is produced by an exudate due to epididymitis, orchitis, trauma, torsion, and most important of all, testicular tumors.

Due to elevation of scrotal temperature, if left untreated hydroceles can lead to oligozoospermia or other disorders of spermatogenesis and, thus, to infertility (Schirren 1972; Ludvik 1976). More than 15 ml hydrocele fluid, may lead to reduction of testicular blood circulation and, thus, to atrophy of the testis or to a disturbance of the thermoregulatory function of the scrotal skin (Schirren 1972).

17.1.2 Symptoms

Symptoms vary according to the size of the hydrocele. Small hydroceles are asymptomatic whereas larger ones may cause a feeling of heaviness or a painless increase in the size of the scrotum with expansion of the scrotal skin (Fig. 1). Large hydroceles may cause discomfort while walking. Some patients have the impression that one testis is larger when in reality this apparent "enlargement" is due to a hydrocele.

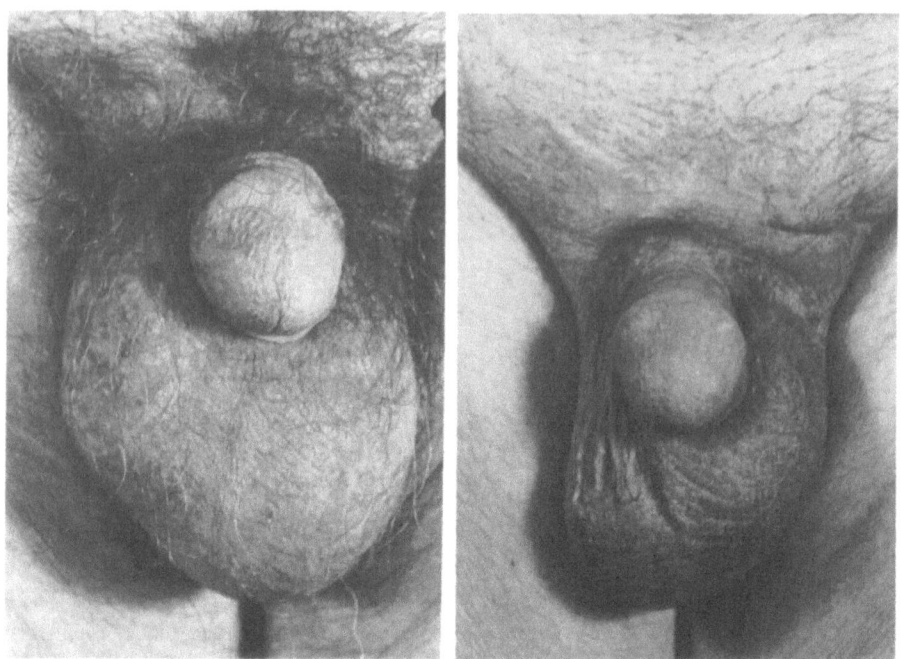

a   b

Fig. 1. a Hydrocele on the left side: Preoperative appearance. **b** Appearance 2 weeks after surgery. Operation was performed through a left-sided "infrapubic" incision. Left scrotum clearly smaller in size. Scrotal skin, no longer under tension, shows almost normal appearance

17.1.3 Diagnosis

The diagnosis is made by palpation and exploration. By putting the third and fourth finger below and the index finger and the thumb above the scrotum, the scrotal mass is palpated bimanually. It is also important to palpate the cord and the inguinal region: the feeling can either be cystic or solid. Often the testis or other scrotal contents cannot be felt if a hydrocele is present. Transillumination in a dark room may also indicate fluid collection. Although aspiration of this fluid allows better palpation, it is not a curative procedure. New techniques, like ultrasonography, may help detect pathological conditions of the scrotal contents (Miskin and Bain 1978; Sample 1979), but the best diagnostic and curative approach is still the exploration of the scrotal contents. Through this approach the appropriate treatment of the hydrocele, as well as other possible pathological disorders, can be performed in one session.

17.1.4 Hydrocele and Testicular Tumors

Of testicular tumors, 25% are accompanied by a hydrocele. Since the presence of a hydrocele makes an exact palpation of the testis difficult, it is recommended that every patient with a hydrocele be explored, so that a testicular tumor will not be overlooked.

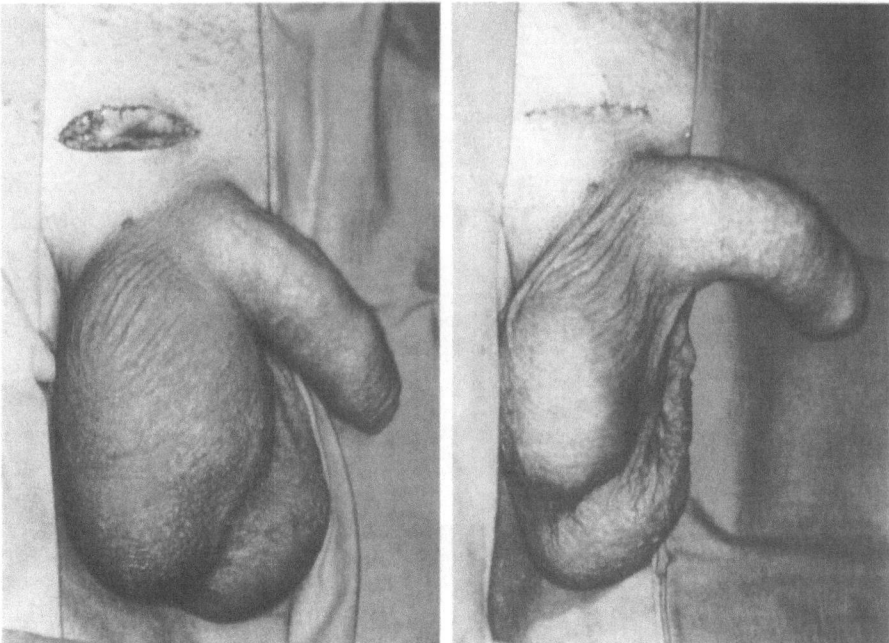

a   b

Fig. 2. a Right-sided hydrocele and "infrapubic" approach: Preoperative appearance. **b** Appearance right after surgery. "Infrapubic" incision is sutured subcuticularly, right scrotum clearly smaller than before surgery

17.1.5 Treatment

The method of choice in the treatment of hydrocele is to excise the distended tunica vaginalis and to suture its margin in a continuous, locked manner to insure hemostasis (von Bergmann, cited by Bramann 1885). As suture material, 3×0 absorbable synthetic is used. The infrapubic approach (Kelâmi 1978a, b, c). (Figs. 1b, 2a, b), especially in bilateral cases, is preferred to scrotal (Stewart 1979) or scrotoinguinal (Major and Zingg 1973) incisions. No drainage is done. A pressure dressing for 24 h serves both the hemostasis and the prevention of edema. In cases of large hydroceles the fluid should be evacuated before eventeration of the scrotal contents through the same incision. In secondary hydroceles, the primary disease must be treated appropriately as well. The operation leads to pressure relief and, thus, to improved spermatological findings (Schirren 1972).

17.2 Spermatocele

17.2.1 Definition and Etiology

Partial obstruction of the vasa efferentia (due to inflammation) on the caput epididymidis leading to a cystic dilation (Fig. 3a) and containing spermatozoa is

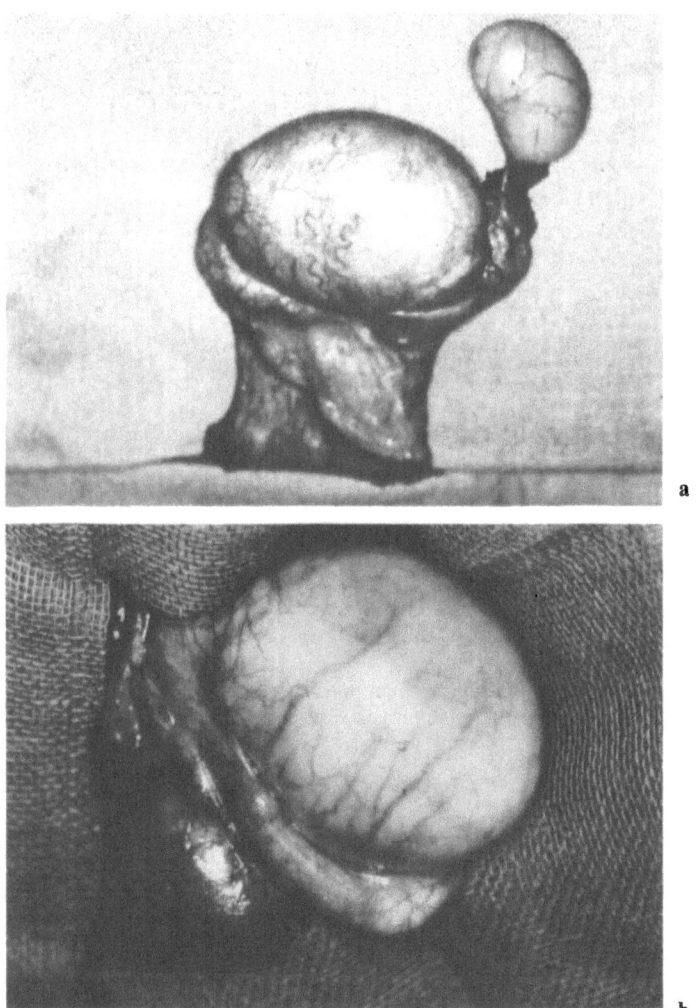

Fig. 3. **a** Spermatocele of caput epididymidis. **b** Cystic tumor of corpus epididymidis

called spermatocele (Whitaker 1976). Spermatoceles, which occur after puberty in 1%–7% of healthy men, contain fluid varying from colorless to yellowish or milky to creamy. Although they are usually multilocular, they may be unilocular. Large spermatoceles may implair epididymal sperm transport and sperm maturation.

17.2.2 Symptoms

Spermatoceles can vary in size, but are smaller than hydroceles. Small spermatoceles are not usually apparent on inspection, but may be felt by the patient himself or by his partner. Occasionally large spermatoceles are called "the second testis." Rarely do they grow larger than a testis and even then do not cause pain, only a feeling of heaviness.

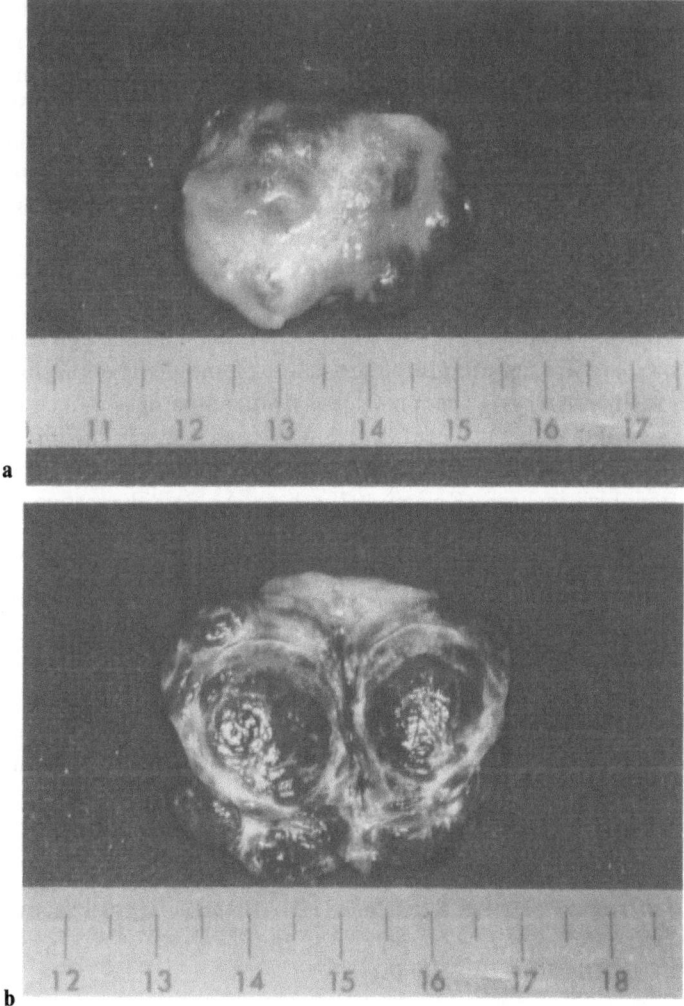

Fig. 4. a Adenomatoid tumor of epididymis. **b** The same adenomatoid tumor, opened

17.2.3 Diagnosis

Diagnosis is made by palpation and transillumination, but in comparison to hydroceles, spermatoceles can usually be felt separately from the testis. Ultrasound as a new noninvasive technique can also be helpful in the diagnosis (Miskin and Bain 1978; Sample 1979).

17.2.4 Spermatocele and Epididymal Tumors

All other enlargements of the epididymis are considered to be epididymal tumors. There are two different types: (1) cystic tumors, which are solitary or multilocular cysts containing water-clear or yellowish translucent fluid without spermatozoa

(Fig. 3b); (2) noncystic tumors, which can be benign [53% of all epididymal tumors are "adenomatoid" tumors (Fig. 4), 10% leiomyomas] or malignant (17% sarcomas, 10% carcinomas). The noncystic tumors are shown by Elsässer (1977) as 25% adenomatoid, 25% rhabdomyosarcoma, 25% leiomyoma, and 25% metastatic tumors.

Epididymal tumors are accompanied by a hydrocele in 25% of the cases. Benign tumors show less occurrence of hydrocele than malignant tumors (Elsässer 1977). Diagnosis can be made either by palpation (in 80%), by ultrasound, or by exploration. The latter combines diagnoses and treatment in one session.

17.2.5 Treatment

To avoid overlooking epididymal tumors, all enlargements of the epididymis (cystic or solid) are indications for surgical exploration. There is no "nonsurgical" way of exactly diagnosing spermatoceles or differentiating between cystic or noncystic benign and malignant epididymal tumors or chronic inflammation. Spermatoceles, cystic, and noncystic benign tumors should be locally excised through an "infrapubic" incision (Kelâmi 1978a, b, c). An epididymectomy is not necessary. Aspiration of the cyst fluid, the collection of which recurs, is only a palliative procedure and should not replace surgery. A recent study shows that 50% of the patients after an operation for spermatocele have reduced fertility, compared with preoperative semen analyses (Chiari and Drujan 1980). The authors suggest not to treat spermatoceles surgically in subfertile patients once a solid tumor is ruled out.

Malignant tumors are best treated with high epididymo-orchidectomy. Through an "infrapubic" incision the cord is cut into two portions at the level of the external inguinal ring and suture-ligated with absorbable synthetic suture no. 1. No drainage is done.

17.3 Peyronie's Disease (Induratio Penis Plastica)

17.3.1 Definition and Etiology

Peyronie's disease was first described in 1743 by François de la Peyronie (Murphy 1972). It is a fibrotic change of the tunica albuginea of the corpus cavernosum penis due to an inflammation. The cause of this condition is yet unknown. It is suggested that repeated minor trauma, especially in patients with a tendency to abnormal production of fibrotic tissue, can lead to this disorder (Hinman 1980). This change leads to hyalinization of the elastic connective tissue and the area becomes a fibrous scar. It can be associated with other collagenoses and occurs primarily between the ages of 30 and 70 years. The erectile tissue is not involved. The plaques are mostly localized on the dorsum penis (77%) (47% are on the coronal area, 36% on the midshaft, and 17% on the penile root). The plaques can be solitary or multiple (6%) (Burford 1951). Of the patients with Peyronie's disease, 10% have Dupuytren's contracture and 3% of the patients with Dupuytren's contracture have Peyronie's disease (Devine 1979). There is no evidence that the disease has a familial tendency (Byström and Rubino 1976). Without treatment the disease can either disappear, remain silent, or progress.

17.3.2 Symptoms

In the beginning a plaque is palpable without pain, curvature, or signs of erectile failure. As the disease progresses erections become painful and the patient avoids having them. The curvature of the erect penis is due to unequal distension of the corpus cavernosum penis. The site of the plaque cannot distend, remains short and causes the penis to bend. In this condition, penetration into the vagina is extremely difficult and sometimes even impossible. Although primary erectile failure does not usually exist, these patients may develop psychogenic impotence secondary to their organic disease.

17.3.3 Diagnosis

The presence of the plaques can easily be diagnosed by palpation. Before starting any treatment, an X-ray of the penis is necessary to rule out possible calcification. In cases of curvature the patients are asked to bring self-made photographs of the erect, bent penis to demonstrate the clinical appearance.

17.3.4 Nonsurgical Treatment

Nonsurgical treatment should be used only in patients without plaque – calcification, massive curvature, or painful erection. In these cases it is best to simply observe for at least 1 year. The least invasive and best tolerable medicine can also be given as an adjuvant therapy (100 mg vitamin E three times daily), (Devine 1979). All other advocated procedures, such as potassium-para-aminobenzoate, steroid infiltrations into the plaques, radiotherapy, and ultrasonic vibrations, should be avoided as results are not satisfactory. The patients are assured that this is not a cancerous disease, and are assessed every 3 months to check the condition of the plaques which may remain clinically silent. These patients are not candidates for surgery. For all other cases, surgery is the best treatment today.

17.3.5 Surgical Treatment

In the past 8 years two, different ways of surgical treatment have been advocated: (1) excision of the plaques and replacement of the tunica albuginea with dermal graft or lyophilized human dura; (2) implantation of penile prostheses.

17.3.5.1 Excision of the Plaques

The excision of the plaques and the replacement of the tunica albuginea with dermal graft was introduced by Devine and Horton (1974). They report 70% success rate in 50 patients 1.5 years after surgery.

It is my practice to excise the plaques and replace the tunica albuginea with lyophilized human dura in patients under 50 years of age (general status should be decisive) (Kelami 1975, 1977a,b, 1978a,b,c). Young patients should be given a chance to manage the Peyronie's disease in the first instance without a prosthesis, since it would be a life-long implant. Lyophilized sterile human dura is an allo-

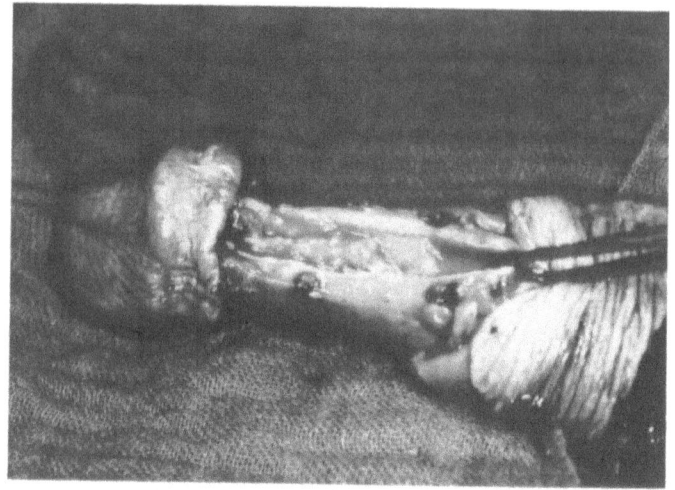

a

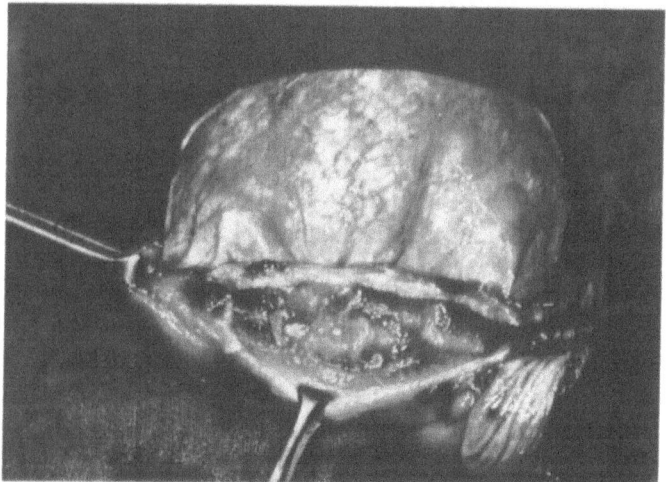

b

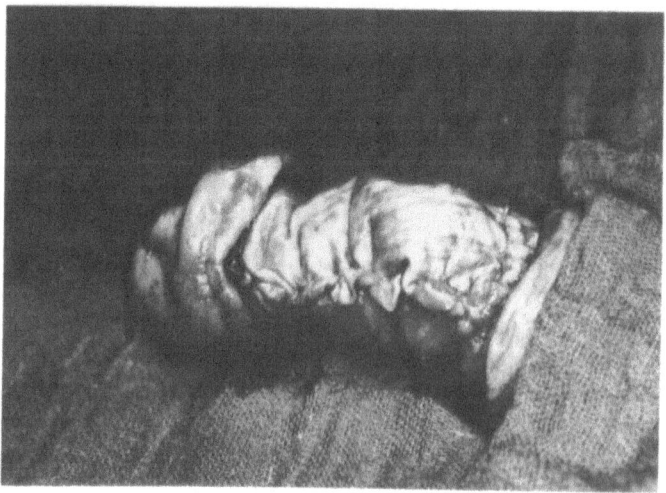

c

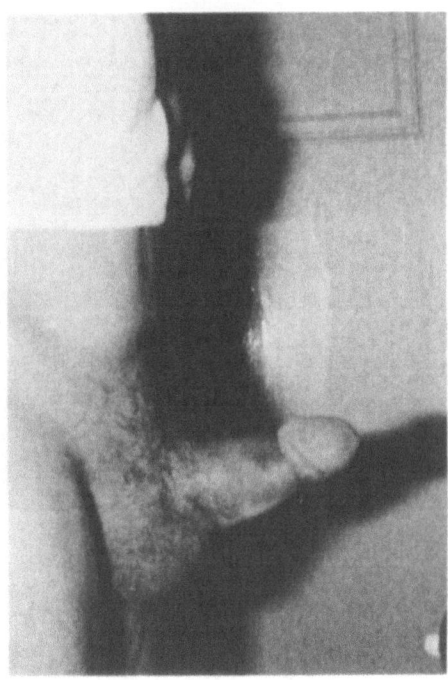

Fig. 6. The same patient 2 months after surgery, penis in erect position. The photograph was taken by the patient himself

plastic material with known advantages over autoplastic materials. By using dura, removal of an autoplastic material from the same organism is avoided. Dura is absorbed after 6–12 weeks and the inner surface entirely epithelized. After a circular incision, the penile skin is retracted, the dorsal nerve and vascular bundle dissected, and the plaques entirely excised. A corresponding piece of the lyophilized human dura with an extra 0.5-cm margin is sutured onto the defect with 2×0 absorbable synthetic suture material (Fig. 5). Erections during the first few weeks are weak, but become firm after 2–3 months (Fig. 6). In 5 years, nine patients have been operated on with completely satisfactory results. Five patients after duraplasty with good results up to 1.5 years have also been reported (Stadie 1979).

17.3.5.2 Implantation of Penile Prosthesis

Some authors have combined the implantation of penile prostheses with various modifications of "plaque-surgery." This has included incision of the plaques (Raz et al. 1977), excision without grafting (Subrini 1979), and excision of the plaques with subsequent covering of the defect with dermis (Furlow 1979, personal communication). Since 1975, it has been my practice to implant penile prostheses *without incision or excision* of the plaques in elderly patients (over the age of approximately 50

Fig. 5. a Excision of the Peyronie plaque. After a circumcision the penile skin is drawn back and the plaque entirely excised. **b** The defect is covered partly with lyophilized human dura. **c** Operation terminated. Appearance before closing the penile skin

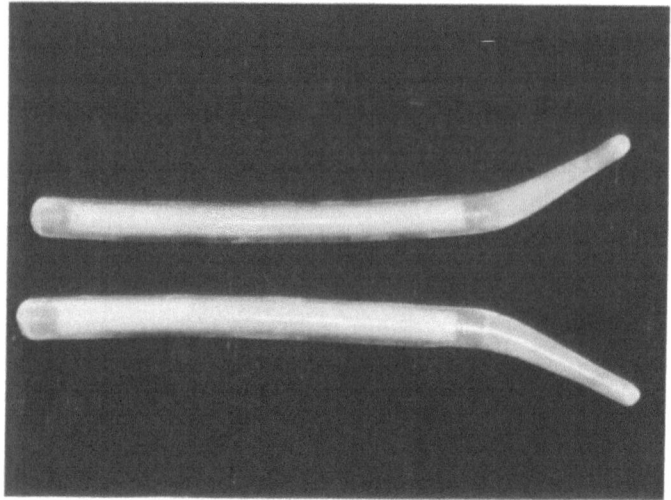

a

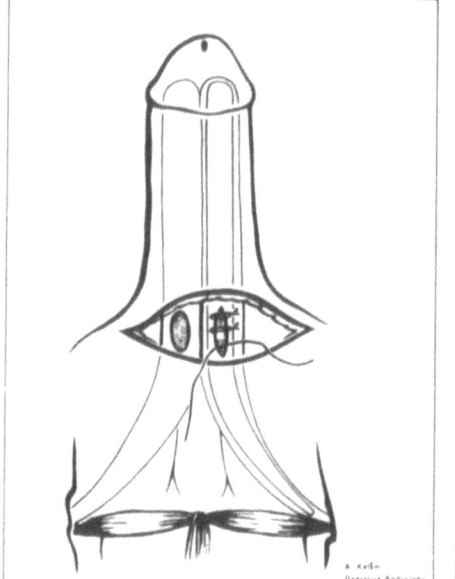

b

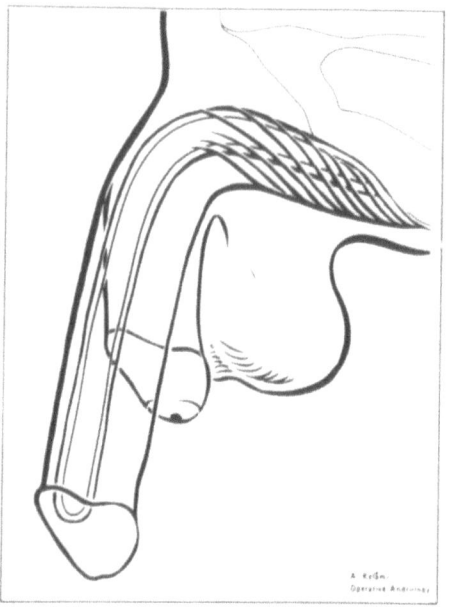

c

Fig. 7. **a** Small-Carrion penile prostheses. **b** Through an infrapubic incision, the tunica albuginea is incised and the Small-Carrion prosthesis inserted (Kelâmi 1980b). **c** After the implantation, the penis hangs down in a semirigid and extended condition compared with the penis without an implant (Kelâmi 1980b)

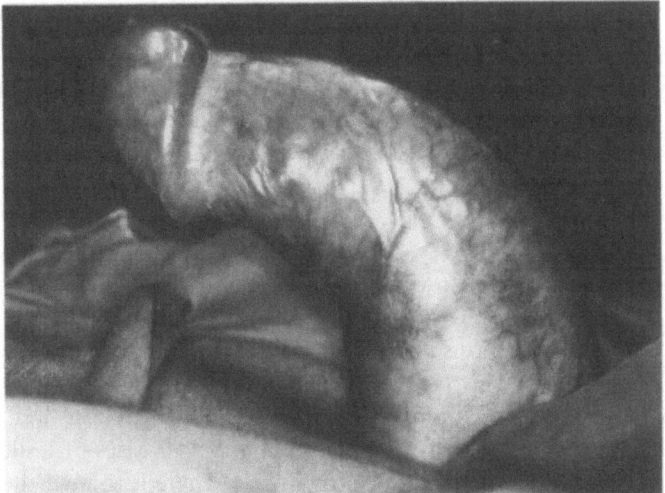

a

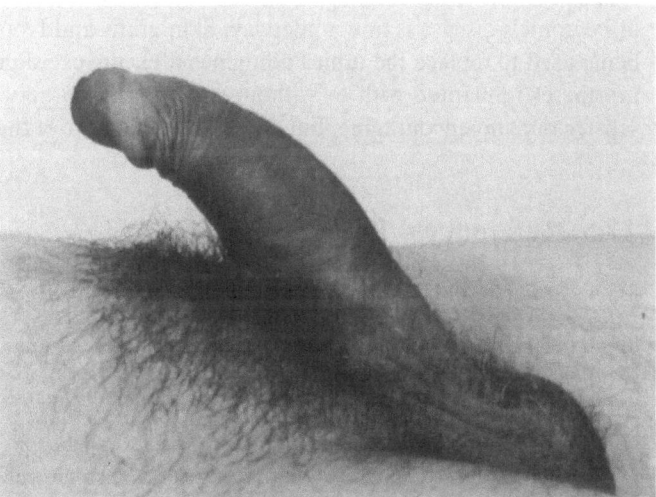

b

Fig. 8. a Patient with Peyronie's disease on the operating table after artificial erection. Notice the massive curvature. **b** The same patient 2 months after implantation of a Small-Carrion prosthesis without incising or excising the plaques. Notice the straight line of the penis compared with preoperative appearance

years) (Kelami 1977 a, b, 1978 a, b, c, 1980 a, b). It is not necessity to incise or excise the plaques if penile prosthesis (Small-Carrion) are implanted (Fig. 7). It is possible to achieve a straight penis in all cases (Fig. 8). In 3–4 months the plaques soften and, in spite of their presence, the penis straightens. All 16 patients operated upon during the last 5 years enjoy normal sexual function.

17.4 Conclusion

Although a number of diagnostic methods exist, these do not necessarily reveal the factor causing a hydrocele.

Exact diagnosis and treatment of hydroceles can only be made through surgical exploration. This procedure combines the diagnosis of the hydrocele, the possible causative factor, and the treatment of the hydrocele, as well as any other pathological disorders. This is especially important in cases of testicular tumors, as 25% of them are accompanied by a hydrocele. There is some evidence that hydroceles are associated with infertility.

Spermatoceles are also diagnosed and treated by surgical exploration. Recent investigations show that infertility may result after excision of spermatoceles.

In addition to the existing conservative treatment, large-scale surgical treatment of Peyronie's disease is now underway. Skin grafts and lyophilized human dura are being used to replace the tunica albuginea after the excision of the plaque or penile prostheses implanted with or without any "plaque surgery". The results are so far satisfactory and encouraging, but time is needed to prove their effectiveness.

17.5 References

Bramann F (1885) Die Volkmannsche Radikaloperation der Hydrozele. Berl Klin Wochenschr 14:209–211
Burford DH (1951) Therapy of Peyronie's disease. Urol Cutan Ref 55:337–341
Byström J, Rubino C (1976) Peyronie's disease. Scand J Urol 10:12–14
Chiari R, Drujan B (1980) Spermatozelenoperation und Fertilität. Urologe A 19:268–271
Devine CJ jr (1979) Peyronie's disease. In: Harrison JH, Gitters RF, Perlmutter AD, Stamey TA, Walsh PC (eds) Campbell's urology. Saunders, Philadelphia London Toronto, p 2432
Devine CJ jr, Horton CE (1974) Surgical treatment of Peyronie's disease with the dermal graft. J Urol 111:44–47
Elsässer E (1977) Epididymyal tumors. In: Grundmann E, Vahlensieck W (eds) Tumors of the male genital system. Springer, Berlin Heidelberg New York (Recent results in cancer research, vol 60, pp 163–175)
Hinman F jr (1980) Etiologic factors in Peyronie's disease. Urol Int 35:407–413
Kelâmi A, Gross U, Fiedler U, Richter-Reichhelm M, Tsaussidis N (1975) Replacement of tunica albuginea of corpus cavernosum penis using human dura. Urology 6:464–467
Kelâmi A (1977a) Surgical treatment of Peyronie's disease using human dura. Eur Urol 3:191–192
Kelâmi A (1977b) Erectile impotence: Small-Carrion prosthesis and the infrapubic approach. Eur Urol 3:299–302
Kelâmi A (1978a) Die Bedeutung der operativen Behandlung bei der erektilen Impotenz. Extr Urol 1:271–281
Kelâmi A (1978b) Operative procedures on male genitalia using a new infrapubic approach. Eur Urol 4:468–470

Kelâmi A (1978c) Infrapubic approach in operative andrology. Urology 12:580–581
Kelâmi A (1980a) Peyronie's disease and surgical treatment: A new concept. Urology 15:559–561
Kelâmi A (1980b) Atlas of operative andrology. De Gruyter, Berlin
Ludvik R (1976) Andrologie. Thieme, Stuttgart, S 130
Mayor G, Zingg E (1973) Urologische Operationen. Thieme, Stuttgart, S 451
Miskin M, Bain J (1978) Use of diagnostic ultrasound in the evaluation of testicular disorders. In: Bain J, Hafez ESE, Barwin BN (eds) Progress in reproductive biology, vol 3. Karger, Basel, pp 117–130
Murphy LJT (1972) The history of urology. Thomas, Springfield Ill., p 485
Raz S, De Kernion IB, Kaufman J (1977) Surgical treatment of Peyronie's disease: A new approach. J Urology 117:598–601
Sample FW (1979) Ultrasonography of the scrotum in ultrasonography in urology. In: Resnick MI, Sanders RC (eds) Ultrasound in urology. Williams & Wilkins, Baltimore, p 251
Schirren C (1972) Doppelseitige Hydrozele. Z Allgemeinmedizin/Landarzt 48:1053
Stadie G (1979) Die operative Behandlung der Induratio penis plastica. Z Urol 72:499–505
Stewart BH (1979) Hydrocelectomy. In: Harrison JH, Gitters RF, Perlmutter AD, Stamey TA, Walsh PC (eds) Campbell's urology. Saunders, Philadelphia London Toronto, p 2495
Subrini LM (1979) The Peyronie's disease: New physio-pathological and therapeutical concepts. Paper presented at the 18th Congress of International Society of Urology. Paris, June 1979
Whitaker RH (1976) Cysts of epididymis. In: Blandy J (ed) Urology. Blackwell, Oxford London, p 1198

IV. Cryopreservation and Insemination

18 Cryopreservation and Pooling of Spermatozoa

J. Barkay and H. Zuckerman

Donor artificial insemination (AID) was a response to the need for treatment of infertile couples in whom there was irreversible or untreatable infertility in the male. AID or heteroinsemination is now the alternative chosen by an increasing number of couples.

The need to efficiently preserve an unlimited number of spermatozoa for an unlimited period of time has led to the search for improvement of cryopreservation techniques. Cryopreservation enables the collection and storage of large numbers of ejaculates and provides an opportunity to choose the most suitable sample for immediate use from available stock. The sperm freezing procedure itself imposes a secondary selection, since only the most resistant spermatozoa survive, enhancing the availability of good quality motile spermatozoa. The future of artificial insemination on a widespread basis depends on preservation and banking of frozen semen.

18.1 History

Spallanzani (1776) was the first to report the freezing of spermatozoa. He froze specimens in snow and, upon thawing, found that motility was retained. Mantegazza (1866) proposed a sperm bank as a practical means for transportation of frozen semen to cattle. He suggested that the method might also be applied to the storage of human spermatozoa to be used to inseminate, for example, wives of soldiers killed in war. Jahnel (1938) noted that a certain number of sperm cells stored at $-79\,°C$ in glass tubes for as many as 40 days and then thawed retained motility. He also showed that survival of spermatozoa is a function of the rate of freezing. Shettles (1940) stored spermatozoa in capillary tubes at $-196\,°C$ and the survival rate in his experiments did not exceed 10%. He found no differences in motility when using thawing baths at temperatures of $20\,°C-37\,°C$. Hoagland and Pincus (1942) froze spermatozoa by different methods with and without pretreatment in plasmolyzing solutions plus liquid nitrogen and the retained motility was 20%–40%. They also noted that human spermatozoa was more resistant to freezing than spermatozoa of any other mammalian species. Survival at $-196\,°C$ was higher when larger quantities were frozen in ampules rather than in capillary tubes, and freezing appeared to have no effect on the degeneration of genes (Parkes 1945). An important advance was the introduction of glycerol for the conservation of spermatozoa (Polge et al. 1949).

Freezing of spermatozoa was neglected until Sherman (1954) reported his experiments using a protective medium containing glycerol. He was the first to try slow freezing and ampule storage in CO_2 at $-79\,°C$, obtaining 67% survival even after 3 months of storage.

The first normal deliveries after inseminations by frozen semen were reported in Japan and the USA between 1954 and 1958 (Bunge et al. 1954; Iizuka and Sawada 1958; Keettel et al. 1956). Egg yolk added to the protective medium, containing glycerol, increased the chances of fertilization (Sherman 1964).

A system which consisted of suspending ampules containing semen over the vapors of liquid nitrogen was proposed as a method of freezing (Sherman 1963): Perloff et al. (1964) used the vapor system proposed by Sherman and results showed a survival rate of 45%–100% and six conceptions. They also found that freezing caused no genetic changes. Cassou (1964) and Jondet (1964) described the use of straws which were first frozen in the vapors of nitrogen at $-80\,°C$ and then passed over to $-196\,°C$ in liquid nitrogen.

Particularly impressive was the revolutionary system presented by Nagase and Niwa (1964), which involved the rapid freezing of semen in pellet form on dry ice at $-80\,°C$. This simple method was quickly adapted throughout Europe and is still in use today, particularly for veterinary purposes.

We have developed a simple semiautomatic apparatus that freezes semen in pellets or straws and uses liquid nitrogen vapors, shortening the procedure to 5 min (Barkay et al. 1974; Barkay and Zuckerman 1978 a, b, 1979 c). This method, together with other methods of freezing, makes the use of sperm conservation and AID therapy simpler and more popular. There are approximately 40 cryobanks in operation throughout the world today and thousands of babies have been born since 1954 as a result of insemination from cryopreserved semen (Sherman 1978, 1979). The percentage of abnormal children born by AID using cryopreserved spermatozoa is far below (1%) the general population (6%), providing evidence against the adverse effects of cryopreservation (Sherman 1973).

18.2 Application of Cryobanking

Sperm freezing solves various problems related to fertility, and each problem in itself can be considered important enough to justify all efforts invested in cryobanking. Among the most humanitarian uses of sperm freezing is the collection and conservation of spermatozoa prior to radiation therapy, chemotherapy, or in cases of tumors in the reproductive system or other malignancies, where therapy may cause irreversible damage to the gonads. Sperm freezing permits the patients to retain hope for children after radiation or castration therapy, which is important from a psychological point of view.

Sperm freezing is also used when prostatectomy or vasectomy are indicated (Sherman 1978). On this point, however, opinions differ. Some believe that a man who is considering vasectomy should recognize that the procedure is basically irreversible and question the wisdom of preparing him psychologically for the possibility of future fertility; however, in such an instance, the man might be better served by being encouraged not to have a vasectomy, but to use a reversible contraceptive method.

Cryobanking is advised as a prophylactic measure for insuring male fertility in professions of high risk; for example, astronauts who are exposed to radiation, workers in atomic reactors and X-ray laboratories, men in dangerous military positions, aircraft pilots, commando unit men, etc. (Barkay and Zuckerman 1979 a). Early collection and banking of spermatozoa might be invaluable for family procreation in cases of fatal injuries. One could object to the idea of encouraging people to "bank" on their death. This may be unnecessary in a peaceful country, but in Israel we have an extra cryobank for such cases, and we are witness to the demand made by people from the above-mentioned jobs who wish to make use of this facility (Barkay and Zuckerman 1979 b).

Sperm conservation may be advised in cases of progressive damage of the reproductive system, paraplegia or progressive muscular dystrophy, myasthenia gravis, multiple sclerosis, etc., where diminution of fertilizing capacity is expected.

A sperm bank permits storage of several donors' semen bearing desired genetic characteristics for unusual blood types, thereby avoiding Rh incompatibility, for example, in cases where conception by the husband's spermatozoa would result in the formation of antibody and stillbirth (Sherman 1964; Amelar et al. 1977).

The use of cryopreservation is preferred in cases in which spermatozoa from the same donor is needed for prolonged therapy or desired for a subsequent pregnancy.

In cases where the semen is of poor quality, banking of many portions of pooled split ejaculates can be very useful, especially if, on the required date of ovulation, the fresh semen of the husband is not sufficient for insemination. By using cryopreserved, pooled split ejaculates it is possible to reverse the consequences of oligozoospermia by delivering more normal numbers of spermatozoa for inseminations (Sherman 1978).

In cases where artificial homologous insemination (AIH) has failed, it is often suggested to the couple that frozen semen from the husband be mixed with conserved donor's semen from the "bank." This is found to be more impersonal than immediate donor insemination. However, according to our experience, the method has a great psychological effect, and even the most intelligent of our patients cling to this hope (Barkay and Zuckerman 1979 a). But, it may be argued that good quality donor sperm should not be diluted with the oligzoospermic husband's semen, because this can affect the results of the insemination.

18.3 The Biological Process of Cryopreservation

The process of sperm freezing depends largely on maximal control of molecular movement. If that movement can be arrested by careful control and later reactivated without injury, the cell will retain its viability and progenative activity.

In cryopreservation, there are a number of problems that should be overcome if a viable and active cell is to survive; cell damage due to dehydration; ice formation within the cell; and electrolyte abnormalities outside the cell. To solve these major problems, methods of controlled-rate freezing and thawing and addition of cryopreservative agents have evolved.

When cooling semen from body temperature to freezing point, there is usually no damage due to temperature shock, although there is some disagreement on this point (Sherman 1977). The problem starts with rates of cooling below the freezing temperature: too fast a rate will cause formation of small intracellular ice crystals which, upon thawing, will merge to form larger crystals and disrupt the cell. If the freezing rate is too slow, cell dehydration and extracellular electrolyte concentration will cause cryoinjuries (Mazur 1970). The optimal rate of sperm freezing is $1°-25°C$ per minute.

The addition of cryoprotectants is extremely important to cryosurvival. One of the two additives most commonly used is egg yolk containing lecithin, which is supposed to give excellent protection in cases of temperature shock (Ackerman 1968). It also plays a great part in long-term storage and is believed to reduce the rate of oxygen loss after thawing (Sawada et al. 1967). The other protectant added is glycerol, whose exact mechanism of protective action is not fully understood. Although it is not clear if glycerol plays a part in water binding, ice formation, buffering, or membrane stabilization, the evidence suggests that its action involves cell wall preservation (Sherman 1977). The fact is that it helps achieve a maximal survival rate. In practice, egg yolk and sodium citrate extender with 5%–10% glycerol give the best results.

We find that, for long-term preservation, the survival of thawed spermatozoa is better using the egg yolk-sodium citrate-glycerol medium than glycerol alone. The best way to freeze the semen is to lower the temperature in two steps; first freezing at $-80°C$, and then $-196°C$. This second step does not injure the spermatozoa. When the spermatozoa have been frozen, they are maintained at $-196°C$ in liquid nitrogen. At this temperature they can be kept up to 15 years (Sherman 1979).

The final step is thawing. Quick thawing is of vital importance since it minimizes the damage to cells caused by the enlargement of ice crystals upon heating.

Freezing in pellet form, utilizing a rapid freezing rate, and the addition of 40% egg yolk (versus the commonly used 20%) causes no more harm than when utilizing the optional slow rate ($1°-24 °C/min$). The pellet's small size (0.1–0.15 ml each) also aids in maintaining survival (Barkay and Zuckerman 1978c). There is evidence suggesting that human spermatozoa are generally more resistant than other mammalian spermatozoa to injury by cryopreservation (Sawada et al. 1967).

18.4 Sperm Freezing and Insemination Techniques

18.4.1 Freezing Methods

The development of the modern sperm freezing technique is largely dependent on the work of Sherman (1963). According to his method, cooling is carried out by vapors of liquid nitrogen step by step (slow-rate freezing). Cans with ampules containing semen mixed with a protective medium (glycerol plus sodium citrate plus glucose plus antibiotics, or only 5%–10% glycerol) were suspended 20–30 cm over the vapors of a liquid nitrogen container (Fig. 1) until their temperature was gradually lowered to $-75°C$ ($16°-25 °C/min$). After reaching this temperature, the cans were submerged into a liquid nitrogen container at $-196°C$ for storage. This method

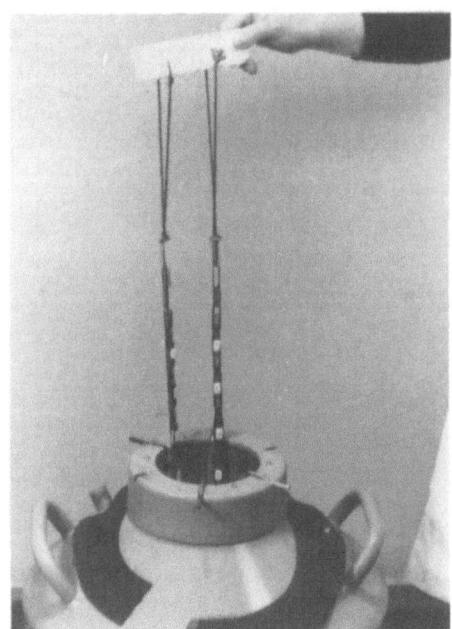

Fig. 1. The original Sherman's freezing method (1963): Cans with ampules containing semen are suspended over the vapors of liquid nitrogen

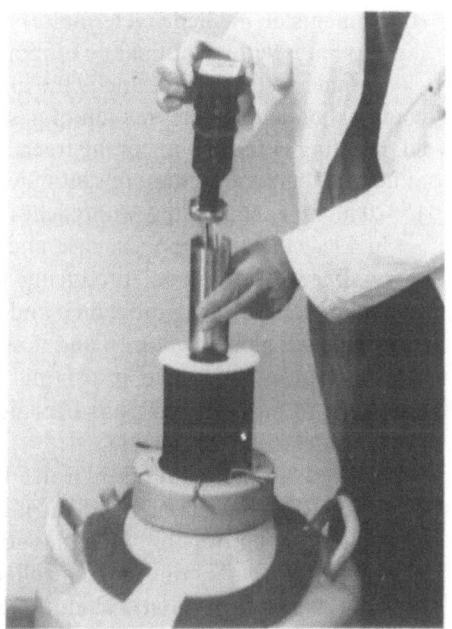

Fig. 2. Sherman's modification BF 5 biological freezer (accessory part to the duer LR 30): **a** the neck tube plug; **b** freezer core assembly; **c** receptacle for straws and ampules are placed in the container over the liquid nitrogen level

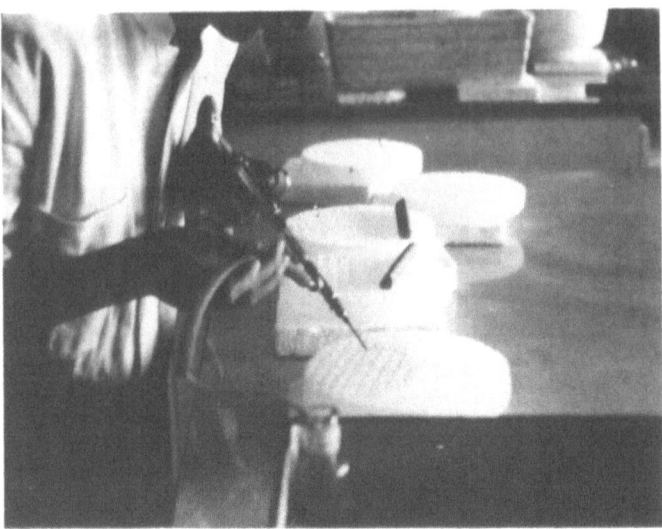

Fig. 3. Rapid rate freezing of semen in pellet form on dry ice blocks (Nagase and Niwa 1964)

is still in use, with certain modifications (Fig. 2). Some centers use an elevator system to lower the ampules or straws containing semen to the level of the liquid nitrogen, where they are able to monitor the temperature and cooling rate of the spermatozoa. Ampules have now been replaced by plastic straws.

In 1961, Union Carbide began to develop a fully automatic biological freezing system, using cold nitrogen vapors to freeze biological samples such as spermatozoa at precisely controlled rates between $0.5\,°C$ to $30\,°C$ per minute. The French I.M.V. (Instruments de medicine veterinaire) also has a similar nitrogen vapor deep freezing apparatus with an automatic programmer.

Another system of freezing is the air-cooled freezing box. Using the principle of compression and decompression of gas in a closed (sealed) system, heat is dissipated, resulting in the cooling of the freezing chamber. The ampules or straws of semen at normal temperatures are put into the cooling box for a minimum of 30 min. After 15–20 min the temperature approaches $-80\,°C$.

In 1964, the Japanese (Nagase and Niwa 1964) made a major advance in the sperm freezing technique, producing frozen semen in pellet form. They used a simple process, dripping the semen and the protective medium mixture into recesses impressed upon dry ice blocks, and thus freezing them to $-80\,°C$ within 60 s (Fig. 3). The pellets are also stored in a liquid nitrogen container at $-196\,°C$. This simple technique of rapid freezing has become popular and is used today by most of the veterinary centers in the world.

A new kind of cryofreezing device for human sperm freezing was developed in 1974 by Barkay, Zuckerman and Ricor Ltd., and was improved in 1978 (Fig. 4). The aim of this system was to utilize the advantages of both the Nagase-Niwa and the Sherman systems. Thermostat-controlled, this device uses the evaporation of liquid nitrogen as a refrigeration technique. Rapid freezing can be performed for pellet production, but it is also possible to use slow rates for freezing in straws (Fig. 5). By

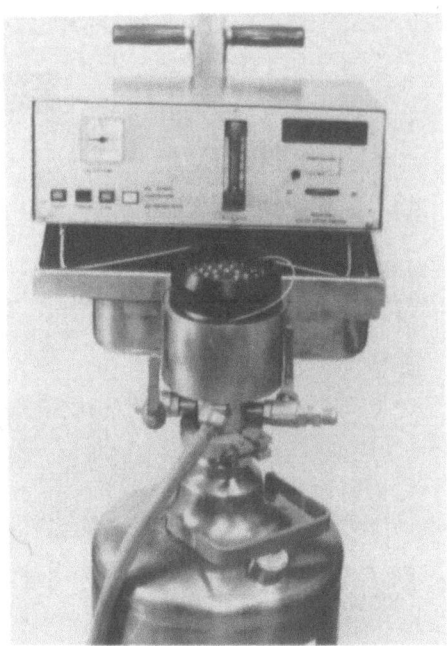

Fig. 4. The semiautomatic sperm freezing device (model CSF 16 Ricor DTD, Kibutz Ein Harod, Barkay and Zuckerman 1978 c)

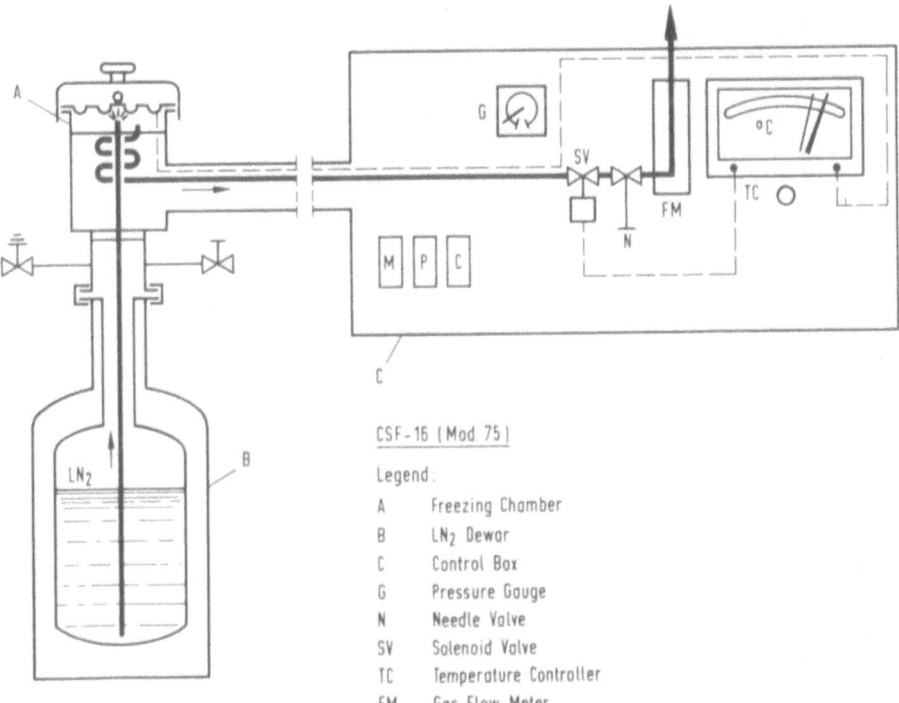

CSF-16 (Mod. 75)

Legend:

A   Freezing Chamber
B   LN$_2$ Dewar
C   Control Box
G   Pressure Gauge
N   Needle Valve
SV   Solenoid Valve
TC   Temperature Controller
FM   Gas Flow Meter

Fig. 5. The freezing chamber: **a** rests on a liquid nitrogen container; **b** controlled flow of liquid nitrogen is forced through the pipe into the freezing chamber; **c** where the freezing plate is being cooled. The control box regulates the rate of freezing and the temperature is indicated on the control panel **d**

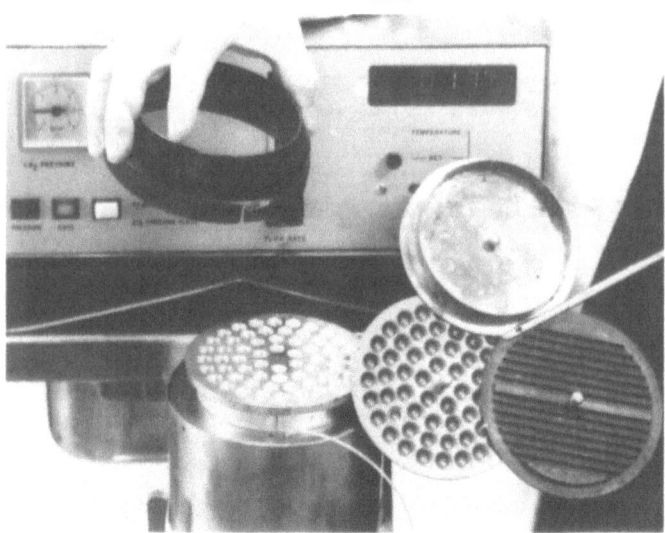

Fig. 6. Interchangeable plates for freezing in pellet form or straws and in alcohol bath (model CSF 16)

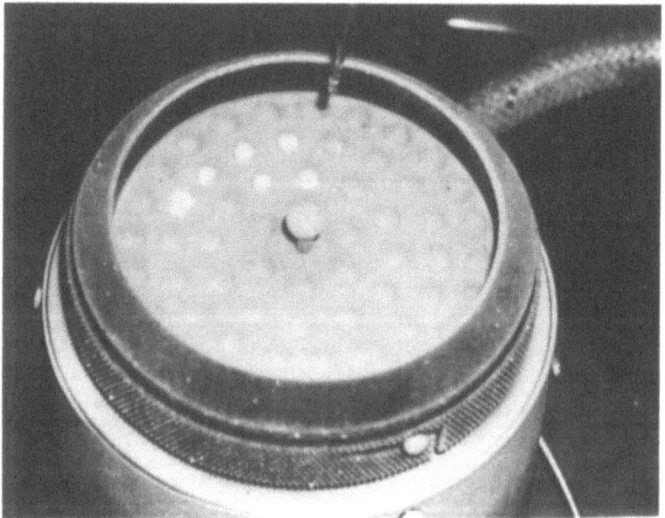

Fig. 7. Rapid freezing in pellet form by dropping mixture of semen and protective medium into the recesses of the freezing plate (model CSF 16)

freezing in pellet form, a high degree of isolation of the samples is maintained by easily interchangeable freezing plates (Fig. 6). The mixture of semen and protective medium is dropped by means of a pipette into the recesses (Fig. 7). Within 60 s, frozen pellets of volume 0.1 ml are obtained. This procedure takes 5 min from obtaining the semen sample until its storage in pellet form in liquid nitrogen containers.

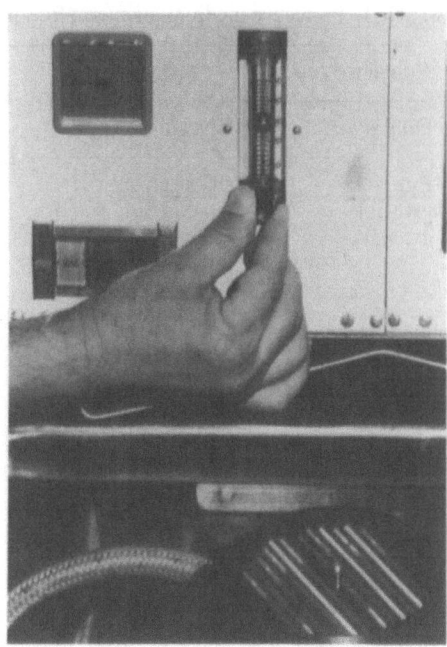

Fig. 8. Slow freezing in straws by regulation of freezing rate with a flowmeter (model CSF 16)

In cases of slow-rate freezing of spermatozoa in straws which contain 0.5 ml of the semen mixture, we use the freezing plate with slots (Fig. 8). The same procedure of freezing is used in the alcohol bath, though the straws have to be put into the "alcohol bath freezing plate".

18.4.2 Preparation for Freezing

The preparation used for freezing in most methods is based on a mixture of semen and protective medium which have been frozen together. In general, there are two kinds of protective media; the first uses glycerol only, and the other is composed of egg yolk plus glycerol extender (Table 1). The ratio between the semen and the egg yolk extender is usually 1:0.66 to 1:1 ml. In order to simplify the procedure, K. Bregulla (1975, personal communication) recommended that the protective medium be stored in plastic syringes in a regular freezing box at –20 °C. When a quantity of medium is needed, it is then thawed in a 36 °C water bath together with semen, but in separate "eprouvettes." The next step consists of mixing the protective medium drop by drop with the semen to prevent the destructive effect of the glycerol on the spermatozoa.

18.4.3 Storage of Semen

The already frozen semen specimens in pellets or straws are transferred to an eprouvette containing liquid nitrogen which lowers the temperature to –196 °C. The frozen spermatozoa are stored in a liquid nitrogen container, where they can stay for

Table 1. Protective medium for sperm freezing

Contains			Semen : medium ratio
Only glycerol	Glycerol		10 : 1
Egg yolk glycerol extender	40% egg yolk (Difco Lab)	= 4.0 ml	
	40% sodium citrate	= 4.0 ml	
			1 : 0.66 to 1 : 1.0
	5%–10% glycerol Streptomycin solution 0.4 mg in	= 0.5 ml = 0.1 ml	
Egg yolk glycerol-glucose extender	20% egg yolk	= 2.0 ml	
	20% glucose 5%	= 2.0 ml	
	40% sodium citrate	= 4.0 ml	10 : 1
	5%–10% glycerol Streptomycin solution 0.4 mg in	= 0.5 ml = 0.1 ml	

decades and still preserve their motility. For precise monitoring, each liquid nitrogen container we use for banking has a special apparatus which signals when the nitrogen level falls below the required level.

The recovery index [(post-thaw motility/pre-thaw motility)$\times 100$] is usually 50%–60%.

18.4.4 Insemination with Frozen Semen

The patient is inseminated on 4 consecutive days, starting 1 day before the estimated time of ovulation. Frozen semen is efficient for no more than 24 h, while fresh semen remains efficient for 2 or 3 days (Ackerman 1968). Five pellets or one straw is taken from storage (each pellet contains 5–7 million spermatozoa) and is put in a dry test tube submerged in a 36 °C water bath for 2 min. After thawing, 0.5 ml semen is injected intracervically. The number of inserted spermatozoa is not a determinant of fertilizing ability. It has been found that, instead of thawing five pellets of semen, the very simple method of so-called "cold insemination Bregulla" can be used, whereby only one pellet is inserted into the cervical canal and allowed to thaw naturally (Bregulla 1976). In cases of immunological complications of cervical mucus or because of a poor postcoital test, a special device is used for intrauterine insemination to help the spermatozoa pass the hostile cervical mucus (Kremer 1978).

Insemination using a cervical cap has been recommended (Jondet 1975). The semen is injected into the cap where it remains in contact with the cervical canal and cervical mucus for 10 h before it is removed. This way, the patient does not have to stay in a horizontal position for 15 min after insemination.

From 1974 to 1979, we inseminated 228 patients with frozen semen. There were 127 deliveries in 551 insemination cycles, 85% of the newborns being boys. This might be explained by the theory that the movement of the Y chromosome-bearing spermatozoa is more rapid than the one bearing the X chromosome, which survives longer. Insemination with frozen semen on several consecutive days allows for fertilization of the ovum on the day of ovulation, when the Y chromosome-bearing spermatozoa are favored (Barkay and Zuckerman 1978 b).

18.5 Enhancing Sperm Motility After Thawing

None of the known methods of semen conservation can avoid the decrease in motility of thawed spermatozoa caused by crystallization and respiratory shock during the freezing process. The recovery index of thawed frozen semen is about 50%–60%, i.e., original sperm motility may be reduced from 70% to 35%–45%. Not all the non-motile spermatozoa are destroyed during the freezing process; some are only paralyzed by respiratory shock, as demonstrated by the eosin supra vital test (Makler 1979). The resuscitation of these spermatozoa is one challenge to andrology.

The density of motile spermatozoa can be increased by filtering the semen specimen through a glass wool column before freezing, thereby separating out immobile, dead, and agglutinated spermatozoa and debris (Paulson and Polakoski 1977; Paulson et al. 1978). According to this technique, a 4–6-mm pipette is filled with 40–60 mg (20 mm) of short, glass wool fibers (Fig. 9). The glass wool should be of good quality, otherwise the fiber column can break and result in the passage of the filtered-out spermatozoa. The glass wool technique is also successful in cases of increased viscosity of the semen. After filtration there is some loss of semen volume and a significant decrease in the total count of the spermatozoa, but there is also an impressive increase in the percentage of motile spermatozoa and the quality of the progressive motility, as well as that of the living spermatozoa. This can be shown in

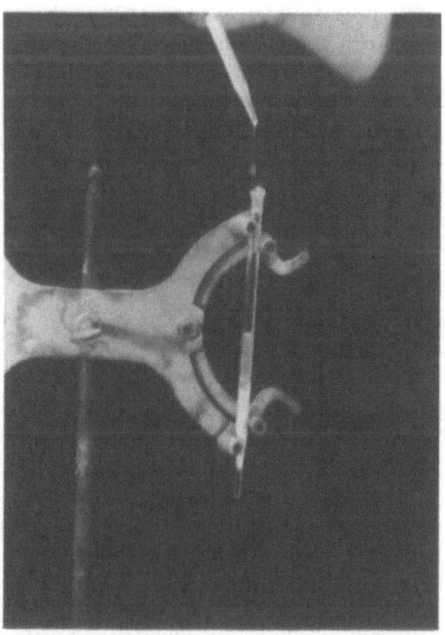

Fig. 9. Paulson glass column filtration: **a** glass wool; **b** semen

the eosin supra vital test. No immunological differences between filtered spermatozoa and spermatozoa which are retained on the fibers are observed.

The filtered semen should be centrifuged (10–15 min, 1000–1200 g) without significant alteration of motility. After resuspension, the spermatozoa are mixed with the protective medium and frozen. By this procedure, good quality thawed semen with good motility and satisfactory density is obtained (Verdaguer et al. 1978).

Ericsson has described a sperm isolation technique using bovine serum albumin (BSA) (Ericsson et al. 1973; Ericsson 1977). An attempt at sex preselection was made by separating Y chromosome-bearing spermatozoa from X chromosome-bearing spermatozoa. In this technique a Pasteur pipette is half filled with BSA of an increasingly dense solution (6% to 10% to 20%), and a layer of washed spermatozoa is added on top. Within 90 min, the fast-moving spermatozoa, which are rich in Y chromosome-bearing spermatozoa, migrate to the distal end of the Pasteur pipette where the concentration of BSA is higher. The high concentration of Y chromosome-bearing spermatozoa can be demonstrated by quinacrine staining. Debris and non-motile spermatozoa remain on the top of the BSA column. The fast moving spermatozoa at the bottom of the BSA column are pipetted, washed, centrifuged, suspended in protective medium, and preserved by freezing.

This technique has been modified. When separated, the highly motile sperm fraction is used for insemination: human serum albumin (HSA), instead of BSA should be used (Broer 1978). The frozen, thawed, and centrifuged spermatozoa should be washed with Tyrode's solution before it is added into the HSA column, which has two different concentrations forming two different layers (7.5%–17.5%); the highly motile spermatozoa migrate to the higher density fraction.

The Evans (L. M. Evans 1978, personal communication) modification involves putting a polyethylene tube with a stopper on the distal end of the pipette (Fig. 10) and opening the stopper to allow the bottom fraction to descend with clearly isolated, progressively moving spermatozoa, without mixing with dead or poor spermatozoa and debris. Evans used only one layer of HSA (10% and, if the semen was viscous, 20%).

Another modification of this technique is the use of a diluent with a composition similar to preovulation tubal fluid, instead of HSA (Lopata et al. 1976).

All these methods are still experimental and not in routine use. The reason for this is that, in severe oligozoospermia, these techniques do not add significantly to motility. There is a critical level of motility below which it is not possible to improve upon by filtration. However, there are pharmacological methods available to improve the quality of sperm motility in certain semen specimens, e.g., caffeine or pancreatic kallikrein, the latter being discussed elsewhere in this book.

Caffeine can be used to stimulate the motility of frozen spermatozoa (Barkay et al. 1977; Schill et al. 1977). The biological effects of caffeine on the motility of the spermatozoa can be explained in terms of hormonal action on the membrane of the target cell, stimulating it to combine with the specific receptor. The combination of hormone and receptor activates the enzyme adenyl cyclase in the membrane, and the portion of the adenyl cyclase that is exposed to the cytoplasm causes immediate conversion of cytoplasmic ATP to cyclic AMP. This initiates a number of cellular functions before it is itself destroyed. The cyclic AMP is destroyed and converted by phosphodiesterase to inactive 5'-AMP. This conversion process is inhibited by caf-

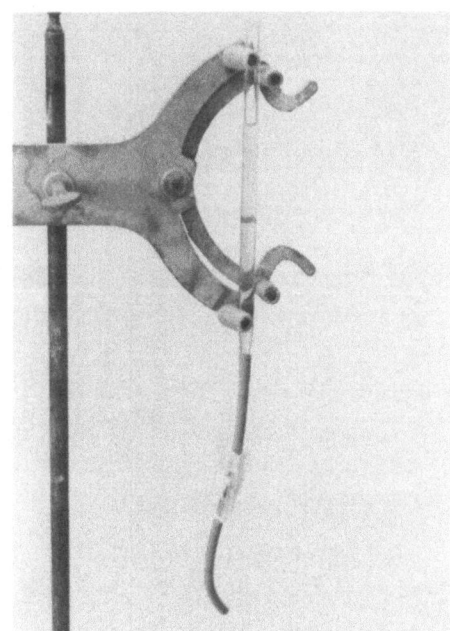

Fig. 10. The modified Ericsson sperm separation method by Evans with HSA **a** and Semen **b**. Spermatozoa of good motility penetrate to the bottom section, while the dead ones remain above the HSA

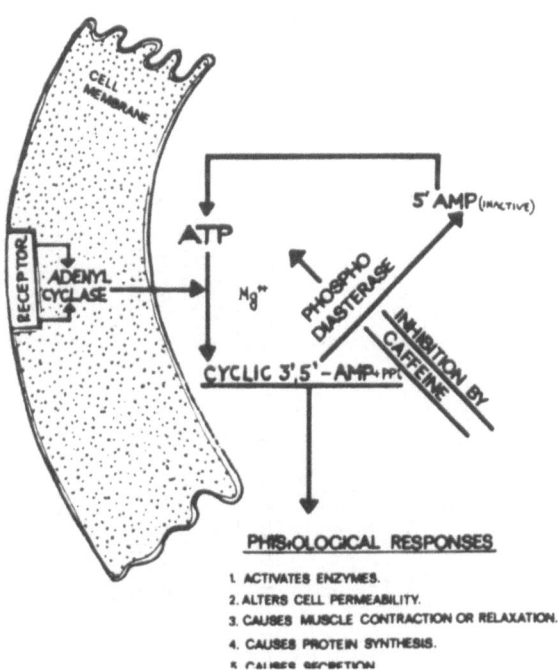

Fig. 11. Improving the motility of frozen spermatozoa by caffeine. The figure shows the role of caffeine as a phosphodiesterase inhibitor, preventing the destruction of the intracellular hormonal mediator cyclic AMP

Table 2. Insemination with frozen semen compared with frozen semen treated with caffeine (Male Fertility Institute of Central Emek Hospital, Afula)

	Type of insemination	No. of patients	Delivery		Abortion		Total pregnancies		
			No. of patients	Cycles of insemination	No. of patients	Cycles of insemination	No. of patients	Cycles of insemination	Percent pregnancies
1974–1979 without caffeine	AID	76	40	225	5	31	45	256	59.2
	AIH	17	4	32	3	24	7	56	41.1
	Total	93	44	257	8	55	52	312	55.9
1976–1979 with caffeine	AID	110	74	249	9	35	83	284	75.4
	AIH	25	9	45	2	11	11	56	44.0
	Total	135	83	294	11	46	94	340	69.6

feine, which thereby increases the endogenous cyclic AMP concentration, which in turn activates all the above physiological responses (Barkay and Zuckerman 1978 b) (Fig. 11). The works of several authors (Haesungcharern and Chulavatnatol 1973; Schill 1975, Schoenfeld et al. 1975; Homonnai et al. 1976) have shown the increase in motility of fresh spermatozoa treated with caffeine, and this has lead to attempts to improve the post-thaw motility of frozen sperm according to the technique of Barkay and Zuckerman (1979 b), where 80 mg pure caffeine is mixed with 10 ml Hartman solution, with a final concentration of 7 mmol/liter. The caffeine solution is frozen into pellet form and stored. In case of insemination, one caffeine pellet is added to five semen pellets, which are thawed together in a 36 °C water bath. The result is a significant increase in motility ranging from 40% to 50% (Makler 1980). According to our clinical experience (Table 2) from 1974 to 1979, the total number of the frozen AID- and AIH-treated patients without caffeine addition were 93, 52 of them becoming pregnant (55.9%) with 312 insemination cycles. From 1976 to 1979, 135 patients were treated by frozen AID and AIH with the addition of caffeine, with results of 94 pregnancies (69.5%) in 340 insemination cycles. According to these data, the addition of caffeine to frozen semen raised the fertilizing capacity by more than 10%. The first "caffeine babies" were born in our hospital in Afula (Barkay and Zuckerman 1978 b): Each of the 84 newborns was healthy, with no malformation or teratogenic changes. Paz et al. (1978) carried out investigations with caffeine-treated epididymal spermatozoa of rats inseminated into four generations of rats and proved that no teratogenic malformations of embryos occurred. Additionally, in work done on guinea pigs, it was shown that the fertilizing capacity of epididymal spermatozoa treated with caffeine increased without any teratogenic signs. This technique makes it possible to freeze human semen samples which are otherwise unsuitable for cryobanking.

18.6 Conclusions

18.6.1 Pooling and Storing of Semen

The pooling and storing of semen is suggested as a method of treatment in severe oligozoospermia, although there is no general agreement as to its efficacy. It is suggested that as many samples of the first fractions of split ejaculates from the oligozoospermic husband as possible be collected over a period of several months and that they should be freeze-preserved to obtain enough material for high concentration; i.e., from 1 ml oligozoospermic thawed semen with the density of 5×10^6 spermatozoa/ml, one should obtain 0.1 ml concentrated semen with 50×10^6/ml density. The same effect can be achieved if the collected samples are first concentrated and then freeze-preserved.

Successful treatments using the method of intracervical as well as intrauterine insemination have been reported (Behrman and Sawada 1966; Barwin 1974; Tyler 1973). The criticism of these techniques relates to the fact that this treatment can only be successful in those cases where the only reason for the infertility is due to a reduced number of spermatozoa. Unfortunately, in cases of oligozoospermia, other factors could also be responsible for infertility, i.e., the problem of "quality of spermatozoa" due to asthenozoospermia, a high percentage of pathologic sperm deformations, and low resistance of oligozoospermic samples to cryoinjury, all of which may make post-thawing survival unsatisfactory. These handicaps limit the therapeutic results of the pooling and storing treatment of oligozoospermic semen (Sherman 1964, 1973, 1978; Gasser et al. 1978; Keswani 1978). Despite these disadvantages, this method should be considered, especially in combination with the in vitro-improving method of caffeine or kallikrein treatment to improve motility and fertilizing capacity.

18.6.2 Suggested Freezing Methods

There are several different freezing methods, each suitable for a specific purpose. We, therefore, recommend various freezing methods for different purposes, i.e., cryobanking, scientific investigation, clinical practice, etc., taking into account local circumstances, as well as practical and economic factors.

Larger research centers carrying out investigation on biological effects of cryopreservation and in the field of reproduction would be well served by one of the large automatic freezing devices. With such devices it is possible to program the freezing procedure, and also to obtain an permanent display of temperature during freezing.

For those research institutes which freeze semen in great quantities and which prefer freezing to be carried out in straws, there are practical automatic devices available which fill and seal the straws, greatly increasing the capacity of production.

In small laboratories, or in clinical practices, the original Sherman method (Sherman 1963) with the cooling of the semen is recommended, whether in ampules or straws, over liquid nitrogen vapors. It is recommended that the Union Carbide container system Linde L 30 with BF 5 "Biological Freezer" accessory with a neck tube plug and freezer core assembly be used. Its receptacle for straws or ampules is put into the container over the liquid nitrogen level. The disadvantages of this method lie in the fact that the system does not have a temperature display, so that exact regulation of the freezing rate is not possible. In addition, filling and sealing of ampules or straws are more complicated than the simple freezing in pellet form.

The method of Nagase and Niwa (1974), which uses freezing in pellet form on dry ice, is not suitable for human sperm freezing. In the process of freezing on dry ice, the residual of the first frozen semen samples is retained in the recesses of the dry ice. This results in an inadequate isolation between the consecutive semen samples. Another disadvantage of this method is that the dry ice blocks are constantly evaporating. The supply of the dry ice must be programmed exactly on the days of freezing. For these reasons, dry ice freezing has not been accepted and has become popular almost exclusively for veterinary use.

In smaller medical centers or hospitals in suburban settings, where research is performed and the sperm bank is used for human semen insemination, the semi-automatic freezing device is practical (Barkay and Zuckerman 1978 c). With this method, rapid freezing in pellet form is very quick and simple. It takes just 5 min from the delivery of the semen to its preservation in nitrogen containers. With the aid of the interchangeable freezing plates, all the samples are completely isolated.

The freezing of straws is also possible and regulation of the temperature of the instrument makes it suitable for scientific investigation. Its low cost makes it possible for every clinical practice to obtain this system, and it is small enough to be easily stored, so that a special room is not necessary.

Different freezing techniques are available for every type of laboratory, but the success of any one system depends on the motility and survival rate of the spermatozoa and the consequent rate of fertilizing capacity of the cryopreserved spermatozoa.

18.6.3 The Future

In 1978, the American Association of Tissue Banks was established in order to standardize the efficiency of cryobanks and to exchange clinical research data. The same facility is in operation in Belgium and France, where, since 1973, CECOS (Centre d'Etude et de Conservation du Sperme) has co-ordinated cryobanking activities (David 1975). The coordination and establishment of these kinds of international corporations in cryobanking for the future was the aim of the international symposium of human artificial insemination and sperm preservation in Paris, 1979.

The increasing use of the electron microscope in the study of frozen spermatozoa (Schill and Wolff 1974) will also increase our future knowledge of cryoinjury and will help achieve improvement in sperm survival and fertilizing capacity.

The spreading of semen banks will attract governmental attention, thus, introducing licensing and the maintenance of strict standards for materials and operational methods for the protection of the public. There is a rising demand for treatment by heteroinsemination. This will hopefully contribute to the incentive for the development of institutionalized fertility centers.

18.7 References

Ackerman DR (1968) The effect of cooling and freezing on the aerobic and anaerobic lactic acid production of human semen. Fertil Steril 19:123–128

Amelar R, Dubin L, Walsh P (1977) Male infertility. Saunders, Philadelphia, pp 238–239

Barkay J, Zuckerman H (1978a) Effect of caffeine on the fresh and frozen sperm motility. In: Emperaire JC, Audebert A (eds) Proceedings of First International Symposium on artificial insemination homologous and male subfertility. Institut Aquitain de Recherches sur la Reproduction Humaine, Bordeaux, pp 236–241

Barkay J, Zuckerman H (1978b) Further-developed device for human sperm freezing by the 20 minute method. Fertil Steril 29:304–307

Barkay J, Zuckerman H (1979a) Role of cryobanking in artifician insemination. Arch Androl [Suppl 1] 2:Abs. No. 238

Barkay J, Zuckerman H (1979b) Presentation of AID treatment and development of sperm bank in Israel. In: David G, Price WS (eds) Human artificial insemination and semen presentation. Plenum Press, New York London, pp 45–50

Barkay J, Zuckerman H (1979c) Quick freezing method with caffeine stimulation of human sperm. International symposium on human artificial insemination and semen preservation (Abstr), Paris, p 50

Barkay J, Zuckerman H, Heiman M (1974) A new practical method of freezing and storing human sperm and a preliminary report on its use. Fertil Steril 25:399–406

Barkay J, Zuckerman H, Sklan D, Gordon S (1977) Effect of caffeine on increasing the motility of frozen human sperm. Fertil Steril 28:175–177

Barwin BN (1974) Intrauterine insemination of husband's semen. J Reprod Fert 36:101–106

Behrman SJ, Sawada Y (1966) Heterologous and homologous insemination with human semen frozen and stored in liquid nitrogen refrigerator. Fertil Steril 17:457–466

Bregulla K (1976) Aufarbeitung und Applikation von Kryosperma in Pelletform. Fortschritte der Fertilitätsforschung III. Grosse, Berlin, S 266–272

Broer KH (1978) Improvement of motility and morphology of human spermatozoa by filtration assay. In: Emperaire JC, Audelbert A (eds) Proceedings of First International Symposium on artificial insemination homologous and male subfertility. Institut Aquitain de Recherches sur la Reproduction Humaine, Bordeaux, pp 188–195

Bunge RG, Keettel WC, Sherman JK (1954) Clinical use of frozen semen. Fertil Steril 5:520–529

Cassou R (1964) La méthode des paillettes en plastique adapter à la généralisation de la congélation. Proceedings of Fifth International Congress on Animal Reproduction and Artificial Insemination. Trento 4:540–546

David G (1975) Les banques de spermeen france. Arch France Ped 32:401–404

Ericsson RJ (1977) Isolation and storage of progressively motile human sperm. Andrologia 9:111–114

Ericsson RJ (1978) Isolation of progressively motile human sperm to select for Y sperm or to improve fertility. In: Emperaire JC, Audebert A (eds) Proceedings of First International Symposium on artificial insemination homologous and male subfertility. Institut Aquitain de Recherches sur la Reproduction Humaine, Bordeaux, pp 176–185

Ericsson RJ, Langevin CN, Nishino M (1973) Isolation of fractions rich in human Y sperm. Nature 246:421–424

Gasser G, Ita H, Mossig H, Schmid R, Schneider W (1978) Experience with AIH of native and frozen human semen. In: Emperaire JC, Audebert A (eds) Proceedings of First International Symposium on artificial insemination homologous and male subfertility. Institut Aquitain de Recherches sur la Reproduction Humaine, Bordeaux, pp 151–156

Haesungcharern A, Chulavatnatol M (1973) Stimulation of human spermatozoal motility by caffeine. Fertil Steril 24:662–665

Hoagland H, Pincus G (1942) Revival of mammalian sperm after immersion in liquid nitrogen. J Gen Physiol 25:337

Homonnai T, Paz G, Soffer A, Peretz F, Kraicer PF, Harel A (1976) Effect of caffeine on the motility, viability, oxygen consumption and glycolytic rate of ejaculated human normokinetic and hypokinetic spermatozoa. Int J Fertil 21:163–170

Iizuka R, Sawada Y (1958) Successful insemination with frozen human semen. Jpn J Fertil Steril 3:4–9

Jahnel F (1938) Über die Widerstandsfähigkeit von menschlichen Spermatozoen gegenüber starker Kälte. Klin Wochenschr 17:1273

Jondet R (1964) Congelation rapide du sperme de taureau conditionné en paillettes. Proceedings of Fifth International Congress on animal reproduction and artificial insemination. Trento 4:463–468

Jondet M (1975) Adaptation d'une cape cervicale pour l'insémination artificielle humaine. J Gynecol Obstet Biol Reprod 4:141–144

Keettel WC, Bunge RG, Bradbury JT, Nelson WO (1956) Report of pregnancies with frozen semen in infertile couples. JAMA 160:102

Keswani SG (1978) AIH for sub-fertility with frozen and fresh sperm concentrates. In: Emperaire JC, Audebert A (eds) Proceedings of First International Symposium on artificial insemination homologous and male subfertility. Institut Aquitain de Recherches sur la Reproduction Humaine, Bordeaux, pp 138–141

Kremer J (1978) A new technique for intrauterine insemination. In: Emperaire JC, Audebert A (eds) Proceedings of First International Symposium on artificial insemination homologous and male subfertility. Institut Aquitain de Recherches sur la Reproduction Humaine, Bordeaux, pp 43–48

Lopata A, Patullo MJ, Chang A, James B (1976) A method for collecting motile spermatozoa from human semen. Fertil Steril 27:677–684

Makler A (1979) Simultaneous differentiation between motile, non-motile, live and dead human spermatozoa by combining supra-vital staining and MET procedures. Int J Andrology 2:32

Makler E, Itzkovitz J, Brandes MJ (1980) Factors affecting sperm motility. Effect of caffeine, kallikrein and other metabolically active compounds on human spermatozoal motility and viability. Fertil Steril 33:624–630

Mantegazza J (1866) Fisiologia sullo sperma umano. Rend R Ist Lomb 3:183

Mazur P (1970) Crybiology: The freezing of biological systems. Sci Mag 168:3934, 939–949

Nagase H, Niwa T (1964) Deep freezing bull semen in concentrated pellet form. Proceedings of Fifth International Congress of animal reproduction and AI treatment. Trento 4:410–415

Parkes AS (1945) Preservation of human spermatozoa at low temperatures. Br Med J 2:212–213

Paulson JD, Polakoski KL (1977) A glass wool column procedure for removing extraneous materials from the human ejaculate. Fertil Steril 28:178–181

Paulson JD, Polakoski KL, Leto S (1978) Glass wool column filtration. In: Emperaire JC, Audebert A (eds) Proceedings of First International Symposium on artificial insemination homologous and male subfertility. Institut Aquitain de Recherches sur la Reproduction Humaine, Bordeaux, pp 158–168

Paz G, Kaplan R, Yedwab G, Homonnai T, Kraicer PF (1978) The effect of caffeine on rat epididymal spermatozoa motility, metabolism, and fertilization capacity. Int J Androl 1:145–152

Perloff WH, Steinberger E, Sherman JK (1964) Conception with human spermatozoa frozen by nitrogen vapour technique. Fertil Steril 15:501–504

Polge C, Smith AU, Parkes AS (1949) Revival of spermatozoa after vitrification and dehydration at low temperatures. Nature 164:666

Sawada Y (1958) Studies on the freeze preservation of the human spermatozoa. Jpn J Fertil Steril 4:1–11

Sawada Y, Ackerman DR, Behrman SJ (1967) Motility and respiration of human spermatozoa after cooling to various low temperatures. Fertil Steril 18:775–781

Schill WB (1975) Caffeine- and kallikrein-induced stimulation of human sperm motility: A comparative study. Andrology 7:229–236

Schill WB, Wolff HH (1974) Ultrastructure of human sperm acrosome and determination of acrosin activity under conditions of semen preservation. Int J Fertil 13:217–223

Schill WB, Pritsch W, Preissler G (1977) Effect of kallikrein and caffeine on frozen human semen. Fertil Steril 28:312

Schoenfeld CY, Amelar D, Dubin L (1975) Stimulation of ejaculated human spermatozoa by caffeine. Fertil Steril 26:158–161

Sherman JK (1954) Freezing and freeze drying of human spermatozoa. Fertil Steril 5:357–371

Sherman JK (1963) Improved methods of preservation of human spermatozoa by freezing and freeze drying. Fertil Steril 14:49–64

Sherman JK (1964) Research on frozen human sperm. Fertil Steril 15:485–499

Sherman JK (1973) Synopsis of the use of frozen human semen since 1964: State of the art of human semen banking. Fertil Steril 24:397–412

Sherman JK (1977) Cryopreservation of human semen. In: Hafez ESE (ed) Techniques of human andrology. Elsevier/North-Holland, Amsterdam Oxford New York, p 399

Sherman JK (1978) The role of cryobanking of human semen in AIH for male subfertility. In: Emperaire JC, Audebert A (eds) Proceedings of First International Symposium on artificial insemination homologous and male subfertility. Institut Aquitain de Recherches sur la Reproduction Humaine, Bordeaux, pp 132–137

Sherman JK (1979) Historical synopsis of human cryobanking. In: David G, Price WS (eds) Human artificial insemination and semen presentation. Plenum, New York London, p 95

Shettles LB (1940) The respiration of human spermatozoa and their response to various cases and low temperatures. Am J Physiol 128:408–415

Spallanzani L (1776) Opuscoli di fisca. Animale e vegetabile, opuscola. II. Osservazioni e sperienze intorno ai vermicelli spermatici dell'uomo e degli animali. Modena 1776

Tyler ET (1973) The clinical use of frozen semen banks. Fertil Steril 24:413–416

Verdaguer S, Emperaire JC, Audebert A (1978) Modification du sperme après filtration sur laine de verre. In: Emperaire JC, Audebert A (eds) Proceedings of First International Symposium on artificial insemination homologous and male subfertility. Institut Aquitain de Recherches sur la Reproduction Humaine, Bordeaux, pp 169–175

19 Enhancement of Sperm Motility: Selecting Progressively Motile Spermatozoa

F. Comhaire, L. Vermeulen, and F. Zegers-Hochschild

The reported success rates in terms of pregnancies after various forms of treatment of the infertile male remain unsatisfactory; therefore, the idea of stimulating sperm motility, selecting, concentrating, and eventually preserving the motile spermatozoa, and pooling the "good" spermatozoa harvested from several ejaculates for artificial insemination, remains attractive. Here, we report our experience with different techniques of motility stimulation, cryopreservation of stimulated spermatozoa, and selection and concentration of motile spermatozoa.

The application of such techniques will be restricted to selected cases, mainly characterized by isolated oligozoospermia with reasonable sperm morphology.

Patients with oligozoospermia of less than 2 million/ml or total sperm count per ejaculate inferior to 5 million/ml will probably not benefit form sperm manipulation. The same can be said if more than 90% of spermatozoa present morphological abnormalities of either the head, middle piece, or end piece. Even where sperm motility can be stimulated in these situations, no pregnancies have ever been obtained due to the poor structural quality of the spermatozoa.

19.1 Techniques

19.1.1 Caffeine Stimulation of Motility for Cryopreservation

The major problem of spermatozoa cryopreservation is in the loss of fertilizing capacity due to loss of sperm motility. Even when a glycerol egg yolk cryoprotective medium is added, a significant decrease in motility (approximately 25%–50%) is commonly registered (Smith and Steinberger 1973; Barkay et al. 1977).

The addition of caffeine to fresh semen results in stimulation of sperm motility (Schoenfeld et al. 1973) and the same phenomenon is observed when caffeine is added to cryopreserved spermatozoa (Barkay et al. 1977; Schill et al. 1977).

The best results in terms of motility recovery are seen when pellets of caffeine solution (final concentration 7,2 mmol/l) are added to thawing semen (Barkay et al. 1977). It has been suggested that caffeine may cause alterations in the electron-microscopic appearance of spermatozoa (Harrison and Sheppard 1978).

We have studied the influence of caffeine on the motility and the detailed light-microscopic morphology of spermatozoa (Vermeulen et al. 1978), comparing the effect of addition of this substance before freezing or after thawing (Vandeweghe et al. 1979).

Preparation of the Semen-Cryoprotective Medium Mixture. An aliquot of 0.66 ml cryoprotective medium (Appendix A) is added to 1 ml freshly liquefied semen, with a final glycerol concentration of 0.68 mol/l. To this mixture, 0.2 ml caffeine solution is added, the final caffeine concentration being 7.2 mmol/l. The caffeine solution is prepared by adding 13 mg caffeine to 1 ml Ringer lactate buffer. The semen and cryoprotective medium are thoroughly mixed for 10 min at 37 °C in a shaking water bath. The semen mixture is aspirated in 0.25 ml straws which are sealed with special sealing powder.

Freezing and Thawing Procedure. The straws are cooled to −120 °C by leaving them for 8 min in nitrogen vapor, after which they are submerged into the liquid nitrogen for storage. Thawing is performed by allowing the straws to remain at room temperature.

19.1.2 Selection of Motile Spermatozoa

19.1.2.1 Glass Wool Filtration

Glass wool filtration of semen makes use of a column which is slightly modified from that described by Paulson and Polakowski (1977). The glass wool column was originally designed for the treatment of ejaculates with disturbed liquefaction or increased threadiness.

Preparation of the Glass Wool Column. Industrial yellow glass wool for isolation is used. It should be carefully cleaned with methanol on either a Büchner filter or a Soxhlet apparatus. On the Büchner filter, the glass wool is superfused until it is completely colorless; the cleaning is performed on the Soxhlet apparatus over a period of 1 h. Cleaning glass wool using acid solutions, e.g., diluted HCl, is contraindicated since these solutions change the structure of the glass wool fibers. Indeed, after washing with acid solutions, the glass wool fibers are fractioned and have sharp cutting edges which can damage the spermatozoa.

A fine Pasteur pipette (I.D. 5 mm, length 40–50 mm) is used to manufacture the filter column and 10–15 mg, cleaned glass wool is inserted into this pipette. The glass wool is tightly compressed using a glass rod with a smooth end. The Pasteur pipette tapers over a distance of ±5 mm, the tapering part is filled with the glass wool cylinder (Fig. 1). The point of the pipette should have a diameter of about 1 mm and a length of about 10 mm.

Filtration Procedure. Between 0.5 and 0.7 ml freshly liquefied ejaculate is aspirated into a disposable 2-ml plastic syringe together with 0.2 ml caffeine solution. The caffeine solution contains 13 mg caffeine diluted in 1 ml Ringer lactate buffer. The ejaculate is thoroughly mixed with the caffeine solution by gentle shaking of the syringe.

A 1.2×38 mm disposable needle is inserted onto the syringe and the sperm-caffeine mixture is injected into the column. After 10–30 s, the filtered ejaculate starts to drip out of the pipette. If greater volumes of ejaculate are to be filtered, several columns can be used in parallel. Indeed, injection of more than 1 ml sperm-caffeine solution on one single filter column results in a considerable loss of spermatozoa due to saturation and obstruction of the filter.

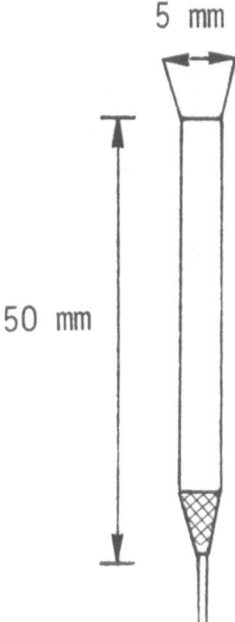

5 mm

50 mm

Fig. 1. Schematic drawing of glass wool column used in this study

19.1.2.2 Active Selection of Motile Spermatozoa in Biggers, Whitten and Whittingham (BWW) Medium

Whereas the glass wool filter technique passively selects the motile spermatozoa through binding of the immotile spermatozoa on the glass wool filaments, the BWW technique actively selects motile spermatozoa through their capacity to move from the semen into a layer of BWW medium. This movement is performed against gravity.

The procedure is performed in a Falcon dish made of transparent plastic. First 1 ml BWW medium (Appendix B) is pipetted into a plastic cylinder with diameter of 1 cm. Then 1 ml freshly liquefied semen is aspirated into a disposable plastic syringe. A 1.2×38-mm disposable needle is inserted onto the syringe and the semen is gently ejected beneath the BWW layer. When expression of semen is performed carefully no mixture occurs between the two layers. Finally, a liquid paraffin layer is applied on top of the BWW layer to inhibit evaporation during further manipulation. Thus, the layers are formed with semen at the bottom, covered by BWW, which is itself covered by a thin paraffin film.

The Falcon dish is placed in an incubator at 37 °C with a water-saturated atmosphere. After an incubation period of 2 h, the BWW layer is carefully aspirated.

19.1.2.3 Selection of Motile Spermatozoa on Albumin Columns

Another technique for selection of a population of motile spermatozoa has been de-scribed by Ericsson (1973). By this method, spermatozoa are layered on and allowed to swim into a column of liquid albumin. The method has been found to select not only the most motile and morphologically ideal spermatozoa, but also those bearing the y chromosome. Insemination of these selected spermatozoa has resulted in the birth of 23 males and eight females to date (Ericsson and Glass, to be published).

19.1.3 Techniques for the Concentration of Spermatozoa

Two techniques for the concentration of spermatozoa have been explored. The first uses a Millipore filter to absorb water and the second uses centrifugation.

19.1.3.1 Millipore Filter Absorption of Water

This technique is used to concentrate the filtrate obtained after passing the semen sample over a glass wool filter column. An aliquot of 0.4–0.5 ml filtrate is aspirated into a disposable plastic tuberculin syringe. The syringe is inserted onto a Millex Millipore filter with pores of 0.22 μm diameter and the filtered semen is injected in-to the filter chamber. The semen completely fills the chamber, but is not pressed through the filter membrane. After a few seconds, the semen is reaspirated out of the filter chamber. During its presence in the chamber, the volume of the semen plasma is reduced to roughly two-thirds of the initial volume, due to the absorption of water onto the filter membrane.

19.1.3.2 Centrifugation

Centrifugation is performed with either glass wool-filtered semen or on spermatozoa containing BWW medium. The sample is spun for 15 min at 2000 rpm and the supernatant is then discarded, except for a volume of 0.25–0.5 ml covering the bot-tom pellet. The pellet is resuspended in the remaining aliquot of fluid by gentle shaking.

19.1.4 Techniques of Semen Analysis

19.1.4.1 Motility of Spermatozoa

The motility of the spermatozoa is estimated in a phase-contrast microscope at magnification 400 (objective 40× ocular 10).

Several microscopic fields are visually scanned and all spermatozoa encountered are classified into the following grades: rapid, linear progressive motility (grade 3); sluggish linear or non-linear progressive motility (grade 2); non-progressive motility (grade 1); immotile spermatozoa (grade 0). One hundred spermatozoa are classified.

19.1.4.2 Sperm Density

The concentration of spermatozoa/ml is counted in a Burker hemacytometer after appropriate dilution of the semen in immobilizing fluid. This immobilizing fluid contains one-fifth Hayem's solution diluted in four-fifths physiological saline.

19.2 Results

19.2.1 Caffeine Stimulation and Cryopreservation

The addition of cryoprotective medium without caffeine generally causes a significant decrease ($\pm 10\%$) in sperm motility (Vandeweghe et al. 1979). The addition of cryoprotective medium plus caffeine, on the contrary, significantly stimulates motility (Fig. 2). There is a shift from sluggish (grade 2) to rapid progression (grade 3) and the number of spermatozoa that are either im-motile or motile on the spot decreases.

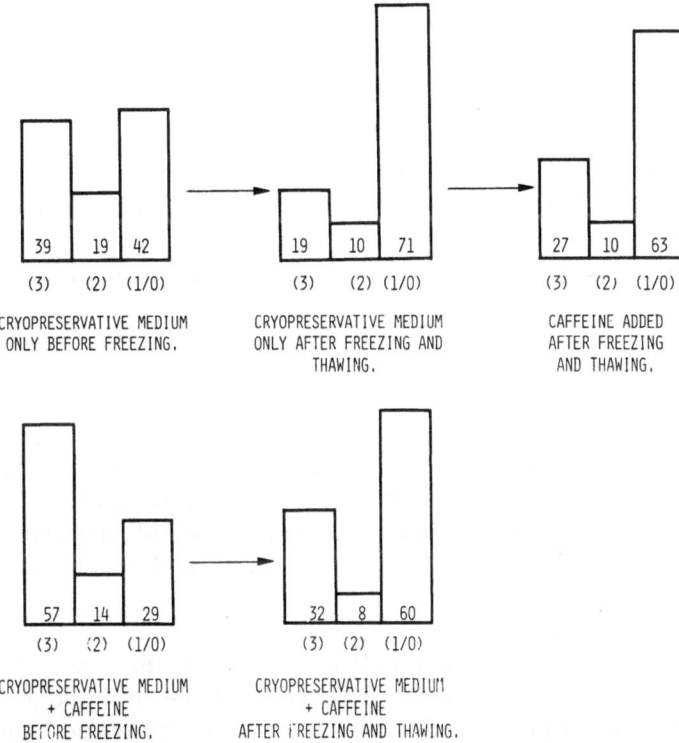

Fig. 2. Influence of caffeine on motility of cryopreserved spermatozoa. Sperm motility before and after freezing and thawing. Mean motility of the spermatozoa as expressed in percentage before and after freezing and thawing in 28 donor semen samples. The semen samples were either frozen without caffeine (*upper panel*) (caffeine was then added after thawing) or frozen with cryopreservative medium containing caffeine (*lower panel*). The figures in boxes indicate the percentage corresponding to the grades of motility indicated under the boxes in parenthesis: rapid progressive motility (grade 3); sluggish linear progression or non-linear progression (grade 2); motile on the spot or immotile spermatozoa (grades 1 and 0, respectively)

The post-freeze recovery of motility in semen without caffeine is about 50%, and significantly less than that if caffeine is added. The addition of caffeine after freezing and thawing has an effect on sperm motility which is almost equal to that of caffeine addition before freezing and thawing.

Sperm morphology after freezing and thawing is not influenced by caffeine. In semen frozen without caffeine the percentage of morphologically ideal spermatozoa was 45 ± 3.1 SEM, as compared to 44 ± 2.8 in semen with caffeine.

It, thus, appears that caffeine addition to semen improves sperm motility after freezing and thawing. Caffeine does not influence the light-microscopic morphological appearance of the spermatozoa.

Due to caffeine addition, some semen samples which are not freezable due to a significant loss of motility become freezable, containing sufficient motile spermatozoa/ml so as to be suitable for insemination. Pregnancy rates calculated on the life table (Schwartz and Mayaux 1980), using caffeine-stimulated spermatozoa, are comparable to pregnancy rates reported by authors not adding caffeine to the cryopreserved spermatozoa. Thus, the increased motility obtained by caffeine addition does not result in an important improvement in fertilizing capacity.

19.2.2 Selection of Motile Spermatozoa

19.2.2.1 Glass Wool Filtration

The volume of the filtrate is 0.2–0.3 ml less than the initial volume of semen poured into the column. Since the same aliquot (± 0.2 ml) of caffeine solution was added to the semen before filtration, the volume of the filtrate is roughly equal to the initial volume of semen. If the initial semen sample is, however, highly viscous or unliquefied, a somewhat greater volume of fluid is lost in the column. The filtrate is perfectly fluid and cleaned of mucus threads, cellular debris, and possible agglutinates or aggregates of spermatozoa. Round cells, such as leukocytes or spermatogenic cells, do pass through the filter.

Sperm Motility. The percentage of spermatozoa with grade 3 or grade 2 motility is doubled in the filtrate (Table 1), whereas the percentage of immotile spermatozoa (grade 0) is reduced to one-third. The glass wool filtration, thus, results in a selection of motile spermatozoa while most of the immotile spermatozoa stay attached to the glass wool fibers.

Sperm Density. In a series of 14 experiments, sperm density was found to be reduced to 44% of the initial value. However, due to the increased percentage motility, the number of progressively motile spermatozoa/ml (grade 3 plus grade 2) remains practically unchanged. Indeed, this number in the filtrate equals 94% of that in the original semen sample. On the contrary, the number of immotile spermatozoa/ml is reduced to 15% of the prefilter value.

The percentage of spermatozoa with ideal morphology is clearly increased in all samples after filtration. All types of morphological abnormalities occurred less frequently in the filtrate than in the original sample, and no morphological alterations were found to be induced by the filtration process.

Table 1. Effect of glass wool filtration on motility, concentration, and morphology of spermatozoa. The table lists the mean values before and after filtration, the number of observations, as well as the statistical significance (Wilcoxon's rank sum test for paired replicates)

	Before	After	Number of ejaculate	Statistical significance (before versus after)
Percentage of grade 3 motile spermatozoa	22.5	50.4	14	<0.01
Percentage grade 3 + 2 motile spermatozoa	34.7	69.2	14	<0.01
Percentage immotile spermatozoa	51.9	19.2	14	<0.01
Sperm concentration (million/ml)	50.2	22.2	14	<0.01
Concentration of progressively motile spermatozoa (grade 3 + 2) (million/ml)	16.8	15.7	14	N.S.
Concentration of immotile spermatozoa (grade 0) (million/ml)	25.4	3.7	14	<0.01
Percentage of ideal spermatozoa	15.5	26.3	6	<0.05

Glass wool filtration was found to be useful in highly viscous or nonliquefied semen samples. Artificial insemination of the filtered ejaculate resulted in pregnancies if the motile sperm count and morphology of the filtered spermatozoa was satisfactory. No pregnancies were obtained in cases with very low motile sperm counts (less than 2 million/ml) or disturbed sperm morphology (less than 10%–15% ideal spermatozoa). The method was without success when applied to ejaculates with immunological agglutination. Artificial (intrauterine) insemination of filtrate resulted in no more pregnancies than in noninseminated cases.

19.2.2.2 BWW Selection

Twenty-two semen samples were processed with the BWW technique (Table 2). The sperm concentration in the BWW medium was reduced to 27% of the initial value, however, 88% of the spermatozoa in the medium showed progressive motility. Spermatozoa with rapid progression (grade 3) were selected. Of the grade 3 motile spermatozoa, 52% were recovered in the BWW and only 7% of the grade 1 or grade 0 spermatozoa were found in the medium.

Although incubation took 2 h, very little loss of motility occurs, since the sum of grade 3 plus grade 2 spermatozoa found in the semen plus BWW was only 5% less than the number in the initial sample. Grade 3 plus grade 2 spermatozoa were distributed almost randomly between the semen and BWW layer, therefore, the recovery of motile spermatozoa in the BWW was only 47%.

Table 2. Effect of BWW selection on motility and concentration of spermatozoa. The table lists the mean values in the initial semen sample, the semen layer after incubation, and in the BWW layer as recorded in 22 experiments

	Initial semen	Final semen	BWW
Percentage grade 3 motile spermatozoa	39.9	26.4	77.3
Percentage grade 2 motile spermatozoa	12.6	9.8	10.5
Percentage grade 3+2 motile spermatozoa	52.5	36.2	87.8
Percentage grade 1+0 spermatozoa	47.5	63.8	12.2
Sperm concentration (million/ml)	68.5	50.1	18.4
Concentration grade 3 motile spermatozoa (million/ml)	27.3	13.2	14.3
Concentration grade 2 motile spermatozoa (million/ml)	8.7	4.9	1.9
Concentration grade 3+2 motile spermatozoa (million/ml)	36.0	18.1	16.2
Concentration of grade 1+0 spermatozoa	32.5	32.0	2.2

The BWW selection technique may be useful if semen plasma is believed to unfavorably influence the spermatozoa due to its abnormal composition, pH, or to the presence of toxic substances secreted by pathogenic bacteria. As yet, we have no experience with artificial insemination of BWW-selected spermatozoa.

19.2.3 Concentration Procedures

19.2.3.1 Millipore Filter Concentration

During the short stay of the filtered ejaculate in the Millipore filter chamber, volume is reduced by absorption of water onto the filter membrane. The mean of the ratios of sperm density after Millipore filtration over sperm density before manipulation is 1.67 (range 1.0–3.1). The mean sperm concentration increases from 8.6 million/ml before, to 14 million/ml after manipulation (Fig. 3).

Sperm motility is not significantly influenced by the Millipore concentration procedure. The mean ratio of motility after compared to before the procedure is 0.98 (range 0.58–1.22). The mean recovery of motile spermatozoa is 95%. Concentration using the Millipore technique is valuable for semen samples with moderate oligozoospermia which are to be cryopreserved. Indeed, the dilution effect of cryoprotective medium addition is neutralized by previous concentration of the semen sample on the Millipore filter. This technique is utilized for the cryopreservation of semen from patients suffering from Hodgkin's disease and who are to undergo treatment with cytostatic drugs. Such patients commonly present moderate oligozoospermia before the initiation of the chemotherapy, due to changes in general health.

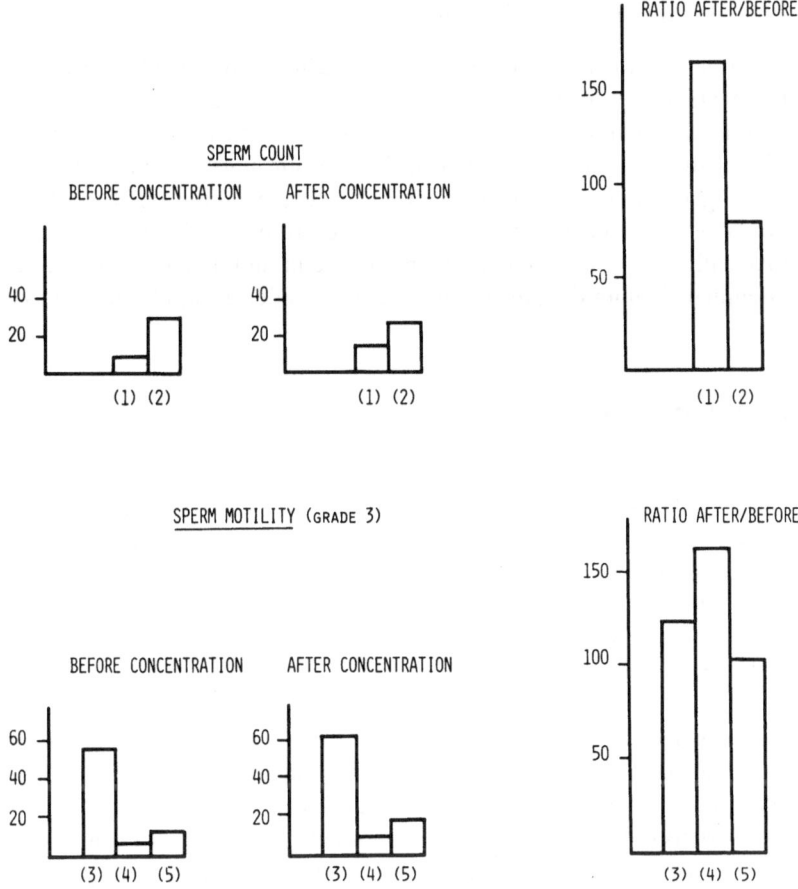

Fig. 3. Millipore filter technique for semen concentration. The *upper panel* represents the mean sperm count/ml (1) and sperm content per ejaculate (2) before and after concentration on the Millipore filter. The *upper right* box represents the ratio of sperm count after and before concentration expressed as percentage for (1) sperm concentration, (2) total sperm content per ejaculate. The *lower panel* presents the mean of grade 3 motile spermatozoa before and after concentration. The grade 3 sperm motility is expressed as: (3) percent; (4) number of grade 3 motile spermatozoa/ml; (5) number of grade 3 motile spermatozoa per ejaculate. The *lower right* box represents the ratio of grade 3 motility after and before concentration

19.2.3.2 Centrifugation

Centrifugation results in stronger concentration. The mean of ratios of sperm density after centrifugation over density before centrifugation equals 3.33 (range 1.34–6). However, the percent motility decreases slightly, since the mean of ratios of percent motility after concentration over percent motility before concentration is 0.86. The recovery of motile spermatozoa is reduced to 72%.

Centrifugation, thus, will be elected as a method for concentration in ejaculates with a large volume and dilution oligozoospermia, but with a total sperm count in the ejaculate in excess of 10 million.

19.2.3.3 BWW Plus Centrifugation

In a small number of samples spermatozoa recovered in BWW were concentrated by means of centrifugation. The centrifugation procedure was performed on the spermatozoa harvested on several cylinders. It was possible to concentrate about 80% of the spermatozoa present in the medium into a volume of 0.5 ml, thus, increasing the concentration three- to six-fold depending on the volume of BWW available for concentration. This technique can be considered in cases suspected of toxic influence of the seminal plasma on sperm motility. The concentrate should be inseminated either directly into the uterus or under the application of a cervical cap.

19.3 Discussion

Glass wool filtration is reasonably effective in discarding immotile, agglutinated, or aggregated spermatozoa. The procedure cleans the ejaculate of mucus threads and cellular debris and is very efficient in reducing increased viscosity. Artificial insemination of filtered ejaculate results in pregnancies only if the motile sperm count and morphology of the filtered spermatozoa is adequate. The method should be elected for infertility cases with poor postcoital test results, highly viscous ejaculate, but normal sperm concentration and morphology.

The BWW method actively selects the spermatozoa with progressive motility. With this technique, it is possible to separate an almost pure population of motile spermatozoa. These may be concentrated by means of centrifugation, though recovery is rather poor. Selection and washing of spermatozoa with the BWW technique, therefore, is only useful in cases of abnormal seminal plasma composition of heavy bacterial contamination, but satisfactory sperm concentration and morphology.

Glass wool-filtered spermatozoa may be concentrated by centrifugation. The centrifugation effect is strong, but recovery is suboptimal. Therefore, this method should be elected for ejaculates with pseudo-oligozoospermia due to dilution of the spermatozoa in a high volume of seminal fluid. The method is applicable if the total sperm content of the ejaculate is more than 10 million.

The use of the Millipore filter results in a less pronounced concentrating effect, though recovery of motile spermatozoa is almost complete. This method, therefore, is useful for the concentration of ejaculates with moderate oligozoospermia and relatively small volume. The Millipore filter concentrating procedure may be used for ejaculates to be frozen, especially before chemotherapy in the case of patients with malignant diseases. The diluting effect of the addition of the cryoprotective medium to the semen can be neutralized by previous filtration of the ejaculate through the Millipore filter.

Addition of caffeine to the ejaculate improves sperm motility and enhances the recovery of motile spermatozoa in subsequent selection procedures. The addition of caffeine to semen for cryopreservation equally enhances the postfreeze motility, however, without influencing the pregnancy rate.

Thus, each of the methods described has advantages and disadvantages. The usefulness of these methods in clinical practive needs further evaluation.

Appendix A. Cryoprotective Medium

1.32 g glucose
1.15 g citrate
66.0 ml water
14.0 ml glycerol
20.0 ml egg yolk

Heat at 56 °C for 30 min, add 2 g glycine,
adjust pH to 7–7.4, freeze in small aliquots, and maintain at –20 °C

Appendix B. BWW Medium

This medium is a modified Krebs-Ringer solution.
It contains:

Stock solution		
	NaCl	5.540 g/l
	KCl	0.356 g/l
	CaCl$_2$	0.189 g/l
	KH$_2$PO$_4$	0.162 g/l
	MgSO$_4$ · 7 aq	0.601 g/l
	NaHCO$_3$	2.100 g/l
	Optional: phenol red (0.5%)	1.0 ml/l
	(dilute in 800 ml Aq dest.)	

To a 8 ml aliquot of the stock solution is added:

	Na lactate (50.6%) syrup	2.0 µl
	Na pyruvate	14.0 µl
	Glucose	10.0 mg
	Human or bovine serum	3.3 %
	albumin (1.65 ml HSA 20%)	
	Adjust to 10 ml	

Sterilize or press through Millex Millipore filter (0.22 µm)

19.4 References

Barkay J, Zuckerman H, Sklan D, Gordon S (1977) Effect of caffeine on increasing the mo-
tility of frozen sperm. Fertil Steril 28:175–177
Ericsson RJ, Glass RH (to be published) Implications for artificial insemination with a preselected population of sperm (Abstr 11). IInd Pan American Congress of Andrology,
Mexico City, January 26th–30th 1981
Ericsson RJ, Langevin CN, Nishino M (1973) Isolation of fractions rich in human Y sperm.
Nature 246:421–424
Harrison RF, Sheppard BL (1978) Electron microscopy studies in spermatozoa energized by
caffeine. In: Salvadori B, Semm K, Vadora E (eds) Fertility and Sterility. Proceedings of
the Vth European Congress on Sterility and Fertility. Edizioni Internazionali Gruppo Editoriale Medico, Milano, pp 373–376

Paulson JD, Polakowski KL (1977) Preparation of human semen by glass wool columns. In: Hafez ESE (ed) Techniques of human andrology. Elsevier/North Holland Biomedical Press, Amsterdam Oxford New York, pp 445–446

Schill WB, Pritsch W, Preissler G (1977) Effect of kallikrein and caffeine on frozen human semen. Fertil Steril 28:312

Schoenfeld CY, Amelar RD, Dubin L (1973) Stimulation of ejaculated human spermatozoa by caffeine: a preliminary report. Fertil Steril 24:772–775

Schwartz O, Mayaux M (1980) Mode of evaluation of results in artificial insemination. In: David G, Price WB (eds) Proceedings of International Symposium on human artificial insemination and semen preservation. Plenum, New York, pp 197–210

Smith KD, Steinberger E (1973) Survival of spermatozoa in a human sperm bank: Effect of long-term storage in liquid nitrogen. JAMA 223:774–777

Vandeweghe M, Comhaire F, Vermeulen L (1979) The effect of caffeine on motility and morphology of deep frozen donor spermatozoa (in Dutch). Ann Ver Fertil 6:6–8

Vermeulen L, Comhaire F, Van Egmond J (1978) Ordinator-assisted detailed light-microscopic study of sperm morphology as a routine technique in male infertility diagnosis. In: Cortes-Prieto J, Semm K (eds) Proceedings of IVth European Sterility Congress, Reproduction, Madrid, pp 415–417

20 Artificial Homologous Insemination

M. Glezerman

Fertilization of a properly released ovum requires three basic prerequisites: the availability of a sufficient number of motile and morphologically normal sperm cells, the intravaginal deposition of these cells, and ascent of sperm cells into the higher parts of the female genital tract.

While the production of normal semen results solely from normal functioning of the male reproductive system, the second and third prerequisites require adequate interaction between the anatomic-physiological systems of both partners. Whenever a dysfunction occurs in any of these three prerequisites, fertility may be impaired. When medical, surgical, and other treatment schemes have failed, an attempt may be made to employ artificial insemination procedures.

If artificial homologous insemination (AIH) is used indiscriminately, results may be disappointing. Artificial insemination is not an innocuous procedure and its value has to be weighed carefully against possible adverse effects. Whenever AIH is employed, the possibility of mechanization of the sexual relationship enters into consideration. The process of AIH may not be perceived by the couple as a purely medical procedure, but rather as a corrective measure of performance inability. Consequently, the archaic perception of the connection between sexuality and procreation may be revived and guilt feelings, subconscious accusations, and a severe blow to the ego of the "responsible" partner may ensue. It is not a rare phenomenon to observe previously ovulatory cycles turn anovulatory as soon as treatment with AIH is started and various degrees of impaired sexual response may occur in either partner (Beck 1976). For the male who has to produce an ejaculate on demand at a given time, performance coercion is even more evident and presents the most immediate psychological drawback to AIH. The resulting continuous stress situation for the couple and mounting month to month failures exert a tremendous emotional effect on the marriage in general and sexual relationship in particular. Considering this background, the decision for AIH has to be made very carefully.

20.1 Indications for AIH

Three main areas may be defined within which AIH may be of benefit as a tool to treat infertile couples. These are: subnormal semen, failure to deliver semen properly to a position which allows sufficient contact to the external cervical os, and disturbed migration of sperm cells within the female genital tract. The etiology of the infertility determines the appropriate insemination technique to be used.

20.1.1 Subnormal Semen

When repeated semen analyses have shown subnormal results, it is the intent of AIH to apply what few spermatozoa are present as closely as possible to the external cervical os; however, mere substitution of the natural sperm delivery mechanism by mechanical means (intravaginal insemination) does not ameliorate the decreased fertilizing capacity of a given semen. Only if artificial insemination can provide additional protective, promoting, or corrective features for a given semen sample, will its use be superior to sexual intercourse for procreation purposes. When decision for AIH is taken, some basic physiological facts have to be considered. Out of hundreds of millions of sperm cells which leave the male genital tract during intercourse and reach the vagina, only a tiny minority reach the female endocervix in order to be stored there for continuous release. Settlage et al. (1973) and Insler et al. (1980) reported the total sperm cell content of the endocervical storage space to be around 200,000. The vast majority of spermatozoa is either spilled from the vagina or destroyed there by its acidity within a very short period of time.

20.1.1.1 Oligozoospermia

The term oligozoospermia indicates a condition in which the seminal plasma contains less than the normal concentration of sperm cells per ml; however, no consensus exists as to what should be considered the normal content of sperm cells in a semen sample. Various investigators have proposed different "normal" values and the same authors have proposed different "normal" values at different times (Table 1). For practical purposes, we consider the lower limit of sperm concentration to be 20–30 million/ml measured at at least two consecutive examinations.

In cases of isolated oligozoospermia it would be a rational approach to concentrate as many as possible of the available spermatozoa at the external cervical os while avoiding as far as possible direct contact with vaginal secretions and spilling from the vagina.

Table 1. Proposed normal values for sperm concentration (Lunenfeld and Glezerman 1981)

Reference	Sperm cells/ml (millions)
Macomber and Sanders (1929)	60
MacLeod (1965)	20
van Zyl (1972)	10
Santamauro et al. (1972)	10
Schirren (1972)	40
Schill (1975a)	40
Ludvik (1976)	40
Freund and Petersen (1976)	20
Eliasson (1977)	20
Amelar and Dubin (1977a)	40
Zaneveld and Polakoski (1977)	50

Bedford (1971) demonstrated that, in the rabbit, destruction of all sperm cells 5 min after mating resulted in a 93% fertilization rate. Tredway et al. (1975) showed that the ratio of the number of spermatozoa within the cervical mucus to the number of motile sperm cells inseminated remains relatively constant for 15 min to 24 h after insemination. Thus, one may speculate, that the initial concentration of sperm cells coming into contact with the uterine cervix is of greater importance than the time period of contact. Reduced concentration may be partially compensated for by prolonged contact time. Endocervical and, to a lesser extent, pericervical insemination procedures respond to the demand of optimal semino-cervical contact. However, in both methods, the seminal volume that can be used is restricted. The "cap" method enables the use of the whole semen specimen and allows prolonged "undisturbed" semino-cervical contact. Nevertheless, endocervical, pericervical, and "cap" insemination deal with protection of a given semen sample without attempting to ameliorate its qualities. Fertilization chances of a given semen sample will improve markedly if quality-promoting features are added to the protective ones. Thus, many attempts have been made to concentrate spermatozoa prior to insemination using centrifugation, pooling, etc.; however, one of the most efficient ways of concentrating sperm cells may be found by observing the natural process of ejaculation. MacLeod and Hotchkiss (1942) observed that the first ejaculatory spurt contains a significantly higher concentration of sperm cells than the following spurts. Hartmann (1962) stated that this first portion contains about 90% of all sperm cells destined to leave the male genital tract during a given ejaculation. The first ejaculatory spurt is made up mainly of products from the testes, epididymides, vasa deferentia, and prostate. Thus, the first ejaculatory portion contains the highest concentration of sperm cells. The following ejaculatory spurts consist of secretions from the seminal vesicles which act as a buffering agent, as a source of nutrition (due to the high fructose content), and as a vehicle for spermatozoa. By splitting the ejaculatory spurts into different fractions, one will obtain the highest sperm concentration in the first "split" (Amelar and Hotchkiss 1965; Eliasson and Lindholmer 1972; Farris and Murphy 1960; Harvey 1956). Thus, the use of the first ejaculatory split is uniquely suited for AIH whenever the major seminal problem is reduced sperm concentration. Prior to insemination the different fractions should be examined, since in about 6% of cases sperm concentration is higher in the second ejaculatory spurt and in 5% of cases sperm concentration is equally distributed in the different fractions (Amelar and Hotchkiss 1965). This may be due to a disturbance in the sequence of ejaculatory synchronization.

The use of split ejaculates for AIH in cases of subnormal semen findings may be advantageous also from other points of view. Lindholmer (1973) postulated suppressive factors in the secretions of the seminal vesicles which may have a deleterious effect on sperm survival. MacLeod and Hotchkiss (1942) observed, in addition to increased sperm density, a higher percentage of motile sperm cells in the first split. This observation has since been confirmed by other investigators.

20.1.1.2 Asthenozoospermia

Progressive motility is crucial for the fertilizing capacity of sperm cells. Reduced motility has been more often associated with infertility than reduced sperm concentration or increased percentage of abnormally configurated sperm cells (Glezerman et al. 1980). Usually, 40%–80% of sperm cells in a given semen sample present fast progressive motility. Asthenozoospermia is a condition in which less than 40% of sperm cells move progressively.

In cases of reduced sperm motility, semen may be treated in vitro prior to insemination. Kallikrein (Schill et al. 1974) and caffeine (Schoenfeld et al. 1975) have been used to vitalize sperm cells in vitro. Kallikrein, a proteinase, releases kinins which enhance sperm metabolism. Schill (1975 b) advocates the addition of a source for kininogen, such as human serum. Caffeine inhibits cyclic nucleotide phosphodiesterase, thus, preventing degradation of cyclic nucleotides, which, in turn, may stimulate sperm metabolism. Following correction of the motility problem in vitro, a protective insemination procedure such as endocervical or, even better, cap insemination may then be performed.

20.1.1.3 Teratozoospermia and Debris-Contaminated Semen

Presence of debris or dead and agglutinated spermatozoa in a semen sample may increase its viscosity and influence penetrability of sperm cells through cervical mucus. Paulson and Polakoski (1978) have used glass wool columns to remove the majority of debris and agglutinated and dead sperm cells. Following this filtration procedure the percentage of abnormal sperm cells decreased as well. Samples passed through columns showed increased percentage of forward progression, decreased percentage of abnormally configurated sperm cells, and normal viscosity. Dmowski et al. (1979) used albumin columns to filter debris and abnormally configurated sperm cells. Using a one-layer technique in semen samples of 12 men, a significant increase in the percentage of motile sperm cells and in normally configurated spermatozoa was observed. AIH using filtered semen resulted in four pregnancies.

Hahn (1976, unpublished) performed a study comparing the in vitro fertilization capacity of normal and abnormal sperm cells using rabbit and mice ova. In these experiments no fertilization capacity of abnormally configurated sperm cells could be demonstrated. Although no human study has been reported to date, most investigators recognize the reduced fertilizing potential of a semen sample with increased percentage of abnormally configurated sperm cells (teratozoospermia). In vitro filtered semen may be suitable for AIH.

20.1.1.4 Increased Seminal Viscosity and Delayed Seminal Liquefaction

Increased seminal viscosity has been mentioned as a possible cause for infertility particularly when coinciding with decreased motility (Tjioe and Oentoeng 1968). In these cases the use of the first ejaculatory spurt for insemination may be of value. Amelar and Dubin (1977 b) have proposed to either force the semen specimen through an 18–19-gauge needle several times or to mix the semen with a mucolytic solution such as Alevaire (Breon Laboratories). Both methods yield a semen sample with highly reduced viscosity suitable for AIH.

Non-liquefying semen may be treated in vitro by adding a 4% solution of α-amylase in Locke's solution (Bunge and Sherman 1954). Following this procedure the specimen may be used for AIH. Another possibility is the treatment of non-liquefying semen by the proteolytic enzyme α-chymotrypsin (5 mg/ejaculate) as successfully used by Schill (1973).

20.1.1.5 Hypospermia

Hypospermia is defined as a condition in which repeated semen analyses reveal a seminal volume of less than 2 ml. In cases of severe hypospermia, i.e., seminal volume below 1 ml, infertility may be present due to failure of the small amount of seminal fluid to make contact with the cervical os and its secretions. AIH may be useful in these cases in promoting fertility.

20.1.2 Deposition Failure

20.1.2.1 Impotence and Anejaculation

Occasionally couples are referred with the request for AIH because of erectile failure or premature ejaculation. When erectile failure is due to psychological factors AIH is contraindicated until behavior therapy has been tried and proven unsuccessful. Even then, AIH should be instituted only after marriage counseling has been provided. An additional group of couples may not volunteer or may withhold information about sexual problems while requesting AIH. Repeated negative postcoital tests in the female, concomitant with normal semen analyses and normal sperm penetration tests may reveal the sperm deposition problem (Insler et al. 1977). In cases of organic impotence (paraplegics, diabetic neuropathy) in whom treatment of the cause is ineffective, AIH is the treatment of choice. If indicated, intravaginal insemination is very effective. This may be performed by the couples themselves following appropriate explanation. AIH performed by the male partner in the home will be much more convenient for the couple, relieved from some of the stress connected with the procedure, eliminates the connection between ejaculation on demand and the physician's busy schedule and provide the male partner with a more active role, relieving him of some of the associated emotional stress.

Anejaculation may have a variety of causes (endocrine, anatomic, psychogenic). Following evaluation and treatment, some patients may still require artificial procedures to obtain semen for artificial insemination. Electrovibration may be used for this purpose (Glezerman and Lunenfeld 1976).

One entity, often mistakenly described as anejaculation presents a clear-cut indication for AIH, namely retrograde ejaculation (Glezerman et al. 1976). In this condition, the semen is ejected backwards into the bladder rather than forward through the urethra. The diagnosis of retrograde ejaculation is made by observing sperm cells in the postcoital urine. Attempts to achieve fertility in these patients can be done through procedures to restore antegrade ejaculation (with the use of α-sympathomimetic agents) and through efforts to regain viable and fertile spermatozoa from the urinary bladder after sexual intercourse or masturbation with subsequent artificial insemination. In order to avoid possible damage to the sperm cells by contact with the urine, its acidity is neutralized by administering alkalizing agents prior to intercourse. When the urine is received, it is washed with nutrient solutions (Eagle's solution, Ringer's solution, etc.) centrifuged, and the female partner is inseminated with the sediment using the pericervical or cap technique (Glezerman et al. 1976).

20.1.2.2 Vaginismus

Erectile failure in the male has its female counterpart as vaginismus, i.e., tension within the walls of the vagina preventing penile penetration. The etiology is almost always psychogenic in origin. AIH is generally not indicated in these patients.

20.1.2.3 Deformed Female or Male Genital Organs

Severe hypospadias or epispadias in the male or extreme displacement of the uterus or uterine cervix or severe uterine prolapse in the female may be causative factors for disturbed sperm deposition. The first reported AIH was done in the wife of a patient with severe hypospadias who constantly ejaculated ante portas. John Hunter performed the procedure in 1870 (Shields 1950). Obviously, these conditions require surgical correction, if possible. AIH, performed intracervically or pericervically, has been proven to be a most efficient treatment to restore fertility.

20.1.3 Failure of Sperm Migration

The uterine cervix and its secretions play an important role in the reproductive process. The main element of this function is the transport and preservation of spermatozoa so that sufficient number of sperm cells may be sustained long enough to reach the fallopian tube at a time appropriate for fertilization of the ovum (Insler et al. 1977, 1979 b). It is now generally accepted that ill function of the uterine cervix will impede sperm transport and infertility may ensue. The clinical expression of this dysfunction may be "relative or absolute dysmucorrhea", i.e., inability of the uterine cervix to produce sufficient amounts of cervical mucus of adequate physical and chemical properties, and "penetration dysmucorrhea", i.e., inability of the cervical mucus to permit penetration of sperm cells. On the other hand, migration failure may be due to an "inherent penetration inability" of sperm cells which seem normal on routine semen analysis (Insler et al. 1979 a). It is beyond the scope of this paper to discuss the evaluation of the cervical factor of infertility (Insler et al. 1977, 1979 b). Any of the disturbances mentioned will require the artificial bypassing of the uterine cervix by introducing semen directly into the uterine cavity.

Problems arising using intrauterine insemination will be discussed later. The split insemination is uniquely suited to intrauterine insemination. Also in cases of the so-called "immunological infertility", namely, the presence of antisperm antibodies on either sperm cells or within the cervical mucus, intrauterine insemination using the split fraction may be effective.

20.1.4 Cryopreserved Semen

During the past decade, semen banking has received much public attention because of its potential as fertility insurance for men whose professional activity may affect fertility and in men contemplating vasectomy. Cryopreserved semen is in use for artifical insemination. Intracervical, pericervical, or cap insemination may then be employed.

In men with subnormal semen, mainly oligozoospermia, many attempts have been made to freeze semen samples for consequent pooling and artificial insemination. Subnormal semen sustains further loss of quality during the freezing and thawing process, so that this technique may not offer any advantage. Various aspects of cryopreservation of semen are discussed elsewhere in this book.

20.2 Technique of Artificial Insemination

By means of semen deposited into the vagina, about the cervix, into the cervix or into the uterus, artificial insemination may be performed. Special insemination instruments, such as cervical caps, are available.

20.2.1 Intravaginal Insemination

Intravaginal insemination is easily performed by means of a plastic syringe using the whole semen specimen. This method does not require exposure of the cervix and may be performed by the couple. The female partner is in the supine Trendelenburg's position. If the procedure is performed by the couple at their home the pelvis may be elevated slightly by means of a pillow. The position should be maintained for about 20 min following insemination. Extreme care has to be taken not to inject air into the vagina and cervix, since this could cause air embolism.

20.2.2 Pericervical and Intracervical Insemination

Usually, pericervical and intracervical insemination are used concomitently. The patient is placed in Trendelenburg's position, 0.2–0.5 ml semen is injected slowly into a depth of approximately 1 cm into the cervical canal by applying the blunt tip of a plastic syringe to the external os. The rest of the specimen is placed in the anterior vaginal fornix. The patient remains in the supine position for approximately 20 min.

20.2.3 Cap Insemination

While the small amount of semen deposited intracervically will be stored there for further release to the fertilization site, the major part of the specimen, which is deposited in the vagina will pour out very soon following insemination. Remaining spermatozoa will be inactivated quickly by vaginal acidity. Furthermore, all insemination techniques mentioned require that the patient remain supine for almost 30 min following insemination. This may tie up rooms in a busy practice. The cervical cap technique overcomes these drawbacks. Although a variety of caps have been designed, most systems do not provide close contact to the cervix and dislocation of the cap may occur following placement. In addition, merely applying the cap to the cervix will protect only part of the semen from the vaginal environment while a large part will still be spilled. The vacuum cap as developed by Fikentscher and

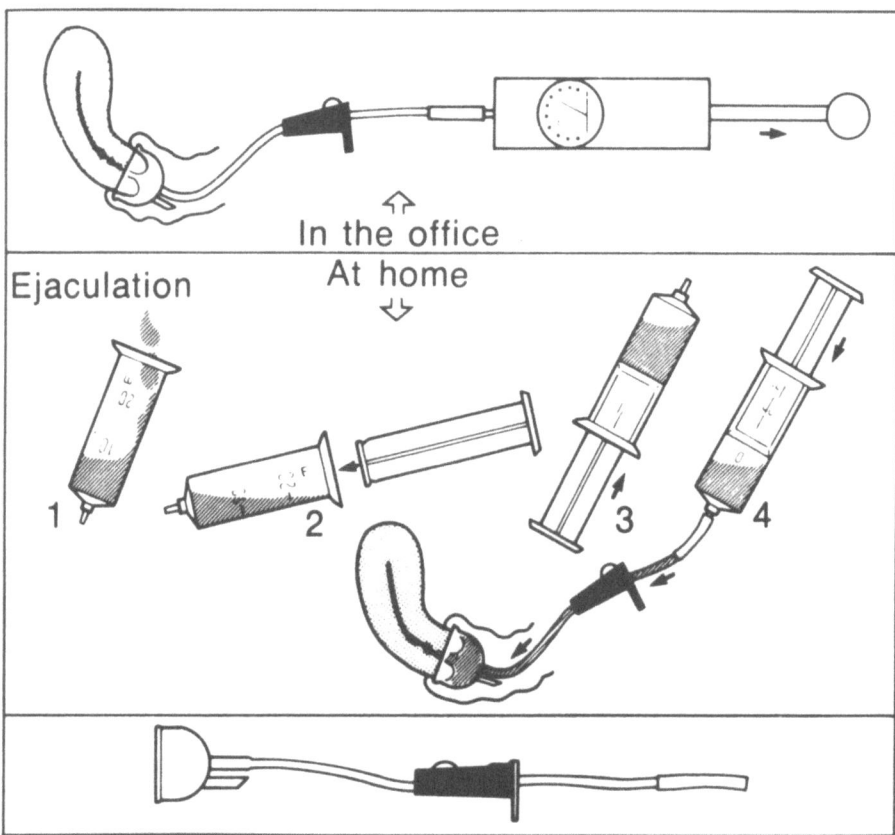

Fig. 1. Application of the vacuum cervical cap. The *upper part* of the figure shows the application of the cap to the uterine cervix and the production of vacuum by a hand pump. The *middle part* shows the filling of a syringe with semen and the application of the syringe to the cap tubing. This procedure may be performed by the couple themselves at their home if, for any reason, the husband cannot produce an ejaculation at a pre-set time. The *lower part* of the figure shows the vacuum cervical cap (Semm et al. 1976)

Semm guarantees close contact with the cervix and makes superfluous the sometimes tedious task of filling the adapted cap in situ with semen. This cap consists of a plastic hood, available in two sizes, connected to a flexible plastic tubing which may be closed by a "roll-on" clamp (Fig. 1). Following exposure of the cervix by a speculum and cleansing of the vagina and cervix, the cap is placed on the portio vaginalis using a grasping instrument. Vacuum is produced either by a commercially available, small hand pump or simply by evacuating air by means of a 10 ml syringe. During this process the application to the cervix is controlled visually. The clamp is then closed and the semen-containing syringe is attached. The clamp is now opened and the semen is visibly injected. The speculum is withdrawn and the patient may leave the table immediately. The cap remains in situ for 8–16 h. The patient is advised to open the clamp the next morning and to remove the cap by simply pulling the plastic tubing.

For some patients the production of an ejaculate on demand presents a serious problem. In these cases one should not exert further pressure on the patient, but offer the vacuum cap as an alternative. The instrument is fixed to the uterine cervix by the physician just prior to the time when ovulation is expected (Semm et al. 1976). Within the next 16 h the male partner may, at his leisure, fill the syringe with semen and complete the insemination procedure at a time convenient for him and his partner (Fig. 1).

20.2.4 Intrauterine Insemination

By means of intrauterine insemination the uterine cervix is bypassed and seminal fluid is injected directly into the uterine cavity. This may be done by the use of an infant feeding tube or the plastic tubing of an "intracath," attached to the sperm-containing syringe. Intrauterine insemination is not physiologic, in that spermatozoa are introduced into the uterine cavity together with seminal fluid (Asch et al. 1977). This may pose some unique problems. Firstly, uterine spermatozoa leave the female genital tract quickly via the uterine tubes and disappear into the peritoneal cavity, while no supply from the endocervical storage space replaces the loss. There is, therefore, a decreased chance that spermatozoa will be able to meet a short-lived fresh ovum on their way through the oviduct. More frequent insemination (e.g., daily) compensates only partially for this drawback.

Secondly, the bactericidal properties of the endocervix are excluded by intrauterine insemination (Pommerenke 1946). The risk of infections may, thus, increase (Russel 1960). Meticulous cleansing of vagina and cervix by use of ample amounts of, e.g., lactated Ringer's solution, prior to insemination and strictly sterile handling of the seminal specimen, obtained in a sterile jar, is of paramount importance. In addition we advocate prophylactic antibiotic treatment during the insemination period. Doxycycline (100 mg daily) in a single dose results in good penetration into the secretions of the female genital tract and is, thus, suitable for this purpose (Whelton et al. 1980). Thirdly, intrauterine insemination may lead to very painful uterine cramps due to the effect of the prostaglandin content of humen semen (Taylor and Kelly 1974). Most authors advocate, therefore, restriction of the inseminated volume to 0.3 ml (White and Glass 1976). Prostaglandins are secreted by the seminal vesicles which contribute to the last ejaculatory spurts. Thus, the first ejaculatory portion, consisting mainly of epididymal and prostatic contributions, contains relatively little prostaglandin but a high concentration of spermatozoa. It is, thus, uniquely suited for intrauterine inseminations and we have exclusively used the first split fraction for this purpose, injecting up to 0.8 ml/insemination without observing any sideeffects.

20.3 Timing of Insemination

Before initiating artificial insemination, the average midcycle can be calculated from the observation of three basal body temperature charts. However, this preliminary observation period is not sufficient to be the sole basis for consequent therapy. The fertility status of the female partner has to be assessed thoroughly and the

Table 2. Artificial homologous insemination using whole semen: techniques, indications and pregnancy rates

Reference	Indications	Definition	No. of patients	Technique	No. pregnancies (Rate)	Remarks
Whithelaw (1950)	Oligozoospermia	$<60 \times 10^6$/ml	32	Cap	14 (43.8%)	Range of sperm count/ml: $19 - 60 \times 10^6$
Kaskarelis and Comninos (1959)	Oligozoospermia	$7 - 40 \times 10^6$/ml $>40 \times 10^6$/ml	36 50	Para-intra-cervical, Intrauterine	0 13 (26%)	No pregnancy when count 40×10^6/ml, motility $<50\%$, normal cells $< 70\%$
Russel (1960)	Oligozoospermia	$<10 \times 10^6$/ml	34	Intracervical	2 (5.8%)	Eight women conceived later without AIH
	Cervical factor	PCT negative	10	Intracervical	3 (30%)	Two women conceived later without AIH
	Impotence Hypospadias Vas deferens occlusion		7 2 2	Intracervical Intracervical Intracervical	6 (86%) 2 (100%) 0	Semen retrieved from epid. cysts ($<10 \times 10^6$/ml)
Heuer (1971)	Oligozoospermia	Not given	70	Cap	31 (44.3%)	No details for indications cited
Barwin (1974)	Oligozoospermia	$<10 \times 10^6$/ml $10 - 20 \times 10^6$/ml	8 12	Intrauterine Intrauterine	3 (38%) 8 (66%)	Frozen-thawed semen
	Impotence Cervical factor	7 male, 1 female PCT negative SPT	8 18	Intrauterine Intrauterine	5 (63%) 13 (70%)	PCT = postcoital test; SPT = Sperm penetration test
	Retrograde ejaculation Before radiotheraphy (seminoma)		1 3	Intrauterine Intrauterine	0 2 (66%)	

Author (year)	Indication	Criteria	n	Technique	Result	Comments
Speichinger and Mattox (1976)	Oligozoospermia	$<10 \times 10^6$/ml	7	Intracervical + cap	0	
		$11 - 20 \times 10^6$/ml	5		0	
		$21 - 40 \times 10^6$/ml;	6		0	
	Cervical factor	PCT negative; immunol. tests	1		0	
Weller (1976)	Asthenozoospermia	Motil. <50%	1	Intrauterine	0	Thirty-two cases of male indications, 21 cases of male and female indications, and 7 cases of female indications. Total of female indications included among others: tubal occlusion, corpus lut. insufficiency, anorgasm, retroflexio, hyperanteversio, anovulation, etc.
	Hypospermia	<1 ml semen	3	Intracervical + cap	1 (33%)	
	Oligoastheno-teratozoospermia	Not given	43		4 (9.3%)	
	Viscosipathia	Not given	3		0	
	Impotence		6		4 (66.6%)	
	Hyperspermia	Not given	1		0	
	Female factors	Not given	7		2 (28.6%)	
Steiman and Taymor (1977)	Oligozoospermia	$<40 \times 10^6$/ml	29	Intracervical	7 (24%)	
	Impotence		3		2 (66.6%)	
	Cervical factors	PCT negative	25		8 (32%)	
Nunley et al. (1978)	Oligozoospermia	$<22 \times 10^6$/ml	15	Intracervical + cap	2 (13.3%)	Nine males had more than one indication
	Hypospermia	<3.1 ml	14		2 (14.3%)	
	Hyperspermia	>4 ml	14		0	Of 53 women, 43 had additional factors for infertility
	Cervical factor	Not given	6		2 (33.3%)	
	Polyzoospermia	$>100 \times 10^6$/ml	5		0	
	Retrograde ejaculation		2		1	
	Infrequent coitus		1		0	
	Patient request		1		0	

periovulatory period has to be identified as clearly as possible. The survey should include a complete cycle evaluation with ovulation detection and timing by means of basal body temperature, progesterone levels, and observation of the cervical score (Insler et al. 1972).

The life-span of the human ovum is believed to average 6–24 h, while motile human sperm cells have been observed in the cervical mucus for periods up to 205 h following intercourse. Thus, three inseminations per cycle on alternating days will usually suffice to "cover" the periovulatory period and ensure that sufficient sperm cells are available at the fertilization site when the ovum arrives.

Serial scoring of the cervical mucus, i.e., observation of its amount, spinnbarkeit, ferning, and the appearance of the external cervical os, has been very useful as an adjunct in scheduling repeated inseminations.

20.4 Contraindications for AIH

Absolute or relative contraindication for AIH is present

1. whenever pregnancy is contraindicated for medical or psychic reasons,
2. in cases of incompatibilities (e.g., Rh factor),
3. if either partner carries a hereditary disease,
4. in cases of severe systemic diseases in either partner (such as syphilis, severe forms of diabetes mellitus, malignant disease, etc.),
5. when recently cytostatic or immunosuppressive treatment has been applied (up to 1 year before attempted AIH),
6. when either partner has received therapeutic X-ray (up to 4 months before attempted AIH),
7. when acute genital infection is present in either partner.

20.5 Results of AIH

The success rate of AIH varies widely according to the indication and not all ensuing pregnancies are easily attributable to the AIH procedure. In 8 of 34 oligozoospermic patients treated by Russel (1960) with AIH, pregnancies occurred when the insemination scheme was discontinued while only 2 of these 34 patients reported pregnancies during the treatment scheme. In the same study, ten females with apparent cervical hostility were treated with AIH and three pregnancies ensued. However, two women conceived spontaneously after discontinuation of inseminations. Generally, comparison of data is difficult, since multifactorial infertility is treated by AIH, equivocal indications are sometimes used and data are not always completely reported (Table 2). In the series reported by Nunley et al. (1978) only in 10 of 53 patients treated by AIH were no additional causes for infertility present: in nine women, more than one additional cause for infertility was known. Weller (1976) treated 60 couples with AIH: There were 32 male indications, seven female indications, and 21 couples in whom both partners were considered to pose indications for AIH. Some of the indications cited in the female partners seem to be equivocal.

All indications were given as terms without definitions (i.e., oligozoospermia, asthenozoospermia, etc.).

Cervical hostility has been mentioned by many investigators as an indication for AIH. However, most authors define cervical hostility when repeated postcoital tests show poor results (Barwin 1974; White and Glass 1976; Nunley et al. 1978; Steiman and Taymor 1977). Considering that results of postcoital tests do not necessarily indicate cervical hostility, and correlation to occurrence of pregnancy has not been found by some investigators (Gibor et al. 1970; Giner et al. 1974), it seems that poor postcoital tests do not pose sufficient evidence for cervical hostility. Insler et al. (1977) observed poor postcoital tests in 10 of 75 cases with normal in vitro penetrability of sperm cells through cervical mucus while 5 of 77 cases with abnormal in vitro sperm penetration tests showed normal postcoital tests.

Oligozoospermia has often been cited as an indication for AIH. Again, comparison of data is difficult due to the frequent coexistence of other factors of infertility and to the fact that the condition is either not defined at all (Heuer 1971) or defined arbitrarily.

AIH in cases of severe oligozoospermia (less than 10 million sperm cells/ml), asthenozoospermia (less than 40% progressive sperm motility), or teratozoospermia (less than 50% normally configurated sperm cells) has rarely produced pregnancy rates in a range which might be considered clearly beyond the rate of chance. We, too, have not been able to demonstrate the benefit of simple protective AIH in these cases. However, if the quality of semen is improved before insemination, treatment success is considerably higher. We have employed AIH in 21 patients in whom reduced sperm concentration was due to high seminal volume (dilution-oligozoospermia). The mean spermatozoal concentration was 12.4 ± 4.8 million/ml. The mean volume of seminal fluid was 4.9 ± 1.1 ml. In 11 cases the first ejaculatory spurt

Table 3. Artificial homologous insemination using the split fraction: techniques, indications and pregnancy rates

Reference	Indications	No. of patients	Pregnancy rate	Technique
Farris and Murphy (1960)	Oligozoospermia	100	13%	Intrauterine
Amelar and Hotchkiss (1965)	Oligozoospermia	23	56%	?
Perez-Pelaez and Cohen (1965)	Oligozoospermia	38	26.3%	Intracervical/uterine
Steiman and Taymor (1977)	Oligozoospermia	29	24.1%	Intracervical
Moghissi et al. (1977)	Oligozoospermia Deposition Failure	62	32.1%	Intracervical
Glezerman et al. (1980)	Oligozoospermia	21	76.2%	Intra-pericervical split intercourse
David (1979)	Oligozoospermia Asthenozoospermia	72	62.5%	Intracervical split intercourse

contained at least twice as many sperm cells per milliliter than the following spurts. These males were advised to perform "split intercourse" during the periovulatory period. The method consists of a modified coitus interruptus during which only the first ejaculatory spurt is allowed to enter the vagina while the following spurts are ejaculated "ante portas". Five of these eleven patients reported difficulties in performing split intercourse and split AIH was applied using the first ejaculatory spurt. The wives of all 11 men conceived within 7 months. In ten males the first ejaculatory spurt contained less than twice the spermatozoal concentration than the following spurts. Split intercourse or split AIH resulted in five pregnancies in this group. Thus, the total pregnancy rate in these 21 couples was 76.2% following either split intercourse or split AIH.

The highest success rates for AIH are certainly observed in couples in whom normal spermatozoa exist which cannot be delivered properly to the uterine cervix during intercourse. Pregnancy rates are reported as high as 86% (Barwin 1974). Pregnancy rates reported for other indications vary largely with no apparent relation to the insemination technique used (Table 2), although split insemination seems to be more successful (Table 3). If following six consecutive cycles, no pregnancy ensues, the couple should be re-evaluated.

20.6 The Value of Split Insemination

With the exception of sperm deposition failure and severe teratozoospermia and ejaculatory disturbances the use of the split fraction of the ejaculate is indicated whenever AIH has to be performed. The split fraction contains a significantly higher concentration of sperm cells with better motility. Since during pericervical and intracervical insemination procedures the seminal volume which may be used is restricted, the higher concentration of qualitatively better spermatozoa achieved by the use of the split fraction will markedly improve the chances for fertilization. In cases in which intrauterine insemination is indicated, the use of the split fraction enables the introduction of higher number of spermatozoa into the uterine cavity containing anti-infectious features of the prostatic secretions while avoiding the introduction of high concentrations of prostaglandins.

20.7 Conclusions

AIH is a valuable tool for promoting fertility; however, AIH is certainly no panacea. If applied indiscriminately, one may expect a placebo effect in many cases rather than therapeutic value. The protective features of AIH seem to be of value in cases of severe hypospermia. Apart from this entity, protective AIH should be applied only if there is sound evidence that its employment surpasses what nature has provided as a very efficient insemination system. This is the case in sperm deposition failure (impotence, deformation of female or male genitals). Males with oligozoospermia, asthenozoospermia, or teratozoospermia may have similar chances to impregnate their partners whether normal intercourse is executed or when AIH is applied. The latter mode may possibly even decrease the chance due to the stress inflicted upon both partners during AIH treatment. If in vitro treatment of semen yields improved seminal qualities (split, in vitro vitalization, filtration, treatment for viscosipathia, etc.), AIH seems to be superior to intercourse for procreation purposes and is a very valuable tool for promoting fertility.

20.8 References

Amelar RD, Dubin L (1977 a) Semen analysis. In: Amelar RD, Dubin L, Walsh PC (eds) Male infertility. Saunders, Philadelphia London Toronto, pp 105–140

Amelar RD, Dubin L (1977 b) Special problems in management. In: Amelar RD, Dubin L, Walsh PC (eds) Male infertility. Saunders, Philadelphia London Toronto, pp 191–214

Amelar RD, Hotchkiss RS (1965) The split ejaculate: its use in the management of male infertility. Fertil Steril 16:46–60

Asch RH, Balmaceda J, Pauerstein CJ (1977) Failure of seminal plasma to enter the uterus and oviducts of the rabbit following artificial insemination. Fertil Steril 28:671–673

Barwin BN (1974) Intrauterine insemination of husband's semen. J Reprod Fertil 36:101–106

Beck WW (1976) A critical look at the legal, ethical and technical aspects of artificial insemination. Fertil Steril 27:1–8

Bedford JM (1971) The rate of sperm passage into the cervix after coitus in the rabbit. J Reprod Fertil 25:211–218

Bunge RG, Sherman JK (1954) Liquefication of human semen by α-amylase. Fertil Steril 5:353–356

David A (1979) Homologous insemination using the split ejaculate. Int J Androl 2:534–548

Dmowski WP, Gaynor L, Lawrence M, Rao R, Scommegna A (1979) Artificial insemination homologous with oligospermic semen separated on albumin columns. Fertil Steril 31:58–62

Eliasson R (1977) Semen analysis and laboratory work-up. In: Cockett ATK, Urry RL (eds) Male infertility. Grune & Stratton, New York San Francisco London, pp 169–188

Eliasson R, Lindholmer C (1972) Distribution and properties of spermatozoa in different fractions of split ejaculates. Fertil Steril 23:252–256

Farris EJ, Murphy PD (1960) Characteristics of the two parts of the portioned ejaculate and the advantages of its use for intrauterine insemination. Fertil Steril 11:465–469

Freund M, Petersen RN (1976) Semen evaluation and infertility. In: Hafez ESE (ed) Human semen and fertility regulation in man. Mosby, St Louis, pp 344–354

Gibor Y, Garcia CJ jr, Cohen MR, Scommegna A (1970) The cyclical changes in the physical properties of the cervical mucus and the results of the post-coital test. Fertil Steril 21:20–27

Giner J, Merino G, Luna J, Aznar R (1974) Evaluation of the Sims-Huhner postcoital test in fertile couples. Fertil Steril 25:145–148

Glezerman M, Lunenfeld B (1976) Zur Therapie der männlichen Anorgasmie – ein Fallbericht. Aktuel Dermatol 2:167–169

Glezerman M, Lunenfeld B, Potashnik G, Oelsner G, Beer R (1976) Retrograde ejaculation: Pathophysiological aspects and report of two successfully treated cases. Fertil Steril 27:796–800

Glezerman M, Brook I, Potashnik G, Ben Aderet N, Insler V (1980) Fertility pattern and reported pregnancies in 333 patients referred to male infertility clinics. In: Salvatori B, Semm K, Vadora E (eds) Fertility and sterility. Proceedings of the Vth ESCO, Venice. Edizioni Internazionali Gruppo Editoriale Medico, Rome, pp 495–496

Hahn J (1976) Extrakorporale Befruchtung. Paper given at: Human-Veterinärmedizinische Gemeinschaftstagung. Hannover

Hartman CG (1962) Science and the safe period: A compendium of human reproduction. Williams & Wilkins, Baltimore

Harvey C (1956) The use of portioned ejaculates in investigating the role of accessory secretions in human semen. Studies on fertility. Proc Soc Stud Fertil 8:3–7

Heuer D (1971) Die Portiokappe als therapeutische Möglichkeit bei Oligozoospermie des Mannes. In: Schirren C (ed) Fortschritte der Fertilitätsforschung, Bd II. Grosse, Berlin, pp 128–130

Insler V, Melmed H, Eichenbrenner I, Serr DM, Lunenfeld B (1972) The cervical score: a simple semi-quantitative method for monitoring of the menstrual cycle. Int J Gynecol Obstet 10:223–228

Insler V, Bernstein D, Glezerman M (1977) Diagnosis and classification of the cervical factor of infertility. In: Insler V, Bettendorf G (eds) The uterine cervix in reproduction. Thieme, Stuttgart, pp 253–265

Insler V, Bernstein D, Glezerman M, Misgav N (1979a) Correlation of seminal fluid analysis with mucus-penetrating ability of spermatozoa. Fertil Steril 32:316–319

Insler V, Glezerman M, Bernstein D (1979b) Die Behandlung des Zervikalfaktors der Infertilität. Arch Gynecol 228:479–490

Insler V, Glezerman M, Zeidel L, Bernstein D, Misgav N (1980) Sperm storage in the human cervix: a quantitative study. Fertil Steril 33:288–293

Kaskarelis D, Comninos A (1959) Critical evaluation of homologous artificial insemination. Int J Fertil 4:38–41

Lindholmer C (1973) Survival of human spermatozoa in different fractions of split ejaculate. Fertil Steril 24:521–526

Ludvik W (1976) Andrologie. Thieme, Stuttgart

Lunenfeld B, Glezerman M (1981) Diagnose und Therapie männlicher Fertilitätsstörungen. Grosse, Berlin

MacLeod J (1965) The semen examination. Clin Obstet Gynecol 8:115

MacLeod J, Hotchkiss RS (1942) Distribution of spermatozoa and of certain chemical constituents in human ejaculate. J Urol 48:225–229

Macomber D, Sanders MR (1929) The spermatozoa count. N Engl J Med 200:981–984

Moghissi KS, Gruber JS, Evans S, Yanez J (1977) Homologous artificial insemination: a reappraisal. Am J Obstet Gynecol 129:909–913

Nunley WC, Kitchin JD, Thiajavajah S (1978) Homologous insemination. Fertil Steril 30:510–515

Paulson JD, Polakoski KI (1978) The removal of extraneous material from the ejaculate. Int J Androl [Suppl] 1:163

Perez-Pelaez M, Cohen MR (1965) Split ejaculate in homologous insemination. Int J Fertil 10:25–30

Pommerenke WT (1946) Cyclic changes in the physical and chemical properties of cervical mucus. Am J Obstet Gynecol 52:1023–1031

Russel JK (1960) Artificial insemination (husband) in the management of childlessness. Lancet III:1223–1225

Santamauro AG, Sciarra JJ, Varma AO (1972) A clinical investigation of the role of the semen analysis and postcoital test in the evaluation of male infertility. Fertil Steril 23:245–251

Schill WB (1973) Probleme der homologen und heterologen Insemination aus andrologischer Sicht. In: Braun-Falco O, Petzoldt D (Hrsg) Fortschritte der praktischen Dermatologie und Venerologie. Springer, Berlin Heidelberg New York, S 187–195

Schill WB (1975a) Moderne Aspekte der andrologischen Therapie. Therapiewoche 25:2762–2770

Schill WB (1975b) Caffeine- and kallikrein-induced stimulation of human sperm motility: a comparative study. Andrologia 7:229–236

Schill WB, Braun-Falco O, Haberland GI (1974) The possible role of kinins in sperm motility. Int J Fertil 19:163–167

Schirren C (1972) Praktische Andrologie. Hartmann, Berlin

Schoenfeld C, Amelar RD, Dubin L (1975) Stimulation of ejaculated spermatozoa by caffeine. Fertil Steril 26:158–161

Semm K, Brandl E, Mettler L (1976) Vacuum insemination cap. In: Hafez ESE (ed) Human semen and fertility regulation in men. Mosby, St Louis, pp 439–441

Settlage DS, Motoshima M, Tredway R (1973) Sperm transport from the external cervical os to the fallopian tubes in women: a time and quantitation study. Fertil Steril 24:655–661

Shields FE (1950) Artificial insemination as related to female. Fertil Steril 1:271

Speichinger JP, Mattox JH (1976) Homologous artificial insemination and oligospermia. Fertil Steril 27:135–138

Steiman RP, Taymor ML (1977) Artificial insemination homologous and its role in the management of infertility. Fertil Steril 146–150

Taylor PL, Kelly RW (1974) 19-OH E prostaglandins as the major prostaglandin of human semen. Nature 250:665–667

Tijoe DY, Oentoeng S (1968) The viscosity of human semen and the percentage of motile spermatozoa. Fertil Steril 19:562–565

Tredway DT, Settlage DSF, Nakamura RM, Motoshima M, Umezaki CU, Mishell DR (1975) Significance of timing for postcoital evaluation of cervical mucus. Am J Obstet Gynecol 121:387–393

Weller J (1976) Ergebnisse und Erfahrungen mit der artifiziellen maritogenen Insemination als Möglichkeit der Behandlung steriler Ehen. Zentralbl Gynaekol 98:151–157

Whelton A, Lucas JB, Carter GC, Craig TJ, Bryant HH, Herbst DV, King TM (1980) Therapeutic implications of doxycycline and cephalotin concentrations in the female genital tract. Obstet Gynecol 55:28–32

White RM, Glass RH (1976) Intrauterine insemination with husband's semen. Obstet Gynecol 47:119–121

Whitelaw MJ (1950) Use of the cervical cap to increase fertility in cases of oligospermia. Fertil Steril 1:33–39

Zaneveld LJD, Polakoski KL (1977) Collection and physical examination of the ejaculate. In: Hafez ESE (ed) Techniques of human andrology. Elsevier/North-Holland Biomedical Press, Amsterdam New York Oxford, pp 147–172

Van Zyl JA (1972) A review of the male factor in 231 infertile couples. S Afr J Obstet Gynecol 10:17

21 In Vitro Fertilization:
Future Treatment for Male Infertility

J. Shuber and J. Bain

Therapy of infertility in the male still remains problematic. Despite increased knowledge of normal physiology, our understanding of the pathophysiology of male reproductive failure is sparse, with the consequence that there are no treatment modes that are known to have a high success rate. There is a multiplicity of therapies, many of them described in this book, but none have dramatically changed our approach to the treatment of the subfertile male. It is because of this background that scientists are constantly in search of new techniques, new understanding, and new approaches to the therapy of male infertility. In vitro fertilization (IVF) and embryo transfer (ET), as tools in the treatment of human reproductive problems, offer another approach in dealing with problems of oligoasthenoteratozoospermia. In vitro fertilization has already been used successfully in cases of human bilateral tubal disease (Steptoe and Edwards 1978; Lopata et al. 1980 b). Whether it can serve as a technique for treating certain cases of male infertility is at present a matter of conjecture and speculation.

21.1 In Vitro Fertilization

21.1.1 Background

Research in IVF and ET has covered a wide span of time and has given new insights into genetic interaction. Successful transfer of rabbit embryos was reported late in the 19th century (Heape 1890). Since then, there have been innumerable reports in which the factors involved in sperm penetration and fertilization of ova in the test tube with subsequent implantation into a host animal have been studied. With in vitro methods, it is possible to directly observe the interaction between egg and spermatozoon and to manipulate their environment so that the factors controlling sperm entry can be better understood.

Conceiving of such experiments and actually performing them posed significant problems for the early researchers in this field. Not only was it necessary to obtain mammalian oocytes, but the next step, oocyte culture, had to be taken. Pioneer work in this area in rabbits (Pincus and Enzmann 1935) and in mice (Moricard and De Fonbrune 1937) opened new vistas in reproductive control that we are only now beginning to realize. Several decades later advances in our understanding of the

Testis   **Ovary**

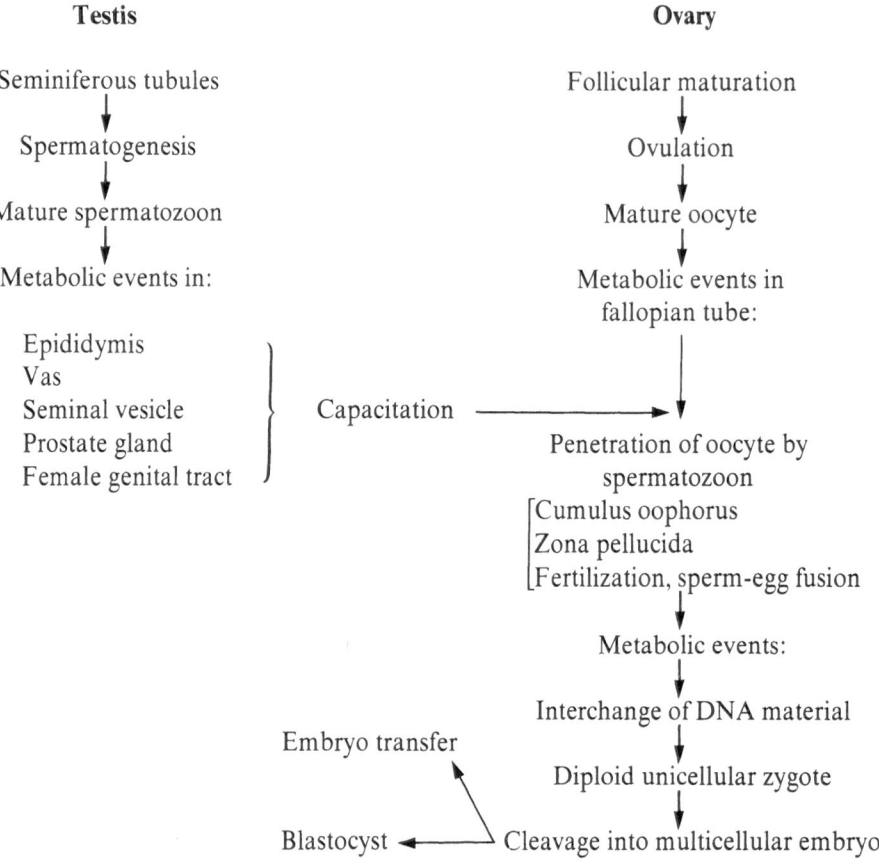

Fig. 1. Major elements of germ cell development and fertilization

metabolism of the pre-implantation mammalian embryo progressed to the stage where a considerable body of knowledge had already been accumulated (Biggers and Stern 1973). In the investigation of oocyte culture techniques, great strides in the metabolic and energy needs for the in vitro development of eggs have been made (Biggers et al. 1967; Donahue 1968; Edwards 1962, 1965 a, b).

Once it became possible to culture mammalian ova in the laboratory, the next logical extension, in vitro fertilization, began to develop. Without invoking the need for practical application, IVF offered the possibility of learning more about the complexities of sperm-egg interaction, including sperm capacitation and penetration of the cumulus oophorus and zona pellucida, entry of spermatozoa into the egg, and the early stages of blastocyst formation. Figure 1 provides a brief overview of the major elements involved in the meeting of spermatozoa and oocytes so that fertilization and subsequent cleavage can take place, and highlights those areas of concern to the scientist studying genetic interaction by IVF: the maturation of spermatozoa and egg, capacitation of spermatozoa (i.e., endogenous and environmentally acquired ability to fertilize), passage of the spermatozoon through the egg coverings and into the ovum, union and interchange of genetic material, appropriate metabolism for mitotic cell division, and finally growth and development of an embryo of sufficient cell number for transfer into the female host for implantation and intrauterine maturation until the time of delivery.

Animal IVF studies have been in progress for many years. Investigation into the difficult steps outlined in Fig. 1 resulted in the birth of normal rabbit offspring conceived by in vitro fertilization (Chang 1959). Work in other animals demonstrated the viability of the technological advances in this man-made in vitro intrusion into reproductive control; for example, Mukherjee (1972) gave details on mice oocyte retrieval and maturation, sperm capacitation, in vitro fertilization, cleavage, intrauterine implantation, and the eventual birth of five normal offspring. The difficulties inherent in this technique became obvious in Mukherjee's work. It is true that five mice were ultimately delivered, but these five were derived from the culture of 325 oocytes, 195 of which showed maturation. After fertilization, 32 normal two-cell embryos were produced from which 11 transfers were made with five resultant offspring.

21.1.2 Human IVF

For its own sake, the IVF of human oocytes by human spermatozoa could provide important information about human genetic interaction, but the clinical application of this technique is of even greater significance. Bilateral disease of the fallopian tubes precludes the possibility of fertility. Retrieval of mature eggs directly from the ovaries, fertilization of the eggs by husband's spermatozoa in an extracorporeal medium, and subsequent implantation of an embryo of only several cells into an appropriately prepared uterus, might be a way of bypassing fallopian tube obstruction and providing fertility in couples where tubal disease is the primary obstacle to pregnancy.

Pincus and Saunders (1939) described a method of human oocyte maturation in vitro using human serum; however, difficulties with finding a suitable culture medium hampered progress in the development of IVF techniques in both animal and human experimentation. Several years later human IVF and subsequent cleavage were described but only in 3 of 138 sperm-exposed oocytes out of a total of the 800 which were recovered (Menkin and Rock 1948). Technological difficulties persisted and, although there was improvement in oocyte retrieval and maturation, IVF either occurred infrequently or, when it did occur, cleavage often appeared to be abnormal (Edwards et al. 1970; Soupart and Morgenstern 1973; Soupart and Strong 1974).

In the interim, Edwards et al. (1966) were gaining extensive experience in in vitro techniques using human ova. In this series, 4 out of 56 mature follicular oocytes became fertilized after exposure to washed spermatozoa. Several others were believed to be fertilized after exposure to spermatozoa that underwent assorted treatment in an attempt to capacitate them. In subsequent reports, Edwards (1970) provided satisfactory evidence that true in vitro fertilization had indeed taken place. Satisfactory evidence of human IVF was provided by Seitz et al. (1971) who observed cleavage beyond the two-cell stage in 7 of 72 follicular oocytes removed at various times in the menstrual cycle.

The theoretical stage had been set for the practical application of a basic science methodology. Edwards (1970) summarized his work on the maturation of human oocytes, the handling of human spermatozoa, IVF, and subsequent growth and cleavage of the fertilized egg. In this paper he demonstrated how the basic science-clinical gap could be bridged. Ovulation had to be predicted, and this could be done by hormonal manipulation. Oocytes had to be readily and easily retrieved from graafian follicles just before ovulation; this could be accomplished by laparoscopy, a technique pioneered by Steptoe (1967).

In a short, but information-filled report, Steptoe (1975) described his experience in attempting "to cure infertility due to irremediable Fallopian tube lesions by the laparoscopic recovery of pre-ovulatory ovarian oocytes, their fertilization in vitro, and their subsequent reimplantation into the uterine cavity." Although three children had reportedly been born 1 year previously as a result of IVF and ET (Bevis 1974), confirmation of these births could not be established (Anonymous 1974). A few short years later, on July 25, 1978, the world received the news of the birth of the first child that had been conceived unequivocally by IVF (Steptoe and Edwards 1978). The normalcy and health of the child were documented (Hilson et al. 1978) and the era of IVF as a method of treating certain cases of human infertility had been introduced to the world. Since then, Steptoe and Edwards have had further success, as have others (Lopata et al. 1980 b).

21.2 IVF and Male Infertility

21.2.1 Rationale

IVF as a method of treating human infertility due to bilateral fallopian tube obstruction is a logical approach, especially since surgical reconstruction of tubes even with the most sophisticated microscopic techniques does not result in a high pregnancy rate. At this point in time, IVF is not yet a highly successful procedure, but it has a rational physiological basis and, as methodology improves, so will our ability to successfully fertilize and reimplant larger numbers of eggs. But IVF may also have potential application in yet another aspect of human infertility, and that is the problem of male infertility.

In order for in vivo fertilization to take place, it is usually necessary that tens of millions of high quality spermatozoa with good motility be ejaculated into the vagina. When oligozoospermia (usually defined as a sperm count less than $20 \times 10^6/$ ml) exists, fertility is reduced; the greater the reduction in sperm count the less the chance of pregnancy. But it has now been demonstrated repeatedly that under ideal circumstances as few as 1–2 million spermatozoa/ml may cause successful IVF (Edwards et al. 1970; Soupart and Morgenstern 1973; Lopata et al. 1980 b; Steptoe and Edwards 1979). This raises the exciting possibility that IVF may have potential value in even very severe oligozoospermia. Not only could consideration be given to IVF as a form of therapy in oligozoospermia, but it is reasonable to consider this technique for teratozoospermia and asthenozoospermia with or without oligozoospermia.

From the theoretical perspective, IVF as a mode of therapy for male infertility might have the following hypothetical advantages:

1. The close juxtapositioning of a mature ovum with spermatozoa in a suitable medium in a Petri dish would overcome or greatly decrease the problem of reduced spermatozoal motility. The need for significant motility would be practically eliminated as long as a spermatozoon in close approximation to an ovum could penetrate that ovum.
2. Cervical mucus hostile to spermatozoa would be bypassed completely.
3. Factors in seminal plasma antagonistic to fertilization could be washed from the spermatozoa prior to addition to the ovum in the Petri dish.
4. Low sperm counts might become inconsequential if the few spermatozoa needed for fertilization were present in the dish.
5. Although a semen specimen had a significant number of abnormal forms, the few spermatozoa with normal morphology might be in close enough approximation to the egg to result in fertilization.

These hypothetical advantages of IVF as a treatment for male infertility presuppose a number of assumptions. The basic assumption is, of course, that within a semen specimen of low numbers of spermatozoa with poor morphology and low motility, there will be found at least one spermatozoon that will fertilize an egg under the right circumstances. This hypothetical situation also presupposes that abnormal spermatozoa will not induce fertilization in the Petri dish at a rate higher than what might occur by chance alone in a conception induced by coitus and intravaginal ejaculation. There are no hard data available to support or reject these assumptions. There is some preliminary evidence that human spermatozoa derived from specimens of greater sperm numbers with better qualitative characteristics will penetrate and subsequently fertilize ova in vitro at a rate higher than spermatozoa derived from specimens of lesser quality (Barros et al. 1979). Whether this is, in fact, the case awaits confirmation.

21.2.2 Ovum Retrieval and Sperm Capacitation

In IVF for spermatozoa related problems, rather than for fallopian tube dysfunction, the retrieval of eggs presents a far less serious problem. This is so because in most instances of oligoasthenoteratozoospermia one would expect to find a relatively healthy pelvis by laparoscopic examination of the patient's female partner. One would not expect pelvic or periovarian adhesions and, consequently, laparoscopic retrieval of preovular ova could be accomplished with much greater ease. Precise timing of ovulation can now be arrived at not only by hormonal assessment, but also by ultrasonography which visualizes the growth and development of the maturing graafian follicle (Lopata et al. 1980 a, b).

There continues to be a controversy regarding capacitation of human spermatozoa in IVF, whether it is needed and, if needed, the factors that are most beneficial. There is evidence that spermatozoa recovered from the oviduct have a greater fertilizing capacity than those recovered from the uterus (Cohen 1975). This suggests that capacitation does occur and is necessary for greater fertilizability. Gonadotropic hormones have been shown to enhance sperm penetration in vitro, which again suggests that, if fertilization can be positively influenced, there is reason to believe that such influence is necessary and is a normal physiological event (Soupart and Morgenstern 1973). Spermatozoa are not immediately able to penetrate eggs after deposition in the female tract, most likely because of the need for a period of time during which capacitation must take place (Chang and Hunter 1975). The capacitation of human spermatozoa for IVF appears to be adequately accomplished by the use of appropriate incubation media (Lopata et al. 1980b; Steptoe and Edwards 1979).

21.2.3 Sperm Characteristics

The potential use of IVF for the treatment of infertiliy due to factors in the male raises a very serious issue. By avoiding the need for passing through the "obstacle course" of cervical mucus, cervix, uterus, and fallopian tubes, will abnormal spermatozoa that would otherwise have been rejected, now be able to fertilize eggs with a resultant increase in abnormal embryos? Under normal conditions, few morphologically abnormal spermatozoa reach the site of fertilization in the fallopian tubes (Ahlgren 1975). Whether the uterotubal junction acts as a barrier to abnormally shaped spermatozoa (Krzanowska 1974), or whether there are other factors which screen out abnormal sperm is not known. Spontaneous abortion of pregnancies achieved by coitus in normally fertile couples are due to chromosome abnormalities in as many as 40% or 50% of cases (Schlesselman 1979). This suggests that when gametes with abnormal genes do cause fertilization, nature intervenes by terminating the pregnancy spontaneously. It is assumed, but currently unknown, that even if abnormal spermatozoa successfully penetrate ova by IVF, a resultant pregnancy would end in a miscarriage. Whether this will, indeed, be the case remains unknown at the present time. The considerable experience now accumulated in animals suggests that IVF does not cause an increase in the number of abnormal offspring (Biggers 1981).

There is some preliminary evidence that human spermatozoa from semen of superior quality have an increased ability to penetrate zona pellucida-free hamster eggs when compared to spermatozoa from oligoasthenozoospermic semen (Barros et al. 1979). This observation remains to be substantiated, but implies that IVF may not increase the chances of fertilization by spermatozoa from a specimen of poor quantity or quality. In this instance, sperm penetration and fertilization might be enhanced by a variety of techniques, including separation of highly motile spermatozoa (Comhaire et al. 1982) or improvement of sperm motility by pharmacological agents (Makler et al. 1980).

21.3 Conclusion

If IVF does prove to be a useful tool in treating male infertility, it will only be used after a number of important steps are first taken. It must be clearly established that there is no remediable cause of the infertility that is amenable to less intrusive therapy. Wherever possible other forms of treatment, even if their usefulness is questioned, should be attempted first in order to effect a change in the quantity and quality of the spermatozoa. Only when these therapeutic modalities have failed and only after the female partner has been judged to be ovulatory can IVF then be considered as a method of treatment. Even then, one must be assured that there are no diseases of the uterus that may prevent normal implantation of a fertilized egg. It may be appropriate to first judge the fertilizing ability of husband's spermatozoa by using the zona pellucida-free hamster egg model prior to undertaking IVF for the couple (Barros et al. 1979).

Whether IVF will ultimately be added to the armamentarium of the andrologist and gynecologist treating male infertility will depend on the further development of this technique, the increased predictability of easily obtaining viable ova by laparoscopy, and the prior demonstration in the research laboratory that IVF is safe and effective for use in male subfertility. Not only do the technological problems require our attention, but so do the ethical and sociological implications of this new inroad into reproductive control. The technique of IVF offers the possibility of overcoming some forms of human infertility, but it is also a technique that is open to the possibility of misuse and even abuse. With the era of genetic manipulation already upon us, we must be watchful and exercise careful control of our new-found resources and techniques.

Acknowledgements. The authors wish to acknowledge with gratitude the assistance in compiling this manuscript given by Morag Smith, Cecelia McHugh, Sari Snyder, and Rona Weist.

21.4 References

Ahlgren M (1975) Sperm transport to and survival in the human fallopian tube. Gynecol Invest 6:206–214

Anonymous (August 7, 1974). Med World News 15:15–16

Barros C, Gonzalez J, Herrera E, Bustos-Obregon E (1979) Human sperm penetration into zona-free oocytes as a test to evaluate the sperm-fertilizing ability. Andrologia 11:197–210

Bevis DCA (1974) Antenatal interference: embryo transplants. Br Med J 3:238

Biggers JD (1981) In vitro fertilization and embryo transfer in human beings. N Engl J Med 304:336–342

Biggers JD, Stern S (1973) Metabolism of the preimplantation mammalian embryo. In: Bishop MWH (ed) Advances in reproductive physiology, vol V/1. Merrimack, Salem NH, pp 1–59

Biggers JD, Whittingham DG, Donahue RP (1967) The pattern of energy metabolism in the mouse oocyte and zygote. Proc Natl Acad Sci USA 58:560–567

Chang MC (1959) Fertilization of rabbit ova in vitro. Nature 184:466–467

Chang MC, Hunter RHF (1975) Capacitation of mammalian sperm: Biological and experimental aspects. In: Hamilton DW, Greep RO (eds) Endocrinology. Male reproductive system. American Physiological Society, Washington D.C. (Handbook of physiology, vol V/7, pp 339–351)

Cohen J (1975) Gametic diversity within an ejaculate. In: Azelius B (ed) The functional anatomy of the spermatozoon. Pergamon, New York, pp 329–339

Comhaire F, Vermeulen L, Zegers-Hochschild F (1982) Enhancement of sperm motility: Selecting progressively motile spermatozoa. In: Bain J, Schwarzstein L, Schill W (eds) Treatment of male infertility. Springer, Berlin Heidelberg New York

Donahue RP (1968) Maturation of the mouse oocyte in vitro. I. Sequence and timing of nuclear progression. J Exp Zool 169:237–250

Edwards RG (1962) Meiosis in ovarian oocytes of adult mammals. Nature 196:446–450

Edwards RG (1965 a) Maturation in vitro of mouse, sheep, cow, pig, rhesus monkey and human ovarian oocytes. Nature 208:349–351

Edwards RG (1965 b) Maturation in vitro of human ovarian oocytes. Lancet 2:926–929

Edwards RG, Steptoe PC, Purdy JM (1970) Fertilization and cleavage in vitro of preovulator human oocytes. Nature 227:1307–1309

Edwards RG, Donahue RP, Baramki TA, Jones HW (1966) Preliminary attempts to fertilize human oocytes matured in vitro. Am J Obstet Gynecol 96:192–200

Edwards RG (1970) Fertilization and cleavage in vitro of human ova. In: Moghissi KS, Hafez ESE (eds) Biology of mammalian fertilization and implantation. Thomas, Springield Il-linois, pp 263–278

Heape W (1890) Preliminary note on the transplantation and growth of mammalian ova within a uterine foster mother. Proc R Soc Lond (Biol) 48:457–458

Hilson D, Bruce RL, Sims DG (1978) Successful pregnancy following in vitro fertilisation. Lancet 2:473

Krzanowska H (1974) The passage of abnormal spermatozoa through the uterotubal junction of the mouse. J Reprod Fertil 38:81–90

Lopata A, Sathananthan AH, McBain JC, Johnston WIH, Speirs AL (1980a) The ul-trastructure of the preovulatory human egg fertilized in vitro. Fertil Steril 33:12–20

Lopata A, Johnston IWH, Hoult IJ, Speirs AI (1980b) Pregnancy following intrauterine im-plantation of an embryo obtained by in vitro fertilization of a preovulatory egg. Fertil Steril 33:117–120

Makler A, Makler E, Hzkovitz J, Brandes JM (1980) Factors affecting sperm motility. IV. Incu-bation of human semen with caffeine, kallikrein and other metabolically active com-pounds. Fertil Steril 33:624–630

Menkin MF, Rock J (1948) In vitro fertilization and cleavage of human ovarian eggs. Am J Obstet Gynecol 55:440–452

Moricard R, De Fonbrune P (1937) Nouvelles études expérimentales sur les mécanismes de la formation du premier globule in vitro chez les mammifères. Arch Anat Microsc Morphol Exp 33:113–128

Mukherjee AB (1972) Normal progeny from fertilization in vitro of mouse oocytes matured in culture and spermatozoa capacitated in vitro. Nature 237:397–398

Pincus G, Enzmann EV (1935) The comparative behaviour of mammalian eggs in vivo and in vitro. I. The activation of ovarian eggs. J Exp Med 62:665–675

Pincus G, Saunders B (1939) The comparative behaviour of mammalian eggs in vivo and in vitro. VI. The maturation of human ovarian ova. Anat Rec 75:537–545

Schlesselman JJ (1979) How does one assess the risk of abnormalities from human in vitro fer-tilization? Am J Obstet Gynecol 135:135–148

Seitz HM jr, Rocha G, Brackett BG, Mastroianni L jr (1971) Cleavage of human ova in vitro. Fertil Steril 22:255

Soupart P, Morgenstern LL (1973) Human sperm capacitation and in vitro fertilization. Fertil Steril 24:462–478

Soupart P, Strong PA (1974) Ultrastructural observations on human oocytes fertilized in vitro. Fertil Steril 25:11–44

Steptoe PC (1967) Laparoscopy in gynaecology. Livingstone, Edinburgh London

Steptoe PC (1975) In vitro fertilisation of human oocytes. S Afr Med J 49:2016–2018

Steptoe PC, Edwards RG, Purdy JM (1971) Human blastocysts grown in culture. Nature 229:132–133

Steptoe PC, Edwards RG (1978) Birth after the reimplantation of a human embryo. Lancet 2:366

Steptoe PC, Edwards RG (1979) Pregnancies following implantation of human embryos grown in culture. Presented at Scientific Meeting of The Royal College of Obstetricians and Gynaecologists. January 26.

V. Closing Remarks

The Last Word – For Now

In this book we have been treated to a potpourri of therapeutic approaches to the difficult problem of male infertility. In the "olden" days there were therapies (used even now) that were hailed as being important tools in our treatment armamentarium. These included vitamin E, triiodothyronine, and others. We have since learned that vitamin E doesn't work because subfertile men are not vitamin E-deficient; triiodothyronine will not work unless thyroidal insufficiency can be proven and even then thyroid treatment may not alter spermatogenesis. It may be that some of the treatments described in this book will fall into the "vitamin E" category – "It may not work, but at least we're doing something." It may be reasonable to raise skepticism about the present or future value of some of the treatments described here. But the editors felt it was important to include those modes of therapy that appear rational and that have been subjected to at least a modicum of scientific critique.

Basic to our search for effective therapies is our need to understand the pathophysiology of male infertility. Our major problem is in this area. Once we begin to know what the fundamental causes of poor sperm formation or function are, the task of developing therapy will become easier and more rational. Until we have further etiological breakthroughs, we must content ourselves with the treatments described in this book or perhaps other therapeutic modalities not discussed here or that may be possible in the near future.

In treating the infertile male, it is important to create a situation in which anything we do will have the optimal chance of success. To assure this, and to increase the possibility of this or that treatment eliciting a positive effect, a few basic principles might be applied. First and foremost, the patient should undergo a careful clinical evaluation including both a thorough medical history and physical examination. It would be an unhappy state of affairs, for example, if a man with modest oligzoospermia and a varicocele was subjected to operation if it were found that he had selective vaginal anejaculation. Clinical evaluation may bring to light a number of treatable conditions.

This leads us to the next important consideration. Before embarking upon what may be empirically based therapy to enhance semen parameters, specific disease entities should be sought for and treated first. Hence, thyroid dysfunction should be treated appropriately, hyperprolactinemia may require surgery or drug treatment or both, and any other specific condition should receive the best available therapy for that condition. Our search for specific disease is usually a frustrating exercise, but because the exercise occasionally yields results it is worth the effort.

Coupled with a search for disease is the acquisition of an awareness of possible noxious influences to which the patient may be exposed. Does the patient smoke heavily? Does he consume an excessive amount of alcohol? Does he work with pesticides or other toxic chemicals or pollutants? The patient's livelihood may depend on continued exposure to potentially harmful substances, but wherever possible they should be minimized prior to initiating therapy due to poor sperm parameters.

One other area of management needs to be emphasized. This is the area of emotional and psychological support for the man and his partner. Too little attention has been paid to this topic in the andrological or infertility literature. The clinician should have an appreciation of the severe emotional difficulty a subfertile man may be experiencing and either help support him through these trying times or direct him to where he might get that support if needed and desired. The man should clearly understand the state of his reproductive capacity and what chance any form of therapy might have in helping him produce a pregnancy.

New information on and, hopefully, more effective medications for male infertility will continue to emerge. This book is but one contribution in that continuum. It is hoped that some or all of the contributions within these covers will spark the imagination of investigators around the world to enlarge upon their search for answers to the difficult questions we have raised regarding male infertility.

The Editors:

Jerald Bain
Wolf-Bernhard Schill
Luis Schwarzstein

Subject Index

Varicocele and Male Infertility

Recent Advances in Diagnosis and Therapy

Editors: E.W.Jecht, E.Zeitler
With the collaboration of numerous experts

1982. 98 figures. XVI, 211 pages.
ISBN 3-540-10727-4

The entire range of problems in the clinical treatment of varicoceles and resultant male infertility is covered in this book. Particular emphasis is placed on the subclinical varicocele and the various forms of its spermiographic assessment. The importance of transcatheter phlebographic radiological examination of the internal spermatic vein for furnishing proof of subclinical varicoceles or postoperative persistence is demonstrated. Phlebographic examinations conducted in various centers are compared and their results correlated with spermatological and clinical findings.

The use of modern diagnostic procedures as well as new therapeutic methods and the technique and results of surgical measures are reviewed. Of particular interest is the detailed description of the indications, risks, limits and results of occlusive treatment of the internal spermatic vein by embolization or sclerotherapy.

Varicocele and Male Infertility will prove an important source of information for physicians and researchers involved in the study and treatment of male infertility, as well as a stimulus for the further exploration of its causes, especially in their early stages.

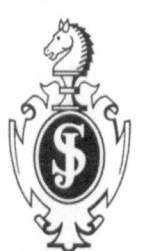

Springer-Verlag
Berlin
Heidelberg
New York

G. Aumüller

Prostate Gland and Seminal Vesicles

1979. 142 figures (some in color) in 181
separate illustrations. X, 380 pages
(Handbuch der mikroskopischen Anatomie
des Menschen, Band 7, Teil 6)
ISBN 3-540-09191-2

A T. K. Cockett, K. Koshiba

Manual of Urologic Sugery

Illustrated by J. Takamoto
1979. 532 color illustrations.
XVIII, 284 pages.
(Comprehensive Manuals of Surgical
Specialities)
ISBN 3-540-90423-9

Disturbances in Male Fertility

By K. Bandhauer, G. Bartsch,
D. M. de Kretser, A. Eshkol, J. Frick,
M. Glezerman, J. B. Kerr, B. Lunenfeld,
W. Pöldinger, H. P. Rohr, F. Scharfetter,
P. D. Temple-Smith
Editors: K. Bandhauer, J. Frick

1982. 153 figures. XXIII, 454 pages
(Handbuch der Urologie/Encyclopedia of
Urology, Volume 16)
ISBN 3-540-05279-8

T. Mann, C. Lutwak-Mann

Male Reproductive Function and Semen

**Themes and Trends in Physiology,
Biochemistry and Investigate Andrology**

1981. 46 figures. XIV, 495 pages
ISBN 3-540-10383-X

Prostate Cancer

Editor: W. Duncan

1981. 68 figures, 67 tables. X, 190 pages
(Recent Results in Cancer Research,
Volume 78)
ISBN 3-540-10676-6

The Ureter

Editor: H. Bergman
With 52 Contributors.

2nd edition 1981. 760 figures.
XVII, 780 pages
ISBN 3-540-90561-8

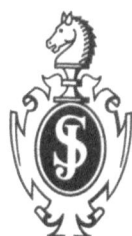

Springer-Verlag Berlin Heidelberg New York